Guidelines for PERINATAL CARE

Second Edition

American Academy of
Pediatrics

American College of
Obstetricians and
Gynecologists

Supported in part by

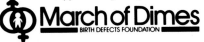

Design: Michael Dodd

Cover Art: John Edwards

Guidelines for Perinatal Care was developed through the cooperative efforts of the AAP Committee on Fetus and Newborn and the ACOG Committee on Obstetrics: Maternal and Fetal Medicine. The guidelines should not be viewed as a body of rigid rules. They are general and intended to be adapted to many different situations, taking into account the needs and resources particular to the locality, the institution, or type of practice. Variations and innovations that demonstrably improve the quality of patient care are to be encouraged rather than restricted. The purpose of these guidelines will be well served if they provide a firm basis on which local norms may be built. The segments related to obstetric practice do not replace the ACOG *Standards for Obstetric-Gynecologic Services,* but rather expand on the principles suggested therein.

Copyright © 1988 by the American Academy of Pediatrics and the American College of Obstetricians and Gynecologists

Library of Congress Cataloging-in-Publication Data
Guidelines for perinatal care. -- Second Edition
        p. cm.
    Developed by the AAP Committee on Fetus and Newborn and the ACOG Committee on Obstetrics: Maternal and Fetal Medicine.
    "Supported in part by March of Dimes Birth Defects Foundation."
    Includes bibliographies and index.
    ISBN 0=915473=08=9 : $30.00
    1. Perinatology—Standards.   I. American Academy of Pediatrics.
Committee on Fetus and Newborn.   II. ACOG Committee on Obstetrics:
Maternal and Fetal Medicine.   III. March of Dimes Birth Defects Foundation.
    [DNLM: 1. Perinatology—standards.   WQ 210 G955]
RG600.G85 1988
618.3'2—dc 19
DNLM/DLC
for Library of Congress   88=16701
                                                                      CIP

ISBN 0-915473-08-9

Quantity prices available on request. Address all orders to AAP; inquiries regarding content may be directed to either organization:

American Academy of Pediatrics
141 Northwest Point Road
P. O. Box 927
Elk Grove Village, Illinois 60204

American College of Obstetricians
    and Gynecologists
409 12th Street, SW
Washington, DC 20024

Editorial Committee

Editors: Fredric D. Frigoletto, MD, FACOG
George A. Little, MD, FAAP

Associate Editors: Roger K. Freeman, MD, FACOG
Ronald L. Poland, MD, FAAP

Managing Editor: Rebecca D. Rinehart

Staff: Jean D. Lockhart, MD, AAP
Harold A. Kaminetzky, MD, ACOG
Shirley A. Shelton, ACOG

AAP Committee on Fetus and Newborn

Current Members,
1987-1988

Ronald L. Poland, MD *(Chairman)*
Allen Erenberg, MD
Bernard H. Feldman, MD
John M. Freeman, MD
John Kattwinkel, MD
Gerald Merenstein, MD
William Oh, MD
Thomas R. C. Sisson, MD

Liaison Representatives
James R. Allen, MD, MPH
Paula Brill, MD
Alfred A. deLorimier, MD
Roger K. Freeman, MD
Dennis Hey, DO
William J. Keenan, MD
James Mardell, MD
Donald McNellis, MD
Gerard Ostheimer, MD
Eugene Outerbridge, MD
Lu-Ann Papile, MD
John A. Van Buskirk, MD
Roberta Gay Williams, MD

CONTENTS

PREFACE

Although the field of perinatal care is typified by rapid advances, one factor remains constant: pregnancy outcome can most effectively be improved by integrating the skills and knowledge of multiple disciplines. This philosophy was the foundation for the original *Guidelines for Perinatal Care* and it has continued to guide the development of the second edition.

The concept of a coordinated, multidisciplinary approach within a regionalized system of perinatal care was first introduced in *Toward Improving the Outcome of Pregnancy,* published by March of Dimes in 1976, for which representatives from ACOG and AAP served as consultants. This document defined the principle of regionalized care and, in broad and general terms, illustrated a system of shared responsibility in providing perinatal services—concepts that were enthusiastically received by most health care professionals and planners.

This coordinated approach created the impetus for further unified efforts to reduce maternal and infant morbidity and mortality. The collaboration focused on the sixth edition of *Standards and Recommendations for Hospital Care of the Newborn,* published by the AAP in 1977 when regionalized care was still a relatively new concept. The result was not merely a revision but rather a new joint publication of ACOG and AAP that incorporated, broadened, and replaced its predecessor. Published in 1983, *Guidelines for Perinatal Care* set a precedent by exemplifying the cooperative efforts of two disciplines dedicated to the improvement of pregnancy outcome.

This multidisciplinary effort has had an impact on perinatal care in three important areas: *1)* improved and expanded understanding of the physiology and pathology of the pregnant woman, fetus, and neonate; *2)* improved health care through risk assessment and regional planning to ensure access to care; and 3) enhanced appreciation of the childbirth experience and the role of the family. These concepts have become fundamental to *Guidelines for Perinatal Care.* The most current scientific information, professional opinions, and clinical practices have been assembled and reviewed in the formulation of this manual, which is intended to offer guidelines, not strict operating rules. Local circumstances must dictate the way in which these guidelines are best interpreted to meet the needs of a particular hospital, community, or system. Emphasis has been placed on the delineation of areas to be covered by specific protocols to be defined locally rather than on promoting more rigid recommendations.

Since the publication of the first edition, new concerns have surfaced: troubling ethical issues have arisen, the liability crisis looms as a serious threat, the AIDS epidemic has appeared, and an increasing awareness of the impact of prematurity and its prevention has altered the long-term approach to improving perinatal outcome. Economic factors have continued to play an increasing role in the provision of health care: Competition is eroding regionalized care, and the practice of early discharge is shortening hospital stays and influencing labor/delivery/recovery room configurations, reimbursement considerations, and perinatal education. All of these factors have shifted the emphasis of services provided and placed new demands on personnel.

To address issues and scientific advances that have emerged since the publication of the first edition, the second edition has grown 20% larger than its predecessor. In some instances, the growth can be attributed to the inclusion of new sections devoted to such topics as Radiation Exposure, Ethics, Standard Terminology for Reporting Reproductive Health Statistics, Fetal Therapy, Tocolysis, and—of course—AIDS. In other cases, more detailed information has been provided in response to increasing recognition of the ramifications of perinatal infections for both mother and baby, preconceptional and antenatal screening, and prenatal and perinatal factors associated with brain disorders. Finally, substantative changes in recommendations regarding controversial areas—fetal monitoring, the role of forceps, and management of herpes—have been introduced.

Consolidating this information into a cohesive document has been a major undertaking. Designed for use by all personnel who are involved with the care of pregnant women, their fetuses, and neonates in both hospitals and medical centers, the manual represents a cross-section of different disciplines within the perinatal community. An intermingling of information of all kinds, in varying degrees of detail, is necessary to address their collective needs. The result is a unique resource that is designed to complement the host of educational documents available from the copublishing organizations that give more specific information on management of high-risk conditions.

In order to obtain a true consensus and to represent the diversity of the audience adequately, the number of those contributing to the second edition and the composition of the group as a whole have been broadened accordingly. The text was written, revised, and reviewed by members of the AAP Committee on Fetus and Newborn and the ACOG Committee on Obstetrics: Maternal and Fetal Medicine, and consultants in a variety of specialized areas have contributed to the content. The pioneering efforts of those who developed the first edition, thus creating the foundation for subsequent revisions, must also be acknowledged. The sheer number of individuals who have participated in this endeavor in some capacity makes it impossible to list them all. Suffice it to say that, without their help, there would be no manual. To each and every one of them our sincere appreciation is extended.

Guidelines for Perinatal Care is in every sense a collaboration. It epitomizes the goal that should be reflected in all efforts directed toward the continued improvement of pregnancy outcome.

Editorial Committee

1
ORGANIZATION OF PERINATAL HEALTH CARE

A regional approach to perinatal care establishes a framework for cooperative efforts to reduce perinatal morbidity and mortality. Regionally coordinated health care systems emphasize professional expertise, consultation, communication, and education for the effective use of resources based on local and individual needs. By ensuring access to services at the appropriate level, such a system facilitates the provision of care to all pregnant women, including those who have problems that may require increased fetal surveillance or maternal and neonatal intervention.

Defining levels of perinatal care within each regional system has proved helpful. New knowledge and technology are improving care, and systems of financial support for perinatal care are evolving. Despite these advances, problems persist. The idealized goal of perinatal health care—an absolute minimum of morbidity and mortality—has not been achieved. Therefore, regional perinatal care cannot remain static; it must continue to undergo refinement and change.

Although outcome is not necessarily influenced by facility or service size, the availability of appropriate equipment and personnel, such as obstetric and pediatric specialists, subspecialists, and experienced nurses, is very important to the effective management of the problems presented by the small proportion of the perinatal population with the highest risks. In the recent past, the outcome for very low birth weight infants (750-1,500 g) has steadily improved. Neonatal intensive care and interhospital transport of high-risk and very ill infants have positively influenced the survival and well-being of small and premature babies.

The outcome is better for high-risk infants born in regional perinatal centers than for those transferred after birth. The benefits of maternal-fetal transport to regional centers are especially apparent when there is a possibility of delivery at less than 32 weeks of gestation. Maternal-fetal referral for those at high risk has also been shown to reduce the overall cost of perinatal care substantially compared with the cost of perinatal care for infants transported after delivery, largely because maternal-fetal transport reduces the length of the infant's subsequent hospital stay.

HISTORICAL CONSIDERATIONS

Maternal Mortality

In the United States, the maternal mortality rate has decreased from 582/100,000 live births in 1935 to 7.8/100,000 live births in 1985. This decrease in maternal deaths is attributable to, in order of importance, the increased safety of blood transfusion, the discovery of antimicrobial agents, the improved ability to control the most severe complications of preeclampsia, and the development of general and regional anesthesia techniques that are safer for both the mother and the fetus. These advances culminated in better management of complicated pregnancies, including labor and delivery, which resulted in the current safety record for both vaginal and cesarean delivery. In fact, 10,000 consecutive cesarean deliveries with no maternal deaths have been reported in one series.

In addition, committees formed by county, state, and regional medical or obstetric-gynecologic organizations have defined preventable events and scrutinized maternal and perinatal deaths according to county, state, and national health guidelines. As an added benefit, these committees established lines of communication between professional groups, which resulted in improved educational programs and services for the mother, fetus, and neonate. In some localities, this led to a positive relationship among professional groups and extended to maternal and child health government agencies, creating a model for other specialties and agencies.

Centers for Premature Neonates

In the 1920s and 1930s, centers designed especially for the care of premature neonates appeared in the United States, fostered in part by the work of Dr. Julius H. Hess in Chicago. Such centers trace some of their origins to the public exhibitions of small babies that Martin Couney organized for fairs and expositions in Europe and the United States at the turn of the century. While criticized for their commercial motivation, the displays attracted the attention of physicians, including Hess. By the 1940s and 1950s, a uniform standard of care based on isolation, thermal stability, proper nutrition, and specialized nursing care had been established at several locations. Academic perinatal study was under way.

The establishment of these centers was followed by the creation of neonatal intensive care units at several locations in the 1950s and 1960s, when the intensive care concept was developed in both adult and pediatric medicine. In fact, early descriptions included discussions of neonatal intensive care provided in conjunction with adult intensive care. During the 1960s, the scope of neonatal care expanded rapidly, resulting in more aggressive medical and surgical care of all neonates; however, the focus remained primarily on the low-birth-weight neonate. The close relationship between neonatal intensive care and the main body of obstetric practice became clear late in the 1960s, although basic concern and preparation for interaction had been evident much earlier.

Maternal-Fetal Assessment

The increasing ability to assess both maternal and fetal risks ushered in a new era of obstetric care in the late 1960s and early 1970s. Not only were there advances in special knowledge and skills for maternal care, but also techniques for the assessment of fetal health, including maturity studies that allow consideration of preterm delivery, became clinical realities. Dialogue between obstetricians and pediatricians became a requirement, not a courtesy, as the parallel development of obstetric and neonatal intensive care resulted in joint centers.

Role of Organizations

Perinatal regional systems have been greatly influenced by professional organizations. After surveying obstetric practices in the United States in 1967, the American College of Obstetricians and Gynecologists defined several problem areas, such as the underutilization of hospital beds, the difficulty encountered by small obstetric services in handling emergency procedures, and deficiencies in the immediate care of the neonate. In 1973, stating that one of its goals was to reduce the perinatal mortality rate in the United States to 10/1,000 births within 10 years, the College emphasized the need for regional education programs and the development of guidelines for a regional perinatal care system. In 1971, a joint committee of the Society of Obstetricians and Gynaecologists of Canada and the Canadian Paediatric Society, as well as the American Medical Association, had also taken positions in favor of the regionalization of perinatal health care. In 1973, The National Foundation-March of Dimes provided financial and administrative support for the ad hoc Committee on Perinatal Health, an interprofessional and multidisciplinary group that included representatives of the American Academy of Family Physicians, the American Academy of Pediatrics, the American College of Obstetricians and Gynecologists, and the American Medical Association. With consultants from various health care professions, government agencies, and consumer groups, the members of this committee developed guidelines for a regional perinatal care system. In order to ensure quality care for all pregnant women and newborns, they proposed maximal use of highly trained perinatal personnel, intensive care facilities, and assurance of reasonable cost effectiveness. The subsequent adoption of these guidelines (published in *Toward Improving the Outcome of Pregnancy*), in principle or with little conceptual modification, by the federal government and by more than 50% of state legislatures, is evidence of their importance, validity, and timeliness. The first edition of *Guidelines for Perinatal Care* confirmed and expanded the principles and approaches to perinatal health outlined in this original document.

The realization that the burgeoning knowledge of perinatology mandated special attention led to the establishment in the 1970s of the Sub-board of Neonatal-Perinatal Medicine by the American Board of Pediatrics and the Division of Maternal-Fetal Medicine of the American Board of Obstetrics and Gynecology.

PROGRAM DEVELOPMENT

A comprehensive regional perinatal care system provides education, evaluation and research, and administration (Appendix A). A three-level system, used by most existing regional health care programs and planning organizations, was originally proposed (Table 1-1). All patients should have access to care at an appropriate level, according to need and regardless of financial status. In most instances, patients have access to the system through a personal physician, such as an obstetrician, pediatrician, or family practitioner.

Table 1-1. Levels of Program Development*

Levels of Basic Perinatal Network	Activity	Locations	Usual Physician Leadership
I	Usual focus of patient entry into system Risk assessment Uncomplicated perinatal care Stabilization of unexpected problems Data collection Sponsor of local education	Community hospital or colocated at level II or level III facility	Primary care physician or specialist
II	Level I activities, plus: Diagnosis and treatment of selected high-risk pregnancies and neonatal problems Patient transport Education efforts for part of network	Large community hospitals with many support services or co-located at level III facility	Specialist or subspecialist
III	Usually level I and level II activities,* plus: Diagnosis and treatment of most perinatal problems Research and outcome surveillance Regional education Regional administration	Large medical centers with comprehensive academic programs	Subspecialist

*Some level III facilities, such as level III neonatal units in children's hospitals, may not provide level I and level II services. Regional resource centers provide specialized knowledge and skills in academic medical centers (level III) at a subspeciality (academic) level.

There are many variations of the three-level system. As previously predicted, level II activity has expanded, sometimes because of newly recognized needs and sometimes because of economic or entrepreneurial initiatives. In addition, although academic institutions have been the principal providers of level III care, an increasing number of sophisticated, nonacademic institutions are now becoming involved in intensive care. The emergence of prepaid health plans and hospital systems for comprehensive care has resulted in the development of many perinatal centers with full-time subspecialists in maternal-fetal medicine and neonatology who provide outstanding maternal and newborn care. When integrated into a regional plan, such centers can be medically responsible and economically desirable.

The failure to integrate a facility that provides any level of care, including level III care, into a regional system is potentially counter-productive. In a flexible system based on levels of program development, professional and lay hospital leaders are obliged to determine their hospitals' roles within a broad regional context. Totally independent activity of an institution obstructs the provision of responsible perinatal care and the attainment of regional goals and objectives.

Goals and Objectives

An organized perinatal care program should be based on goals and objectives designed to meet needs of all perinatal patients. Service, education, and research should be balanced so that care continuously improves through expansion of professional knowledge and skills, proper allocation of resources, and outcome evaluation.

Broad goals for national and regional programs include 1) the reduction of maternal, fetal, and neonatal mortality and morbidity to the lowest attainable levels and 2) the efficient use of available resources to meet patient needs.

National objectives should serve as guidelines for regions, but state or regional planning agencies should alter national recommendations if an assessment of local needs and resources warrants an alteration. The problems and resources of one region may be quite different from those of other regions or from those of the nation as a whole. Rural and economically deprived areas may require special consideration, for example.

A process that limits attention to service needs, such as beds, and does not take into account other factors, such as education or outcome evaluation, is incomplete and can be expected to have less than optimal impact. Also limiting is the concept that there is an irreducible minimum in mortality and morbidity; the ultimate goal should be the well-being of all.

Approaches to Organization

In order to establish and maintain an effective regional perinatal care system, it is necessary to evaluate the existing state of maternal and child health in the region, identify unmet needs, institute a response, and evaluate results. On-site community and hospital surveys of personnel and facilities have been shown to be valuable tools in cataloging resources and examining consumer attitudes toward perceived needs and possible alterations in care practices. Responses to needs will vary, but should be based on the following important considerations: 1) emphasis on local problem-solving by health care providers and consumers, 2) awareness of professional limitations by those responsible for continuing education, 3) continued involvement of personal physicians and other providers in the care of their patients, and 4) outcome evaluation.

State health departments and other health care planning bodies have an obvious interest in perinatal care systems, and their active involvement in the development of regional perinatal care programs is strongly encouraged. Government maternal and child health agencies should provide fiscal support and leadership in the development, management, and evaluation of regional programs.

In many regions, the establishment of a perinatal advisory group charged with the collaborative planning, implementation, and assessment of a comprehensive perinatal care program has been effective. Regardless of the approach to the development and institution of needed improvements in the system, continuity of commitment is essential. Education is the ultimate determinant of improved perinatal outcome. As the regional system of perinatal care evolves, effective communication, appropriate continuing education, and continual and consistent evaluation of data require an ongoing commitment of funds.

Components

All regional organization models for perinatal care have certain identifiable activities that should be integrated into a plan that encompasses the basic components of a system:

I. Patient Care
   A. Ambulatory services
      1. Maternal-fetal assessment and care
      2. Diagnosis of genetic disease and genetic counseling
      3. Laboratory evaluation
      4. Special procedures (eg, amniocentesis, ultrasound examination)
      5. Neonatal follow-up
   B. Inpatient services
      1. Maternal-fetal services, including intensive care and surgery
      2. Neonatal services, including intensive care and surgery
      3. Radiologic, anesthetic, and laboratory services
      4. Ultrasonography
      5. Counseling
   C. Consultation and referral
   D. Transportation
      1. Maternal-fetal
      2. Neonatal
      3. Return

II. Education
   A. Public health information for prevention of disease
   B. Patient awareness and preparation
   C. Professionals
      1. Undergraduate/graduate studies
      2. Postgraduate and continuing education
   D. Institutions
      1. Hospitals
      2. Public service agencies
      3. Regulatory and funding agencies

III. Evaluation and Research
   A. Outcome, including follow-up (maternal and neonatal)
   B. Current therapy and techniques
   C. Systems

IV. Administration
  A. Cost-effectiveness analysis
  B. Resource allocation
  C. Consultation
  D. Systems development and management

The primary component of any systematic approach to quality health care is personnel. Perinatal care is multidisciplinary, involving medical, nursing, paramedical, and nonmedical personnel. Thus, the team concept, with emphasis on leadership and communication, is extremely important. The director or codirector of a perinatal care team should be a physician who has training and experience in perinatal medicine, as well as administrative skills. The team is likely to include not only obstetricians, family physicians, and pediatricians, but also nurses, social workers, and health care administrators.

The obstetrician or family physician, sometimes working with a certified nurse-midwife who practices as a member of a team, is responsible for prenatal care, including risk assessment. Consultation or referral may be necessary for high-risk patients. Pediatricians and obstetricians should collaborate not only in planning but also in specific situations that may affect the fetus and newborn. Labor and delivery should be attended by personnel appropriate to the level of need. (For more information regarding attendance at cesarean births or high-risk deliveries, see Intrapartum Care, Chapter 4.) Postpartum care of the family is also a cooperative effort.

The minimal responsibilities of directors of level III perinatal units (either academic or nonacademic) are to be aware of the community hospitals that provide maternal and child health care in their region, to provide those units with information and education that will improve perinatal care, be it level I or level II, and to ensure the availability of a mechanism of transfer of the maternal-fetal or neonatal patient to a level III unit. These directors should also be aware of new developments in the discipline and provide for the appropriate integration of care within the region.

The role of nurses in perinatal medicine has been expanding. Outpatient and hospital nurses play vital professional roles at all levels of care, and these roles should be identified and structured within a team effort in risk assessment and care. Certified nurse-midwives, obstetric-gynecologic nurse-practitioners, neonatal or perinatal nurse-clinicians or specialists, and pediatric nurse-practitioners make important contributions to the development of regional networks, the management of normal and unanticipated perinatal events, and follow-up. Each regional program should consider employing a perinatal nurse coordinator to assist with educational, service, and administrative endeavors.

Socioeconomic factors are significant determinants of pregnancy outcome, and social workers should be members of perinatal teams. Perinatal services that have a great many high-risk patients require full-time social workers with special skills in solving the problems associated with perinatal risks.

Health care administrators with special expertise in perinatal care should be encouraged to participate in regional programs. Such individuals may represent hospital, government, or private agencies.

Institutions associated with perinatal care systems include hospitals, academic centers, and private and government agencies. Community hospitals should function as integral components of the system coordinating their activities with those of academic medical centers and specialty units (eg, children's hospitals). Faculties at academic centers should play a leadership role in establishing standards for patient care and implementing professional education programs. State and local agencies or foundations should participate actively in the system; their role should not be just supportive.

Transport systems are necessary for each regional system. They require cooperation between institutions, which is best structured by affiliation and transport agreements. Specific arrangements for transport systems differ from region to region, but adjoining regions may agree to share services. Transport services should be available to all perinatal patients, regardless of their point of origin, and should include both maternal-fetal and neonatal services, as well as return services. (Chapter 8 is devoted to this vital subject.)

Funding guarantees are important to most effective regional systems. Although direct and third-party payers can and should be expected to bear the cost of care and transport, these sources seldom provide adequate funding for other activities, such as quality assurance, education, research, and outcome evaluation. Hospitals and academic institutions cannot be expected to subsidize these activities, however. Because such activities benefit the region as a whole, all components of the system should share equitably in their costs. Government agencies may help identify and solve funding problems. Progressive regional programs must anticipate the need for financial support and plan accordingly.

Education and training are essential components of regional programs. Academic centers working with community hospitals often provide these services, or they may be provided by integrated perinatal care committees or associations of professional groups. Experience has shown that it is best to include personnel from as many parts of the system as possible.

Research and outcome surveillance should be integral parts of a regional program. Academic centers, nonacademic institutions that provide tertiary level care, state vital statistics offices, and the Bureau of Maternal and Child Health may share this responsibility. Periodic statistical summaries are very helpful.

Risk Identification

Risk assessment and management, essential elements of comprehensive perinatal care, begin when a patient enters the system and continue as long as the patient is receiving care. For maximum effectiveness, patients must enter the system as early as possible. Preconception care permits prospective selection of patients who might benefit from evaluation or care by another practitioner or institution.

Not all high-risk factors are discernible prior to labor or delivery. Therefore, all facilities that provide perinatal services should have the ability to detect unanticipated maternal, fetal, and neonatal complications and respond with timely, definitive care. For example, all facilities in a perinatal system should have the capability to begin a cesarean delivery within 30 minutes from the time of decision and to resuscitate and stabilize stressed infants.

Physicians in a region must work together to determine factors that constitute additional risk, the most effective ways to deal with that risk, and the best alternatives for present and future care in a region. This coordinated process facilitates acceptance of the resulting system of consultation, referral, and transfer.

Problem Areas

Many regional care systems are experiencing stresses and potential problems. The changes and innovations brought about by expanding knowledge and technology, especially those changes and innovations that result in a seemingly unnecessary proliferation of services, have been sources of uneasiness and ambivalence. In some locales, the present emphasis on a deregulated approach to health care is considered beneficial because services and resources are more plentiful. Concerns have centered on system inefficiency, delayed care resulting from resistance to appropriate referral, and increased cost. In order to respond to these challenges, regional care systems should maintain an integrated approach.

There is increasing concern that free-standing perinatal care units and systems that do not cooperate with other units and systems effectively "deregionalize" care. At best, duplication of services and incomplete evaluation may occur; at worst, different populations may receive a different quality of care. In addition, as the health care system changes, encompassing new arrangements between hospitals, increased use of large prepaid programs, and competition, care must be taken to prevent a decrease in the rate of progress or even an actual regression in the measures of outcome, such as neonatal mortality, because of a two-class system of care.

The increased number and sophistication of level II units have improved the availability of care, shortened transport time or eliminated the need for transport, and enhanced communication in most situations. Such growth of level II units has had disadvantages, however. Some centers are essentially service oriented and neglect educational or scientific activities. Distribution and availability of subspecialist perinatologists and special services, such as pediatric surgery, may be adversely affected, and patients may not be referred appropriately.

The current economics of health care encourage the development of nonacademic advanced level II and level III centers. Many such centers are now recruiting their first neonatal and maternal-fetal subspecialists, and as yet they have no clearly defined job descriptions or expectations other than establishing services. The role of these subspecialists in a community hospital differs from their defined role in an academic setting, however. Thus, both the subspecialist and the institution should prospectively define their goals and objectives. Frank discussions to identify and resolve problems prior to the establishment of these positions are necessary to avoid individual dissatisfaction and duplication of services.

Unequal contributions among hospitals to the care of non-paying patients is a problem in some regions. Purposeful selection of paying patients in an unbalanced manner is counterproductive.

The development of neonatal transport systems has clearly been beneficial, but the lack of an accompanying commitment to maternal referral or transport in some regions has tended to work against the regionalization concept. All but the most seriously ill mothers continue to be delivered in the level I and II community hospitals. A recent report indicated that the risk characteristics of mothers of low-birth-weight infants delivered in facilities at all three levels of care were surprisingly similar, suggesting that there has been no systematic movement of mothers to the proper facility for delivery. In some studies, up to 30% of all neonatal deaths and up to 50% of the deaths of infants weighing less than 1,000 g occurred in the first four hours of life, prior to a time when neonatal transport is likely. Neonatal transport should not be considered a solution to a missed opportunity for maternal transport or referral.

The values and strengths of local individual treatment do not always prevail in systematic and regionalized care. Providers should understand that every part of the system should support personal attention to the patient and that the original primary care physician-patient relationship should resume when referral or consultative care is no longer necessary. Therefore, continuing communication is essential. It should be made clear to patients that the transfer of their trust to another provider is justified and that potential benefits outweigh whatever temporary family and community dislocation is necessary. Impersonal care can exist at any level but is never justified. Return transfer should be routine.

Political divisions and geophysical boundaries are often barriers to regionalized perinatal health care. Similarly, the scattering of maternal and child health programs through multiple departments and agencies at the state and national levels of government has made refinement of developed systems more difficult in some circumstances. Planning and funding for educational activities and transport, particularly maternal-fetal transport, have been inadequate in many regions. Funds for patient care should coincide with patients' needs without concern for county, state, or national boundaries.

THE FUTURE

Perinatology has become increasingly integrated with related subspecialty areas in reproductive medicine, such as genetics and infertility diagnosis and treatment. As more and more concerns are recognized, perinatal programs will evolve to meet the broader needs of maternal and child care.

Accurate data collection will make it easier to identify those specific resources, including primary and specialty medical care, that improve reproductive outcome. With better application of computer technology, a comprehensive perinatal data base should facilitate regional planning and program implementation, as well as efforts to create individual and public acceptance of regionalized care. Concerted efforts will be necessary to interpret mortality and morbidity data and to relate such data to cost factors.

In the future, the concept of levels of patient care will continue to be useful, but program development should be incorporated into the definitions of levels. Program development is a dynamic process of identifying regional needs, allocating resources, initiating activity, evaluating outcome, and then maintaining and adjusting performance accordingly. Each institution within a regional system should go through this process and define its level or sphere of activity within its region. A focus on program development allows for flexibility in defining levels of care and should reflect documented needs and resources. Owing to the highly specialized and costly resources involved, regional resource centers can provide leadership, knowledge, and special skills for each network. These cooperative efforts should be directed toward the cost-effective management of specific specialized problems.

Perinatal medicine will continue to be dynamic and progressive as technology advances and knowledge of pathophysiology and human reproductive behavior increases. The perinatal care system described is flexible enough to accommodate the changes brought about by new developments.

RESOURCES AND RECOMMENDED READING

American Academy of Pediatrics, Committee on Fetus and Newborn: Level II neonatal units. Pediatrics 66(5):810-811, 1980

Aubry RH, Pennington JC: Identification and evaluation of high-risk pregnancy: The perinatal concept. Clin Obstet Gynecol 16(1):3-27, 1973

Backett EM, Davies AM, Petros-Barvazian A: The Risk Approach in Health Care: With Special Reference to Maternal and Child Health, Including Family Planning. Public Health Papers No 76. Geneva, World Health Organization, 1984

Bloom BS: Changing infant mortality: The need to spend more while getting less. Pediatr 73(6):862-866, 1984

Committee to Study the Prevention of Low Birthweight, Division of Health Promotion and Disease Prevention, Institute of Medicine: Preventing Low Birthweight. Washington DC, National Academy Press, 1985

Crenshaw C Jr, Payne P, Blackmon L, et al: Prematurity and the obstetrician: A regional neonatal intensive care nursery is not enough. Am J Obstet Gynecol 147(2):125-132, 1983

Harris TR, Isaman J, Giles HR: Improved neonatal survival through maternal transport. Obstet Gynecol 52(3):294-300, 1978

Hein HA: The status and future of small maternity services in Iowa. JAMA 255(14):1899-1903, 1986

Hobel CJ, Hyvarinen MA, Okada DM, et al: Prenatal and intrapartum high-risk screening: I. Prediction of the high-risk neonate. Am J Obstet Gynecol 117(1):1-9, 1973

Hobel CJ, Youkeles L, Forsythe A: Prenatal and intrapartum high-risk screening: II. Risk factors reassessed. Am J Obstet Gynecol 135(8):1051-1056, 1979

Johnson KG: The promise of referral perinatal care as a national strategy for improved maternal and infant care. Public Health Reports 97(2):134-139, 1983

Kanto WP: Regionalization revisited, editorial. Am J Dis Child 141(4):403-404, 1987

McCarthy BJ, Schulz KF, Terry JS: Identifying neonatal risk factors and predicting neonatal deaths in Georgia. Am J Obstet Gynecol 142(5):557-562, 1982

McCormick MC, Shapiro S, Starfield BH: The regionalization of perinatal services. Summary of the evaluation of a national demonstration program. JAMA 253(6):799-804, 1985

National Foundation—March of Dimes, Committee on Perinatal Health: Toward Improving the Outcome of Pregnancy: Recommendations for the Regional Development of Maternal and Perinatal Health Services. White Plains NY, National Foundation—March of Dimes, 1977

Paneth N, Kiely JL, Susser M: Age at death used to assess the effect of interhospital transfer of newborns. Pediatr 73(6):854-861, 1984

Paneth N, Kiely JL, Wallenstein S, et al: Newborn intensive care and neonatal mortality in low-birth-weight infants: A population study. N Engl J Med 307(3):149-155, 1982

Paneth N, Kiely JL, Wallenstein S, et al: The choice of place of delivery. Effect of hospital level on mortality in all singleton births in New York City. Am J Dis Child 141(1):60-64, 1987

Papiernik E, Bouyer J, Dreyfus J, et al: Prevention of preterm births: A perinatal study in Haguenau, France. Pediatr 76(2):154-158, 1985

Ryan GM Jr, Fielden JG, Pearse WH: Regional planning—Effects on the obstetrician-gynecologist. Obstet Gynecol 59(2):202-205, 1982

Sinclair JC, Torrance GW, Boyle MH, et al: Evaluation of neonatal intensive care programs. N Engl J Med 305(9):489-494, 1981

Williams RL, Chen PM: Identifying the sources of the recent decline in perinatal mortality rates in California. N Engl J Med 306(4):207-214, 1982

2

PHYSICAL FACILITIES FOR PERINATAL CARE

Physical facilities for perinatal care in hospitals should be conducive to care that meets the normal physiologic and psychosocial needs of mothers, fathers, and neonates. Special facilities should be available when deviations from the norm require uninterrupted physiologic, biochemical, and clinical observation of patients throughout the perinatal period. The contiguous location of areas for labor, delivery, and newborn care facilitates the necessary integration of obstetric, anesthetic, nursing, and pediatric efforts.

These recommendations are intended as general guidelines; they should be flexible enough to meet local needs. It is recognized that individual problems of physical facilities for perinatal care may impede strict adherence to the recommendations. Furthermore, not all hospitals will have all functional units described. Provisions for individual units should be consistent with the regionalized perinatal care system involved.

OBSTETRIC FUNCTIONAL UNITS

The inpatient obstetric service should provide a safe and comfortable environment for women to deliver and care for their newborns. The patient's personal needs and those of her newborn and family should be considered when the service units are planned. The service should be consolidated in a designated area that, ideally, is physically separate from the remainder of the hospital (eg, on a single floor or in a special wing).

The obstetric service should have facilities for the following functional components:

1. Antepartum care and testing
2. Fetal diagnostic services
3. Admission/observation/waiting
4. Labor
5. Delivery/cesarean birth
6. Intensive care (levels II and III only)
7. Recovery
8. Postpartum care
9. Visitation

Depending on patient volume and patient care resources available, many of the functional areas can be combined in a single room. For example, an admission/examination room may also serve as a labor room or recovery room, and a family waiting room may be used for sibling visitation. To maximize economy and flexibility of staff and space, many hospitals have successfully combined areas for labor, delivery, recovery, and postpartum care into single areas called labor/delivery/recovery (LDR) or labor/delivery/recovery/postpartum (LDRP) rooms. If functional units are combined, however, care must be taken to ensure that all aspects of each component are retained.

Hospitals that provide level II care should have all the functional units contained in hospitals that provide level I care. Hospitals that provide level I services do not need an intensive care unit. All level III hospitals provide intensive care, as do most level II hospitals.

Antepartum Care

An area should be designated for patients hospitalized before labor because of maternal/fetal conditions or problems.

Fetal Diagnostic Services

A room for performing studies such as nonstress tests, oxytocin challenge tests, amniocentesis, and ultrasound examination should be readily accessible to the delivery area.

Admission/Observation/Waiting

A separate admitting area in the labor and delivery suite should be designated for patient examination and short-term observation of patients who are not yet in active labor or who must be observed to determine whether labor has actually begun. A comfortable waiting area for the family should be adjacent to the labor and delivery suite.

Labor

The number of beds required for labor depends on several factors, including the number of anticipated deliveries, designated usage, and state and local public health regulations. As a general rule, one bed for labor can accommodate approximately 250 deliveries per year. More beds are needed if they are used for antepartum observation and postpartum recovery as well as for active labor.

Local regulations concerning the size of rooms vary; however, private rooms of approximately 180 sq ft floor space are desirable. If multibed labor rooms are necessary, it is preferable that each bed be allotted 100 sq ft floor space. Partitions or curtains are essential to provide privacy in multibed rooms. Labor rooms may be planned so that they can be used for intensive care of high-risk patients in hospitals that have no designated high-risk unit.

An early labor lounge is highly desirable to allow efficient use of space and foster family-centered care.

The components for each labor room are

1. A labor or birthing bed and a footstool
2. A storage area for the patient's clothing and personal belongings
3. One or more comfortable chairs
4. Adjustable lighting that is pleasant for the patient and adequate for examinations
5. An emergency signal and an intercommunication system
6. Adequate ventilation and temperature control
7. A sphygmomanometer, stethoscope, and fetoscope
8. Mechanical infusion equipment
9. Capability for use of electronic fetal monitoring equipment
10. Oxygen and suction outlets
11. Hand-washing facilities in or immediately adjacent to each labor room
12. Conveniently located toilet facilities, which may be shared by two patients in different labor rooms
13. A writing surface for charting
14. Storage facilities

The following additional facilities are needed in the labor room area:

1. Soiled utility room with equipment for cleansing bedpans
2. Clean utility room
3. Secure area for medication storage and preparation
4. Nurses' station
5. Physician and nurse charting area
6. Stretcher/wheelchair storage area
7. Staff lounge
8. Kitchen or pantry for preparing food for patients
9. Conference room
10. Real time ultrasound imaging equipment
11. Auxiliary electrical system

Other supplies and equipment in the labor and delivery room area may include the following items:

1. Stretcher with side rails
2. X-ray film view boxes
3. Equipment and supplies for administering medications and obtaining blood specimens
4. Ice maker

A central area in which medications can be prepared for patients in either the labor or delivery rooms is necessary. All drugs required for emergencies that may arise during labor should be stocked in the labor and delivery area. Cardiopulmonary resuscitation carts should be available to carry the following items:

1. Needles
2. Syringes
3. Emergency drugs
4. Laryngoscope
5. Airways
6. Equipment for delivering positive pressure oxygen
7. Adult cardiac monitor
8. Suction apparatus, if not otherwise provided
9. Defibrillator

Separate lounges with lockers and restrooms nearby should be provided for physicians and nurses near the labor and delivery area. Individual sleeping facilities for physicians on call should also be located near the delivery area.

Delivery/Cesarean Birth

In order to afford easy access and to provide privacy to women in labor, the delivery rooms should be close to the labor rooms. A delivery unit should have no fewer than two delivery rooms. The number of delivery/cesarean birth rooms required depends on the average number of deliveries per day, as well as on the number and use of birthing areas. In traditional labor and delivery units, it is generally agreed that four delivery rooms, with two equipped for cesarean delivery, should be adequate for 3,000 annual deliveries. An obstetric service for 1,000-2,000 deliveries each year requires two to three delivery rooms. Small obstetric services may equip a labor room for alternate use as a delivery room.

A delivery/cesarean birth room is similar in design to an operating room; a room with 350-400 sq ft open floor space and a ceiling height of 9 ft is adequate for normal or cesarean delivery. Room temperature should be controllable so that the chilling of mother and neonate can be prevented. Each room should be equipped with the safeguards necessary for the administration of all forms of anesthesia. At least one delivery room should be equipped with an operating table and instruments necessary for emergency surgical obstetric intervention. It is desirable that cesarean deliveries be performed in the delivery unit and that postpartum sterilization capabilities be available.

Each delivery/cesarean birth room should be maintained as a separate unit with equipment and supplies necessary for normal delivery and for the management of complications:

1. A delivery table that allows variation in position for delivery
2. Instrument table and solution basin stand
3. Instruments and equipment for vaginal delivery, repair of lacerations, cesarean delivery, and the management of obstetric emergencies
4. Solutions and equipment for the intravenous administration of fluids
5. Equipment for inhalation and regional anesthesia, including equipment for emergency resuscitation

6. Heated, temperature-controlled neonatal examination and resuscitation unit
7. Equipment for examination, immediate care, and identification of the neonate
8. Individual oxygen, air, and suction outlets for mother and neonate
9. An emergency call system
10. Mirrors for patients to observe the birth
11. Wall clock with a second hand
12. Equipment for electronic fetal monitoring

In addition, trays containing drugs and equipment necessary for emergency treatment of both mother and neonate should be kept in the delivery room area. Equipment necessary for the treatment of cardiac arrest should also be easily accessible.

The following support facilities should be available:

1. Scrub sinks that have arm, knee, or foot controls and are placed so that, while scrubbing, the physician can observe the patient.
2. A workroom in which instruments are washed and a separate room for preparing and sterilizing instruments. These rooms should be located near the delivery/cesarean birth rooms unless these services are provided by a central supply facility.
3. A room for storing supplies and equipment.
4. A room for the storage and preparation of anesthetics.

Laboratory facilities should be capable of providing blood group, Rh type and cross-matching, blood pH and gas analysis, and basic emergency laboratory evaluations 24 hours/day. Either ABO Rh-specific or type O Rh-negative blood should be available at the facility at all times. Other laboratory procedures, such as serologic testing and determination of rubella titers, should be available.

Intensive Care

Patients who have significant medical or obstetric complications should be cared for in a room especially equipped with cardiopulmonary resuscitation equipment and other monitoring equipment necessary for observation and special care. It is preferable that this room be located in the labor and delivery area and meet the physical requirements of any other intensive care room in the hospital.

Recovery

Larger services should have a specific recovery room for postpartum patients with a separate area for high-risk patients. Generally, the number of recovery beds should equal one-half the number of traditional labor beds. When it is not possible to provide a separate recovery area, designated nursing personnel should observe recently delivered patients in a labor or delivery room.

The equipment needed is similar to that needed in any surgical recovery room and includes equipment for monitoring vital signs, suctioning, administering oxygen, and infusing fluids intravenously. Cardiopulmonary resuscitation equipment should be readily available.

Postpartum Care

The number of beds required in a postpartum unit is calculated by multiplying the number of annual deliveries by the average length of stay and dividing the result by 365 days times the estimated occupancy rate:

$$\frac{\text{Annual deliveries} \times \text{Average stay}}{365 \times \text{Estimated occupancy rate}} = \text{Number of postpartum beds required}$$

This calculation does not allow for use of these beds by antepartum patients. A projected 75% occupancy rate minimizes the risk of a patient load beyond the total bed capacity of the institution. The postpartum unit should be flexible enough to permit comfortable accommodation of patients when the patient census is at its peak and use of beds for alternate functions when the patient census is low. Ideally, not more than two patients share one room.

Each patient unit should accommodate the patient, her newborn, and visitors without crowding. In multibed rooms, the minimum recommended floor area for each patient unit is approximately 100 sq ft. Partitions or curtains are essential in multibed rooms to facilitate privacy. Each unit should provide protection against nosocomial infection, as well as an atmosphere conducive to rest.

Each patient unit should include the following items:

1. Bed with adjustable side rails
2. Adequate lighting
3. Bedside stand
4. Storage space for clothes and personal belongings
5. Signal or intercommunication device

6. Bathing, toilet, and hand-washing facilities that are in or close to the patient's room and are equipped with an emergency call signal

If possible, each room in the postpartum unit should have its own toilet and hand-washing facilities. When this is not possible and it is necessary for patients to use common facilities, patients should be able to reach them without entering a general corridor. When the newborn rooms in with the mother, the room should have hand-washing facilities, a mobile bassinet unit, and supplies necessary for the care of the newborn. Siblings may visit in the mother's room or in a designated space in the antepartum or postpartum area.

In addition to those already mentioned, each postpartum unit should include the following facilities:

1. Nurses' station
2. Staff lounge, lockers, and toilet
3. Washroom for staff use
4. Examination and treatment room
5. Kitchen or pantry for preparing food for patients
6. Separate clean and soiled utility rooms
7. Area for storing and dispensing medication
8. Patient education area
9. Adequate storage areas for clean equipment, linens, and other supplies
10. Conference room
11. Lounge for patients and visitors
12. Sitz bath facilities

The following equipment and supplies should be available:

1. Sphygmomanometers and stethoscopes
2. Intravenous solution and infusion supplies
3. Catheter equipment and supplies
4. Stretcher with side rails
5. Emergency drugs
6. Cardiopulmonary resuscitation cart

Single Room Care

Recently, various combinations of facilities have evolved to accommodate those women who want to deliver their babies in a setting that allows family members or other supporting persons to be present throughout the childbirth process, but who also want to have ready access to modern obstetric facilities. Such units, referred to as LDR or LDRP rooms, should be located in or close to the intrapartum area.

The ideal size of an LDR room is approximately 350 sq ft floor space. Such a room should be able to accommodate six to eight people comfortably during the childbirth process, and it should be equipped for all types of delivery except cesarean delivery. Each room should have a birthing bed that can be positioned for delivery and can be moved to a delivery/cesarean birth room if the need arises. Toilet and shower facilities may be included in each room. The nurse:patient ratio should be the same as that on a traditional obstetric service, even though nurses spend less time transferring patients to different rooms for labor, delivery, and recovery.

The LDRP room is an extension of the same concept to the postpartum period in that the patient remains in the same room, not only for labor, delivery, and recovery, but also for postpartum care. This approach provides single room maternal-neonatal care for all noncesarean deliveries. Nurses are cross-trained in antepartum care, labor and delivery, postpartum care, and neonatal care, making the use of staff more cost-effective and increasing the continuity and quality of care. Most state codes do not currently address this concept.

These rooms should contain the same equipment and supplies that other labor rooms contain, including fetal monitor, infusion pumps, and equipment for anesthesia administration, delivery, and resuscitation. Equipment for neonatal resuscitation and temperature control should also be present. Preferably, equipment is concealed in wall cabinets or behind drapes. It may be necessary to keep expensive equipment in a central location rather than to equip each LDRP room fully, but equipment must be readily available when needed.

PEDIATRIC FUNCTIONAL UNITS

Among the necessary pediatric functional units are areas for the following activities:

1. Resuscitation/stabilization
2. Admission/observation
3. Normal newborn care
4. Continuing care
5. Intermediate care

6. Intensive care
7. Isolation
8. Parent-neonate visitation/breastfeeding/interview

Level I facilities should provide areas for resuscitation, admission/observation, normal newborn care, and parent-neonate visitation. Some level I facilities may provide continuing care for neonates who have relatively uncomplicated problems that do not require advanced laboratory, radiologic, or pediatric consultative services; most level I facilities provide care for convalescing babies who have been transported back to them from level II and III facilities. Hospitals with level II services should have the same areas that hospitals with level I care have, plus areas designated for intermediate care. Some level II hospitals also have intensive care facilities. Level III facilities should have intensive care units, as well as all other pediatric functional units.

A region with 25,000 deliveries annually may require 25 beds for intensive care, 75-100 beds for intermediate neonatal care, and 50 beds for continuing neonatal care. These beds can be distributed among all the qualified facilities in the region. Frequently, level III facilities within a region also admit maternal and neonatal patients from outside their region. The number of beds needed for these perinatal patients generally must be calculated on the basis of historical referral numbers.

It may occasionally be undesirable to establish physically separate neonatal intensive, intermediate, and continuing care areas. For economy of personnel, as well as for primary care nursing, it may be preferable to have a mix of neonatal patients in a single area. Local circumstances should be considered in the design and management of these care areas.

Patient Care Areas

Resuscitation

Immediately after birth, those neonates who require it are resuscitated and stabilized in the resuscitation area. Depending on their condition, neonates are taken from this area to the admission/observation area, the intermediate care area, or the intensive care area in the same hospital, or they are transferred to an intermediate care or intensive care area in a hospital that provides level II or level III care.

The resuscitation area, which should be illuminated to at least 100 foot-candles at the neonate's body surface, should contain the following items:

1. Overhead source of radiant heat that can be regulated to the infant's temperature
2. Thin resuscitation/examination mattress that allows access on three sides
3. Wall clock
4. Flat working surface for charting
5. Table or flat surface for trays and equipment
6. Equipment and medications
7. Oxygen, compressed air, and suction sources that are separate from those for the mother

The resuscitation area is usually within the delivery/cesarean birth room although it may be in a designated separate room. In the latter case, some institutions have found it helpful to have a window between the delivery/cesarean birth room and the resuscitation room through which the neonate can be passed. If resuscitation takes place in the delivery/cesarean birth room, the area should be large enough to ensure that the resuscitation of the neonate does not interfere with the care of the mother. Following stabilization of the neonate, if the mother wishes to hold her newborn, a radiant heater or prewarmed blankets should be available to keep the neonate warm. Also, the room temperature should be increased to a level higher than that customary for patient rooms or operating suites.

A resuscitation area should be allotted a minimum of 40 sq ft floor space if it is within a delivery/cesarean birth room. A separate resuscitation room should have approximately 150 sq ft floor space. The area should have adequate suction, oxygen, and compressed air outlets to resuscitate twins and at least six electrical outlets with a capacity of 15 amp. A separate resuscitation room should also have an electrical outlet to accommodate a portable x-ray machine, if needed. Electrical outlets should conform to the regulations for areas in which anesthetic agents are administered.

Admission/Observation (Transitional Care Stabilization)

The admission/observation area is for careful evaluation of the neonate's condition during the first 4-24 hours after birth (ie, during the period of physiologic adjustment to extrauterine life). This evaluation may take place within one or more functional areas (eg, the room in which the mother is recovering, the LDRP room, the newborn nursery, or a separate admission/observation area). In some hospitals, the newborn nursery is the primary area for transitional care, both for neonates born within the hospital and for those born outside the hospital. No isolation facilities are required for neonates born at home or in transit to the hospital.

The admission/observation area should be near or adjacent to the delivery/cesarean birth room. If it is part of the maternal recovery area, which is preferable, physical separation of the mother and newborn during this period can be avoided.

An estimated 40 sq ft floor space is needed for each neonate in the admission/observation area. The capacity required depends on the size of the delivery service and the duration of close observation. One patient station is needed for each 300 annual births if the neonate's length of stay in the area is 24 hours. Fewer stations are needed if the neonate's stay in this area is of shorter duration, but there should be at least two stations. The admission/observation area should be well lighted, have a wall clock, and contain emergency resuscitation equipment similar to that in the designated resuscitation area. Outlets should also be similar to those in the resuscitation area.

The physicians' and nurses' assessment of the neonate's condition determines the subsequent level of care. Most neonates are taken from the admission/observation area to the newborn nursery or to the postpartum area for rooming-in. Some neonates require transfer to an intermediate or intensive care area.

Newborn Nursery

Routine care of apparently normal full-term or preterm neonates who weigh more than 2,000 g at birth and have demonstrated successful adaptation to extrauterine life may be provided either in the newborn nursery or in the area where the mother is receiving postpartum care. The nursery should be close to the postpartum area. In a multifloor maternity unit, there should be a newborn nursery on each floor.

The number of bassinets in the newborn nursery should exceed the number of obstetric beds by 25% to accommodate multiple births, extended neonatal hospitalization, and fluctuations in patient load. An additional excess of 10% is appropriate for those hospitals that also have intermediate and intensive care facilities. It is also possible to estimate the required capacity of the newborn nursery on the basis of the mean duration of stay and annual number of liveborn, normal, full-term neonates. For example, if these neonates remain in the hospital an average of 3 days, each bassinet has a capacity of 120 neonates per year (365 divided by 3 = 120). If the average annual number of normal live births is 2,000, an average of 17 bassinets (2,000 divided by 120 = 17) are always in use. Adding 25% of these 17 bassinets to allow for fluctuations in patient census indicates that 21 bassinets are required for this unit. The use of LDRPs and rooming-in decreases this requirement substantially, however.

Because a relatively few staff members can provide care in the newborn nursery and because there is no need for bulky equipment, 30 sq ft floor space for each neonate should be adequate. There should be at least 3 ft between bassinets in all directions, measured from the edge of one bassinet to the edge of the neighboring bassinet. The newborn care area may be one room in a small hospital or one or more rooms in larger hospitals. Because one nursing staff member is recommended for each 6-8 neonates, individual rooms should have accommodations for 6-8, 12-16 or 18-24 neonates.

The newborn nursery should be well lighted, have a large wall clock, and be equipped for emergency resuscitation. One pair of wall-mounted electrical outlets is recommended for each two neonatal stations; one oxygen outlet, one compressed air outlet, and one suction outlet are recommended for each five or six neonatal stations. Cabinets and counters should be available within the newborn care area for storage of routinely used supplies, such as diapers, formula, and linens.

Continuing Care

Low-birth-weight neonates who are not sick, but require frequent feeding, and neonates who require more hours of nursing than do normal neonates should be taken to the continuing care area. This area should be close to the intermediate and intensive care areas, as neonates who have received intermediate or intensive care, but no longer require these levels of care, may be transferred to the continuing care area for convalescence. In level II facilities, this area is also used for convalescing babies who have returned from an outside intensive care unit.

Because the care of neonates in this area requires some bulky equipment (eg, rocking chairs and stools), as well as more personnel than are needed in the newborn nursery, more space is needed per patient unit. There should be 40 sq ft floor space for each patient station, with approximately 4 ft between bassinets or incubators.

As in the resuscitation and admission/observation areas, equipment for emergency resuscitation is required in the neonatal continuing care area. It may be most conveniently kept on an emergency cart or in a cabinet, but it should be readily available. There should be four electrical outlets, one oxygen outlet, one compressed air outlet, and one suction outlet for each neonatal station. In addition, the equipment and supplies required in the newborn nursery should be available in the continuing care area. Provisions should be made for the comfort of parents or personnel who feed neonates in both incubators and bassinets.

Intermediate Care

Sick neonates who do not require intensive care, but require 6-12 hours of nursing each day, should be taken to the intermediate care area. Infants requiring complex care, such as assisted ventilation, for more than several hours should be moved to an intensive care area.

The neonatal intermediate care area should be close to the delivery/cesarean birth room and the intensive care area, and away from general hospital traffic. It should have radiant heaters or incubators for maintaining body temperature, as well as infusion pumps, cardiopulmonary monitors, and equipment for ventilatory assistance.

An estimated 50 sq ft floor space is needed for every patient station. Space needed for other purposes (eg, for desks, counters, cabinets, corridors, and treatment rooms) should be added to the space needed for patients. There should be at least 4 ft between incubators, bassinets, or radiant heaters in intermediate care areas. Aisles should be 5 ft wide.

Neonates receiving intermediate care may be housed in a single large room or in two or more smaller rooms. In the latter case, each room should accommodate some multiple of four infant stations, because one nursing staff member is generally required for every three or four neonates who require intermediate care. Large rooms allow greater flexibility in the use of equipment and the assignment of personnel.

Eight electrical outlets, two oxygen outlets, two compressed air outlets, and two suction outlets should be provided for each patient station. In addition, the area should have a special outlet to power the neonatal unit's portable x-ray machine. All electrical outlets for each patient station should be connected to both regular and auxiliary power.

All equipment and supplies for resuscitation should be immediately available within the intermediate care unit. These items may be conveniently placed on an emergency cart.

Intensive Care

Constant nursing and continuous cardiopulmonary and other support for severely ill infants should be provided in the intensive care area. Because emergency care is provided in this area, laboratory and radiologic services should be readily available 24 hours/day. The results of blood gas analysis should be available immediately after sample collection. In many centers, a laboratory adjacent to the intensive care unit provides this service.

The neonatal intensive care area should be near the delivery/cesarean birth room and should be easily accessible from the hospital's ambulance entrance. It should be away from routine hospital traffic. Intensive care may be provided in a single area or in two or more separate rooms.

Not only is the number of nursing, medical, and surgical personnel required in the neonatal intensive care area greater than that required in other perinatal care areas, but also the amount and complexity of equipment required are considerably greater. Therefore, there should be at least 6 ft between incubators, and aisles should be 8 ft wide. The area should have 80-100 sq ft floor space for each neonate, plus space for such things as desks, cabinets, and corridors. In addition, the educational responsibilities of a level III facility require that the design of its neonatal intensive care area include space for instructional activities and office space for data files on the region's perinatal experience.

Each patient station needs 12-16 electrical outlets, 2-4 oxygen outlets, 2-4 compressed air outlets, and 2-4 suction outlets. Like those in the intermediate care area, all electrical outlets for each patient station should be connected to both regular and auxiliary power. In addition, the area should have a special outlet to power the neonatal intensive care unit's portable x-ray machine.

Equipment and supplies in the intensive care area should include all those needed in the resuscitation and intermediate care areas. In addition, equipment for long-term ventilatory support should be provided. Respirators should be equipped with nebulizers or humidifiers with heaters. Continuous on-line monitoring of oxygen concentrations, body temperature, and blood pressure should be available. Supplies should be kept close to the patient station so that nurses are not away from the neonate unnecessarily and may use their time and skills efficiently. A central modular supply system can enhance efficiency.

Isolation

Although most neonates with closed-space infections need not be removed from the newborn nursery, provisions should be made for isolating those neonates who may be harboring certain highly contagious agents (eg, varicella, herpes simplex; see Chapter 6). Because of the inefficiency associated with the use of personnel and space for isolation rooms, neonatal units in smaller hospitals may consider sharing isolation space with another unit of the pediatric service.

Visitation

Parents should have access to their newborns 24 hours/day within all functional units and should be encouraged to participate in the care of their newborns (see Chapter 4). Generally, parents can be with their newborns in the mother's room.

Special provisions may be necessary when neonates are in special care units (ie, continuing, intermediate, or intensive care units). In these situations, mothers are often discharged from the hospital before their newborns and sometimes must travel long distances to be with them. Several systems have been developed to meet the needs of parents and their newborns under these circumstances (eg, rooms for parents in the hospital, adjacent facilities outside the hospital, but provided by the hospital, or motel facilities near the hospital). A period of mother-newborn rooming-in prior to discharge is highly desirable when special care is needed.

Supporting Service Areas

Utility Rooms

Both clean and soiled utility rooms are needed in neonatal care areas. A clean utility room is for preparing formulas, medications, and supplies frequently used in the care of neonates in all functional units. The use of ready-mixed formulas, unit-dose medications, and disposable supplies and equipment has lessened the need for clean utility rooms, however, and they may be replaced by storage areas and clean working surfaces within each functional unit.

A soiled utility room is for storing used and contaminated material before its removal from the care area. This room should contain a counter and a sink with hot and cold running water that is turned on and off by knee or foot controls, soap and paper towel dispensers, and a covered waste receptacle with foot control. A separate deep sink with hot and cold running water should be available for cleaning equipment prior to its return to the central service department for resterilization. Contaminated equipment may be decontaminated in the soiled utility area and transported to the central service department in plastic bags or containers. Contaminated materials should be removed from the care area regularly. Contaminated linen should not be stored in the soiled utility area, but should be taken directly from the care area in plastic or other nonporous containers to appropriate hospital facilities.

Storage Areas

A three-level storage system is desirable. The first storage area should be the central supply department of the hospital. The second storage area should be adjacent to or within the patient care areas. In this area, routinely used supplies, such as diapers, formula, linen, cover gowns, charts, and information booklets, may be stored. Generally, space is required in this area only for the amount of each item used between deliveries from the hospital's central supply department (eg, daily or three times weekly). The third area of storage is for items frequently used at the neonate's bedside.

Bedside cabinet storage should be approximately 8 cu ft for each patient unit in the newborn nursery, 16 cu ft for each patient unit in the intermediate care area, and 24 cu ft for each patient unit in the intensive care area. The newborn nursery requires approximately 3 cu ft/patient for secondary storage of such items as linen and formula. In the resuscitation, admission/observation, continuing care, intermediate care, and intensive care areas, there should be approximately 8 cu ft/patient for secondary storage of syringes, needles, intravenous infusion sets, and sterile trays needed in such procedures as umbilical vessel catheterization, lumbar puncture, and thoracotomy.

Large items of equipment (eg, bassinets, warmers, radiant heaters, phototherapy units, and infusion pumps) should be stored in a clean storage area. Approximately 6 sq ft floor space is required for equipment for each patient in the newborn nursery, 18 sq ft for each patient in the intermediate care area, and 30 sq ft for each patient in the intensive care area.

Treatment Rooms

The development of resuscitation, admission/observation, intermediate care, and intensive care areas in which each patient station constitutes a treatment area has largely eliminated the need for a separate treatment room for the performance of procedures such as lumbar punctures, intravenous infusions, venipuncture, and minor surgical procedures. However, if neonates in the newborn nursery, continuing care area, or the postpartum new family unit are to undergo certain procedures (eg, circumcision), a separate treatment area may be necessary. The facilities, outlets, equipment, and supplies should be similar to those of the resuscitation area. The amount of space required depends on the procedures performed. Equipment, facilities, and supplies for this area, as well as procedures, must conform to or be comparable to those required for similar procedures in the surgical department of the hospital.

Scrub Areas

At the entrance to each nursery, there should be a scrub area that can accommodate all personnel entering the area. It should have a sink that is large enough to prevent splashing and is operated by foot or knee controls. Sinks for hand-washing should not be built into counters used for other purposes. The scrub areas should also contain racks, hooks, or lockers for storing clothing and personal items, as well as cabinets for clean gowns, a receptacle for used gowns, and a large wall clock with a sweep second hand for timing hand-washing.

Scrub sinks with foot-operated or knee-operated controls should be provided for at least every six to eight patient stations in the newborn nursery, for every three to four patient stations in the intermediate care area, and for every two patient stations in the intensive care area. In addition, one scrub sink is needed in the resuscitation area, and one is needed for every three to four patient stations in the admission/observation and continuing care areas.

Newborn Bathing Area

Newborns may be given a bath only after their condition has stabilized and they have demonstrated a satisfactory adjustment to extrauterine life. They may be most conveniently bathed in the admission/observation area or in the newborn nursery. The suggested sink size for newborn bathing is 12 by 24 by 7 inches. The sink should have knee-operated or foot-operated faucets and a flat surface for drying the neonate. There should be no drafts or forced air vents in this area. Large, prewarmed absorbent towels and an overhead radiant heat source help to keep the infant warm. Scales may be placed in this area so that neonates can be weighed after their bath. Daily baths may consist of sponge baths within the bassinet, as necessary.

Nursing Areas

Space should be provided at the bedside not only for patient care, but also for instructional and charting activities. A flat writing surface (eg, a clipboard) is needed.

A nurses' charting area or desk for tasks such as compiling more detailed records, completing requisitions, and handling specimens may be useful. Physicians may also perform charting and clerical activities in this area. Charting should be considered an unclean procedure, and personnel who have been charting should wash their hands before they have further contact with a neonate.

The head nurse should have an office close to the newborn care areas. Preferably adjacent to the lounge, nurses' dressing rooms should contain lockers, storage for clean and soiled scrub attire, toilets, and showers.

Education Areas

A conference room suitable for educational purposes is highly desirable, particularly for level II and level III facilities. It should be in or adjacent to the maternal-newborn areas.

Clerical Areas

The control point for patient care activities is the clerical area. It should be located near the entrance to the neonatal care areas so that the personnel can supervise traffic and limit unnecessary entry into these areas. It should have telephones and communication devices that connect to the various neonatal care areas and the delivery suite. In addition, patients' charts, computer terminals, and hospital forms may be located in the clerical area.

Formula Preparation Area

Recommendations regarding the layout, equipment, and procedures necessary for a hospital formula room have been published by the American Hospital Association. At present, few hospitals prepare their own formulas for the routine feeding of normal newborns, although special formulas may be prepared in formula rooms, diet kitchens, or pharmacies. A recent survey indicated that approximately one-half of children's hospitals or hospitals with large pediatric populations had no formula room. Many states have no regulations for the use of formula rooms.

When a hospital does have a formula preparation area, the area should have:

- One to three rooms
- Scrub sink for hand washing
- Refrigerator dedicated to storage of formula
- Dishwasher
- Adjustable pressure autoclave
- Electronic balance
- Aseptic work area with a laminar flow hood. Such areas can be used for the preparation of infant formulas and enteral formulas for older children and adults. Parenteral nutrition solutions are generally prepared in a separate location.

General Considerations

Illumination

In all newborn care areas, it should be possible to provide approximately 100 foot-candles of illumination for the proper evaluation of subtle skin tones and for the performance of delicate procedures. The lighting system should be designed to permit flexibility of illumination and creation of a diurnal light-dark cycle for those infants who do not require constant observation.

Windows

Solid, windowless walls provide the best temperature insulation for neonatal care areas, but they may have a depressing effect on the staff. If there are windows, they should be insulated with double panes. When possible, it may be preferable to use outside walls for nonpatient care areas (eg, storage, desks, or charting areas).

Interior Finish

Use of the colors off-white or pale beige on the walls minimizes distortion of the staff's color perception in patient care areas. Brighter colors may be used elsewhere. Windows in neonatal care areas should have opaque shades that make it possible to darken the area for procedures such as transillumination.

Oxygen and Compressed Air Outlets

Newborn care areas should have oxygen and compressed air piped from a central source at 50-60 psi. An alarm system that warns of any critical reduction in line pressure should be installed. Reduction valves and mixers should produce adjustable concentrations of 21%-100% oxygen at atmospheric pressure for head hoods and 50-60 psi for mechanical ventilators.

Acoustic Characteristics

The ventilation system, monitors, incubators, suction pumps, mechanical ventilators, and staff produce considerable noise, and the noise level should be monitored intermittently. The construction and redesign of neonatal care areas should include acoustic absorption units or other means to ensure that the sound intensity does not exceed 75 dB and preferably remains below that level (see Nursery Environment Chapter 4). Staff members should take particular care to avoid noise pollution in enclosed patient spaces (eg, incubators).

Electrical Outlets and Electrical Equipment

All electrical outlets should be attached to a common ground. All electrical equipment should be checked for current leakage and grounding adequacy when first introduced into the neonatal care area, after any repair, and periodically while in service. Current leakage allowances, preventive maintenance standards, and equipment quality should meet the standards developed by the Joint Commission on the Accreditation of Healthcare Organizations.

At least some (preferably all in intermediate and intensive care areas) electrical outlets should be connected to the hospital's auxiliary power circuit to maintain life support systems in the event of a power failure. The ground on these outlets should be the same as that for the other outlets.

Personnel should be thoroughly and repeatedly instructed on the potential electrical hazards within the neonatal care areas.

Safety and Environmental Control

Because of the complexities of environmental control and monitoring, it is necessary for a hospital environmental engineer to ensure that all electrical, lighting, air composition, and temperature systems function properly and safely. The environmental temperature in newborn care areas should be independently adjustable, and control should be sufficient to prevent hot and cold spots, particularly when heat-generating equipment (eg, a radiant warmer) is in use. Humidity should be between 40% and 60%; it should be controlled through the heating and air-conditioning system of the hospital.

EVACUATION PLAN

An evacuation policy should be developed for each perinatal care area (ie, antepartum care, labor and delivery, postpartum care, the normal newborn nursery, intermediate care, and intensive care). The policy should specify 1) who orders the evacuation and destination, 2) who designates the assignments, 3) what are the roles and responsibilities of the staff, and 4) what equipment is needed. A floor plan that indicates designated evacuation routes should be posted in a conspicuous place in each unit. The policy and floor plan should be reviewed with the staff at least annually.

RESOURCES AND RECOMMENDED READING

American College of Obstetricians and Gynecologists: Standards for Obstetric-Gynecologic Services, 6 ed. Washington DC, ACOG, 1985

Hager DE, Bajok SG, et al: Perspectives in Perinatal and Pediatric Design. Columbus OH, Ross Laboratories, 1988

Laufman H: Hospital Special Care Facilities: Planning for User Needs. New York, Academic Press, 1981

US Department of Health, Education, and Welfare; Public Health Service; Health Resources Administration; Bureau of Health Facilities Financing, Compliance and Conversion: Minimum Requirements of Construction & Equipment for Hospital & Medical Facilities. DHEW Publication No. (HRA) 79-14500. Washington DC, US Government Printing Office, 1979

3

PERSONNEL FOR PERINATAL CARE SERVICES

The staffing requirements of each hospital depend on its patient care commitments, the nature of the population it serves, and its obligations in education and research.

During the past several years, financial and marketing pressures have encouraged some hospitals to raise their "level designation," primarily in regard to patient care activities. This tendency is inconsistent with the classic concept of regionalization in which tertiary centers not only have the facilities to provide complex patient care, but also assume regional responsibilities for transport, outreach education, research, and quality control. Although there have been some attempts to resolve this dilemma by a sharing of some regionalization responsibilities among hospitals, this approach has resulted in different levels of care for different services at a single hospital. As used in this chapter, the terms level I care, level II care, and level III care encompass the following functions:

Level I

- Surveillance and care of all patients admitted to the obstetric service, with an established triage system for identifying high-risk mothers who should be transferred to a facility that provides level II or III care prior to delivery
- Proper detection and supportive care of unanticipated maternal-fetal problems that occur during labor and delivery
- Performance of cesarean delivery
- Care of postpartum conditions
- Resuscitation of all neonates born in their delivery facilities
- Stabilization of unexpectedly small or sick neonates before transfer to a facility that provides level II or III care

- Evaluation of the condition of healthy neonates and continuing care of these neonates until their discharge

Level II

- Performance of level I services
- Management of high-risk mothers and neonates admitted and transferred

Level III

- Provision of perinatal care services for all mothers and neonates
- Research support
- Compilation, analysis, and evaluation of regional data

MEDICAL STAFF

Level I

The perinatal care program at a level I hospital should be coordinated jointly by the chiefs of the obstetric and pediatric services. In hospitals that do not have separate departments of pediatrics and obstetrics, one physician may be given the responsibility for coordinating perinatal care. This administrative approach requires close coordination and unified policy statements. Responsibilities of the chief(s) of perinatal care at a level I hospital include policy development, maintenance of standards of care, and consultation with staff at those hospitals providing level II and III care in the region.

A qualified physician or a certified nurse-midwife should attend all deliveries. When certified nurse-midwives are involved in patient care, their specific role should be delineated by departmental rules and regulations. At least one person skilled in neonatal resuscitation should be present at every delivery. One or two other persons should be available for an emergency resuscitation. Small hospitals should arrange their staffing schedules to ensure the availability of skilled resuscitation teams. A qualified anesthesiologist or nurse-anesthetist should be readily available to administer appropriate anesthesia and maintain support of vital functions in any emergency.

Level II

A board-certified obstetrician with special interest, experience, and, in some situations, special competence certification in maternal-fetal medicine should be chief of the obstetric service at a level II hospital. A board-certified pediatrician with special interest, experience, and, in some situations, subspecialty certification in neonatal medicine should be chief of the newborn care service. These physicians should coordinate the hospital's perinatal care services and, in conjunction with other medical, nursing, and hospital administration staff, should develop policies concerning staffing, routine procedures, equipment, and supplies.

In order to ensure the safe and effective administration of anesthesia, the director of perinatal anesthesia services should be board-certified and should have training and experience in obstetric anesthesia. An anesthesiologist or nurse-anesthetist with special competence and experience in obstetric anesthesia should be readily available. Policies regarding the provision of obstetric anesthesia, including the necessary qualifications of personnel who are to administer anesthesia and their availability for both routine and emergency deliveries, should be developed. The hospital staff should also include a radiologist and, ideally, a pathologist who are available 24 hours/day. Specialized medical and surgical consultation should be readily available.

Level III

The director of the maternal-fetal medicine service at a level III hospital should be a full-time, board-certified obstetrician who is qualified by training, experience, or special competence certification in maternal-fetal medicine. The director of the regional newborn intensive care unit should be a full-time, board-certified pediatrician with subspecialty certification in neonatal medicine. As codirectors of the perinatal service, these physicians are responsible for the maintenance of standards of care, development of the operating budget, evaluation and purchase of equipment, planning and development of in-hospital and outreach educational programs, coordination of these activities, and evaluation of the effectiveness of perinatal care in the region. They should devote their time to patient care services, research, and teaching, and they should coordinate the services provided at their hospital with those provided at level I and II hospitals in the region.

Other maternal-fetal medicine specialists and neonatologists who practice in the level III facility should have qualifications similar to those of the chief of their service. There should be one neonatologist for every six to ten patients in the continuing care, intermediate care, and intensive care areas. A ratio of one physician (including residents or fellows) to every four or five patients who require intensive care is ideal, but this is practical only in centers with a full complement of personnel. A maternal-fetal medicine specialist and a neonatologist should be available for consultation 24 hours/day.

Obstetric and neonatal diagnostic imaging, provided by obstetricians or radiologists who have special interest and competence in maternal and neonatal disease and its complications, should be available 24 hours/day. Pediatric subspecialists in cardiology, neurology, hematology, and genetics should be available for consultation. Consultant services in renal function, metabolism, endocrinology, gastroenterology-nutrition, infectious diseases, pulmonary function, immunology, and pharmacology are also needed. In addition, pediatric surgical subspecialists (eg, cardiovascular surgeons; neurosurgeons; and orthopedic, ophthalmologic, urologic, and otolaryngologic surgeons) should be available for consultation and care. Pathologists with special competence in placental, fetal, and neonatal disease should also be members of the level III hospital staff.

A board-certified anesthesiologist with special training or experience in maternal-fetal anesthesia should be in charge of perinatal anesthesia services at a level III hospital. Personnel capable of administering obstetric anesthesia should be available in the hospital 24 hours/day. Personnel capable of administering neonatal and pediatric anesthesia should be available as required.

NURSING STAFF

Recommended nurse:patient ratios are shown in Table 3-1. A particular institution may use different staffing systems to meet its specific needs, however, if that system has proved effective. Variables such as type of patient, acuity of patients' conditions, mixture of skills of the staff, environment, types of delivery, and use of anesthesia should be taken into account in determining appropriate nurse:patient ratios. Intrapartum care requires the same level of labor intensiveness and expertise as any other intensive care unit and, accordingly, should be allocated adequate training and fiscal support.

Level I

Although there are significant fluctuations in the number of women in labor at a given time in any hospital that has a low number of

Table 3-1. Recommended Nurse: Patient Ratios for Perinatal Care Services

Staffing Ratio	Care Provided
1:1-2	Antepartum testing
1:2	Laboring patients
1:1	Patients in second stage of labor
1:1	Ill patients with complications
1:2	Oxytocin induction or augmentation of labor
1:1	Coverage of epidural anesthesia
1:1	Circulation for cesarean delivery
1:6	Antepartum/postpartum patients without complications
1:2	Postoperative recovery
1:3	Patients with complications, but in stable condition
1:4	Recently born infants and those needing close observation
1:6	Newborns needing only routine care
1:3	Mother-newborn care
1:1	Newborns requiring multisystem support
1:3-4	Newborns requiring intermediate care
1:1-2	Newborns needing intensive care

annual deliveries, the hospital should ensure that a registered nurse who has both training and clinical competence in perinatal nursing; who can evaluate the condition of the mother, fetus, and neonate; and who can assess the degree of risk to which they are subject during labor, delivery, and the neonatal period is in attendance whenever there are patients in active labor in the hospital. Each hospital should have contingency plans with other hospitals in the regional system for those times in which the patient load is unusually heavy.

A registered nurse should be in charge of the nursing staff of a level I hospital's perinatal facilities. This nurse may be responsible for directing nursing services and implementing policy in the labor and delivery, newborn care, and postpartum care areas.

Nursing personnel assigned to nursery areas in level I hospitals should be under the direct supervision of a registered nurse. Because they oversee the immediate postpartum period, they should understand the environmental requirements of the newborn. They should be able to identify and alert physicians to pathophysiologic processes.

Furthermore, they should be able to perform emergency procedures, such as resuscitation, and to initiate intravenous therapy. If the same nurse is responsible both for the resuscitation of neonates immediately after delivery and for the resuscitation of those in the nursery, these areas should be adjacent.

When the supervising nurse on each shift is directly responsible for nursing care in the labor and delivery area, as well as for resuscitation, neonates in the normal care and the special care areas may be cared for by other nursing staff under the supervising nurse's direction. In smaller hospitals, the same personnel may staff all these areas. In addition to fulfilling the patient care responsibilities associated with each functional area, the nursing staff of the perinatal service should be available to provide emotional support to parents, to make referrals to social services, and to instruct parents in the care of the neonate.

Level II

Each of the obstetric and neonatal patient care areas in level II hospitals should have a head nurse with training and clinical competence in perinatal/neonatal nursing. This nurse is responsible for management of the unit and supervision of the direct nursing care provided. Staffing recommendations are summarized in Table 3-1.

Nursing staff in the labor, delivery, and recovery areas should be able to identify and respond to the obstetric and medical complications of pregnancy, labor, and delivery. Staff requirements for the resuscitation, admission/observation, and newborn care areas are the same as those for hospitals that provide level I care.

The nursing staff of the intermediate care nursery in a level II hospital should be able to 1) monitor and maintain the stability of cardiopulmonary, metabolic, and thermal functions; 2) assist with special procedures, such as lumbar punctures, endotracheal intubation, and umbilical vessel catheterization; and 3) perform emergency resuscitation. Nursing staff in this area should be specially trained and able to initiate, modify, or stop treatment when appropriate—even if a physician is not present—according to established protocols. Medical, nursing, and respiratory therapy staff who have demonstrated ability to intubate the trachea; change the pressure, flow, and frequency of mechanical ventilation; and decompress a pneumothorax by needle aspiration should be available in case a neonate requires assisted ventilation. In such an event, it is appropriate to provide one professional nurse for this neonate. The unit's medical director should supervise the professional activities of these nurses with expanded roles.

Level III

It is highly desirable for the director/supervisor and head nurses of perinatal nursing services in level III hospitals to have not only training and clinical competence in perinatal/neonatal nursing care, but also specialty certification. The obstetric and neonatal patient care areas should each have a head nurse responsible for management of the unit and supervision of direct patient care.

The nursing staff in the labor, delivery, and postpartum care areas should have specialty certification or advanced training and experience in the nursing management of both low- and high-risk patients in labor and their families. Nursing staff should also be experienced in caring for the obstetric and medical complications of pregnancy.

Recommended nurse:patient ratios in the special care nursery areas are indicated in Table 3-1. Additional nurses with special training are required to fulfill regional center responsibilities, such as outreach education and transport (see Chapter 8).

SUPPORT PERSONNEL

All Levels

A blood bank technician should always be available for determining blood type, cross-matching blood, and performing Coombs' tests. The hospital's infection control personnel should be responsible for surveillance of infections in mothers and neonates, as well as for the development of an appropriate environmental control program (see Chapter 6). A radiologic technician should be readily available 24 hours/day to perform chest roentgenograms. The need for other support personnel depends on the intensity and level of sophistication of the other support services provided.

Levels II and III

The following support personnel should be available in the perinatal care service of levels II and III hospitals:

1. At least one full-time medical social worker who has experience with the socioeconomic and psychosocial problems of high-risk

mothers and fetuses, sick neonates, and their families. Additional medical social workers may be required if the patient load is heavy.

2. At least one occupational and one physical therapist.
3. A minimum of one registered dietitian/nutritionist who has special training in perinatal nutrition and can plan diets that meet the special needs of high-risk mothers and neonates.
4. Qualified personnel for support services such as laboratory studies, radiologic studies, and ultrasound examinations. These personnel should be in-hospital 24 hours/day.
5. Respiratory therapists or nurses with special training who can supervise the assisted ventilation of neonates with cardiopulmonary disease. Optimally, one therapist is needed for each four neonates who are receiving assisted ventilation.

The hospital's engineering department should include air-conditioning, electronic, and mechanical engineers, as well as biomedical technicians, who are responsible for the safety and reliability of the equipment in the labor and delivery area and the special care nurseries.

EDUCATION

In-Service and Continuing Education

The medical and nursing staffs of any hospital that provides perinatal care at any level should participate in joint in-service sessions on maternal and neonatal health. These sessions should cover the diagnosis and management of perinatal emergencies, as well as the management of routine problems. The staff of each unit should also have a monthly conference at which the patient care problems that arose during the previous month are presented and discussed.

The staff of regional centers should assist with the in-service programs of other hospitals in their region on a regular basis. Such assistance should include periodic visits to those hospitals, as well as periodic review of the quality of patient care that those hospitals provide. Regional center staff should be accessible for consultation at all times. The medical and nursing staffs of hospitals that provide level I and II care should participate in formal courses or conferences sponsored by a regional perinatal resource center. Regularly scheduled regional conferences should include, as a minimum, coverage of the following areas:

1. Conferences to review major perinatal illnesses and their treatment
2. Conferences to review perinatal statistics, the pathology related to all deaths, and significant surgical specimens
3. Conferences to review current x-ray films and ultrasonographic material
4. Administrative staff conferences to review procedures and policies
5. Teaching seminars for nursing and medical staffs

Perinatal Outreach Education

A program for perinatal outreach education should be designed and coordinated jointly by a neonatal/perinatal physician and a neonatal/perinatal clinical nurse specialist. Their responsibilities should include assessing educational needs, planning curricula, teaching, implementing and evaluating the program, collecting and using perinatal data, providing patient follow-up information to referring community personnel, writing reports, and maintaining informative working relationships with community personnel and outreach team members.

A maternal-fetal medicine specialist, an obstetric nurse, a neonatologist, and a neonatal nurse are the essential members of the perinatal outreach education team. Other professionals (eg, a social worker, a respiratory therapist, or a nutritionist) may also be assigned to the team. Each member should be responsible for teaching, consulting with community professionals as needed, and maintaining communication with the program coordinator and other team members.

Each tertiary care center in a regional system is responsible for organizing an education program tailored to meet the needs of the perinatal health professionals and institutions within the network. Various educational strategies have been found effective, including a series of seminars, media programs, self-instruction booklets, or clinical practicums/rotations. Perinatal outreach education meetings should be held at a routine time and place to allow for continuity of communication among community professionals and regional center personnel.

RESOURCES AND RECOMMENDED READING

American College of Obstetricians and Gynecologists: Standards for Obstetric-Gynecologic Services, 6 ed. Washington DC, ACOG, 1985

Kattwinkel J: Perinatal Outreach Education. In Fanaroff A, Martin R (eds): Behrman's Neonatal-Perinatal Medicine, 4 ed. St Louis, CV Mosby, 1987

Nurses Association of the American College of Obstetricians and Gynecologists: Nurse Providers of Neonatal Care: Guidelines for Educational Development and Practice. Washington DC, NAACOG, 1985

Nurses Association of the American College of Obstetricians and Gynecologists: Standards for Obstetric, Gynecologic, and Neonatal Nursing, 3 ed. Washington DC, NAACOG, 1986

PERINATAL CARE SERVICES

A comprehensive perinatal care program involves an integrated approach to medical care and psychosocial support that begins preconceptionally and extends throughout pregnancy and the perinatal period. It includes counseling, risk assessment, serial surveillance, prenatal education, selective use of specialized skills and technology, delivery, observation of the mother and neonate, preparation for discharge, and follow-up during the postpartum period. In order to achieve optimal results, a comprehensive program should focus on the provision of safe, high-quality care while recognizing pregnancy and childbirth as a family experience.

An important goal of maternal and newborn care is to foster parent-newborn-family relationships. Health care professionals should integrate the concept of family-centered care into every aspect of perinatal services. The process should begin during the first prenatal visit with a review of the parents' attitudes toward the pregnancy, family life, child care practices, stresses in the mother's environment, support systems, and interest in childbirth education classes. It should continue throughout the perinatal period in both the ambulatory and hospital settings.

Most patients are eager to participate in decisions that affect their pregnancy. Prospective parents are usually well-informed and motivated, conscious of their health, and receptive to professional guidance. They should be encouraged to express their preferences regarding decisions that relate to procedures performed during the childbirth process.

The options now available in obstetric care include alternatives in birthing environments, the presence of a supporting person during labor and delivery, early parental interaction with the neonate, and rooming-in. Specific hospital and physician policies, especially those pertaining to a childbirth coach, the presence of the father and other

49

family members during labor and delivery, and visiting should be explained to the patient well in advance of the estimated date of confinement. The appropriate role of the support person throughout the intrapartum and postpartum periods should be clearly defined and understood by all persons involved.

PRECONCEPTIONAL CARE

Preparation for parenthood should begin prior to conception. At the time of conception, the couple should be in optimal physical health and emotionally prepared for parenthood. In order to make an informed decision about parenthood, a couple should have a realistic assessment of their mental and physical status and a thorough understanding of the risks associated with a prospective pregnancy.

When a pregnancy is contemplated, it is desirable for prospective parents to undergo preconceptional counseling. As a part of a comprehensive examination, information that may have a bearing on the couple's health and future pregnancy should be obtained. (Appendix B includes a checklist that may be useful for this purpose.) This information may serve as the basis for a general counseling session focusing on the following areas:

1. Testing for a disease carrier state or other risk factors (eg, Tay-Sachs and hemoglobinopathy screening, blood and Rh type determinations, serologic testing, rubella antibody titer determination, and testing for human immunodeficiency virus infection, if indicated)

2. Problems that can and should be resolved prior to pregnancy (eg, anemia, obesity)

3. Problems that cannot be resolved, but may require extra care prior to and during pregnancy (eg, chronic hypertension, diabetes mellitus)

4. The recurrence of complications experienced in previous pregnancies, including congenital anomalies (eg, neural tube defects)

5. The length of time to wait after use of oral contraceptives (eg, until one normal menstrual period occurs) or following spontaneous or induced abortion

6. Problems associated with potential teratogenic effects of prescribed medications, illicit substances, alcohol, and smoking

7. Exercise and diet in pregnancy
8. The importance of recording the data of each menstrual period and beginning prenatal care as early as possible in the course of pregnancy

The benefits that accrue from preconceptional care are dramatic in the case of phenylketonuria (PKU), which is estimated to affect at least 2,800 women at risk of pregnancy. Maternal blood phenylalanine levels greater than or equal to 20 mg/dl during pregnancy are associated with a high rate of mental retardation, microcephaly, congenital heart defects, and intrauterine growth retardation among non-PKU offspring of women with PKU. Special dietary therapy that restricts phenylalanine intake is the only treatment available that may protect the fetus in a maternal PKU pregnancy. Current evidence suggests that, if the special diet begins before conception and is continued throughout pregnancy, the fetus may not be damaged; if dietary treatment begins after conception, however, protection of the fetus may either be less than optimal or nonexistent. Preconceptional care can be particularly important in identifying conditions that could benefit from early intervention, such as diabetes mellitus, hypertension, and screening for other metabolic and inherited disorders. The results of such screening can be used to formulate a plan for antepartum management.

ANTEPARTUM CARE

In order to enhance pregnancy outcome, a woman should begin antepartum care as early as possible in pregnancy. Early diagnosis of pregnancy is an important factor in establishing a management plan appropriate for the individual. There are three main components of antepartum care: 1) serial surveillance, which begins with a history and physical examination to identify risk factors or abnormalities and to determine uterine size; 2) patient education to foster optimal health, good dietary habits, and proper hygiene; and 3) appropriate psychosocial support.

Serial Surveillance

Antepartum surveillance begins with the first prenatal visit. At this time, the physician should establish an obstetric data base that contains information regarding the patient's last menstrual period, current pregnancy, and past obstetric outcomes, as well as her medical, family, and social history; a dietary assessment (see Chapter 7); physical findings; estimated date of confinement; laboratory tests; and a risk assessment. Early identification of medical conditions that can affect pregnancy outcome (see Risk Assessment, this chapter) can minimize maternal and neonatal morbidity by making it possible for the physician to establish an appropriate treatment plan, to maintain close surveillance, and to plan for delivery.

History

The health history should include a review of all past pregnancies, health status of living children, route of delivery, sex and weight of the newborn, Rho(D) immune globulin (RhIG) administration after earlier pregnancies, and any complications, particularly those resulting in fetal or neonatal deaths. In addition, the history should include important information that helps identify the patient at risk, such as the frequency of alcohol consumption and the use of drugs, cigarette smoking, and exposure to radiation (see Risk Assessment, this chapter). Information on which to base clinical recommendations about environmental hazards is limited. Whenever there is a question of exposure to possibly teratogenic agents, expert consultation and counseling may be helpful.

The history should also address the patient's susceptibility and recent exposure to communicable diseases, including diseases transmitted sexually or through blood transfusions (see Chapter 6). The administration of some vaccines is contraindicated during pregnancy; fortunately, immunization of women during pregnancy is necessary only rarely. If a pregnant woman has been exposed recently or is likely to be exposed to a specific immunizable disease, the physician should evaluate current information about the risks of the disease and the risks and benefits of vaccine administration before selecting a course of action.

The family history should be thorough, including information on metabolic disorders, cardiovascular disease, malignancy, congenital abnormalities, mental retardation, and multiple births. It is important to determine whether the family has a history of congenital anomalies in order to identify the fetus at risk for an inherited disease. If a child with congenital anomalies has already been born to the couple, the history should include the specific details of that pregnancy in anticipation of the need for prenatal genetic counseling and studies (see Antenatal Detection of Genetic Disorders, Chapter 10). A history of repeated midtrimester losses or premature delivery should alert the physician and the parents to the significant risk of recurrence and the possible need for consultation. It should also be remembered that women of high parity are at increased risk for puerperal hemorrhage, multiple gestation, and placenta previa.

The social history should include the patient's occupation and work environment, ethnic origin, and lifestyle.

Establishment of the Expected Date of Confinement

Problems such as intrauterine growth retardation, premature labor, and postterm pregnancy cannot be detected or managed effectively without accurate information on the expected date of confinement. The determination of this date is most likely to be accurate when a patient begins receiving care early in pregnancy and receives regular prenatal care.

Accuracy of the expected date of confinement is confirmed by ascertaining the regularity, duration, and individual character of the menstrual cycle, including changes in bleeding patterns. Errors in pregnancy dating can result from failure to consider menstrual irregularities, longer than average cycle lengths, recent use of oral contraceptives, and the possibility that what appeared to be the last menstrual period was actually implantation bleeding. Whenever there is a doubt about the estimated date of confinement, first or second trimester ultrasonography may be helpful. Third trimester ultrasonography is rarely helpful in establishing gestational age.

Physical Examination

Every pregnant woman should receive a complete physical examination that includes an evaluation of her height, weight, blood pressure, head, neck, breasts, heart, lungs, abdomen, pelvis, rectum, extremities, neurologic system, and current nutritional status. The size and shape of the uterus and adnexal areas, as well as the configuration and capacity of the bony pelvis, should be clinically evaluated and recorded.

The size of the uterus correlates most accurately with the duration of gestation early in pregnancy. The uterus is usually a pelvic organ until the 12th week of gestation. At midpregnancy (20 weeks of gestation), it generally reaches the umbilicus. Uterine size should be measured from the symphysis pubis to the top of the fundus. Between the 18th and 34th week, the uterine height in centimeters approximates the gestational age in weeks. At 18-20 weeks of gestation, fetal heart tones can be heard with a fetoscope, although they may be heard with a Doppler device by 10-12 weeks of gestation or even earlier. With real-time ultrasonography, fetal heart activity can be seen as soon as 1-2 weeks after the first missed menstrual period.

Laboratory Tests

Certain laboratory tests should be performed as early in pregnancy as possible:

    Determination of hemoglobin or hematocrit levels
    Urinalysis for protein and glucose
    Determination of blood group and Rh type
    Irregular antibody screen
    Determination of rubella antibody titer (if previous immunity has
      not been determined)
    Cytologic studies of the cervix
    Serologic testing for syphilis

The additional laboratory evaluations needed are determined by historical factors or findings in the physical examination. For example, the ethnic, racial, and social origins of the patient may indicate the need for special testing. (See also specific recommendations for infection screening, Chapter 6, and maternal serum alpha-fetoprotein screening, Chapter 10.) Because maternal age is associated with diabetes, routine screening for diabetes is recommended for pregnant women aged 30 or older. If any of the following risk factors are present, however, patients should be screened for diabetes irrespective of their age: family history of diabetes; previous delivery of a macrosomic, malformed, or stillborn infant; obesity; hypertension; or glycosuria.

Early in the third trimester, the patient's hemoglobin or hematocrit level should again be determined. A repeat test for syphilis should be performed if the patient belongs to a high-risk population. At some time during the patient's antepartum course, it may be appropriate to repeat an irregular antibody screen. Unsensitized Rh-negative patients should have repeat antibody tests at approximately 28 weeks of pregnancy and receive 300 µg RhIG prophylactically. Repeat administration is necessary after delivery if the newborn is Rh-positive.

Subsequent Visits

The frequency of return visits should be determined by the individual needs of the woman and the assessment of her risks. Generally, a woman with an uncomplicated pregnancy should be examined approximately every 4 weeks for the first 28 weeks of pregnancy, every 2-3 weeks until 36 weeks of gestation, and weekly thereafter, although flexibility is desirable. Women with medical or obstetric problems require closer surveillance; the appropriate intervals between visits are determined by the nature and severity of the problems.

At each follow-up visit, the patient should be given an opportunity to ask questions about her pregnancy or comment on changes that she has noted. Blood pressure, weight, uterine size, and, when appropriate, fetal presentation and heart rate should be assessed during each visit. The patient should be asked about fetal movement at each visit after she reports quickening. Urinalysis should be performed to detect protein and glucose. Any change in the pregnancy risk assessment should be recorded after each evaluation and an appropriate management plan outlined.

Risk Assessment

Continual risk assessment should be a standard part of antenatal care. For most effective clinical use, risk assessment instruments should be simple, rapid, and easy to interpret.

Identification of the high-risk patient is critical to minimize maternal and neonatal morbidity and mortality. As illustrated in Figure 4-1, there is ample evidence that known risk factors can be used to identify high-risk patients early in the antenatal course, as well as intrapartally. Approximately 20% of pregnant women can be identified prenatally to be at risk, accounting for 55% of poor pregnancy outcomes. In addition, 5-10% of pregnant women can be identified to be at risk for the first time during labor, resulting in 20-25% of poor pregnancy outcomes. Thus, a total of 25-30% of pregnant women who are found to be at risk during either the antepartum or intrapartum periods account for 75-80% of poor pregnancy outcomes. It is important to recognize, however, that 20% of perinatal morbidity and mortality arise from the group without identifiable risks.

Risk assessment is influenced by medical and obstetric considerations, as well as by the patient's lifestyle and environmental factors. For example, maternal cigarette smoking and low birth weight are known to be related. The chronic, excessive consumption of alcohol during pregnancy is associated with a variety of congenital malformations and other defects. Because the effects of a pregnant woman's moderate intake of alcohol on the fetus and the threshold at which alcohol damages a developing conceptus in a given individual are unknown, it is prudent to avoid alcohol during pregnancy.

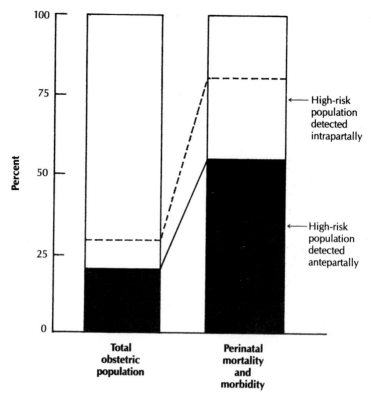

Fig. 4-1. High-risk pregnancy outcome. (Aubry RH: Identification of the high-risk
obstetric patient. In: Ryan GM Jr (ed): Ambulatory Care in Obstetrics and
Gynecology. New York, Grune & Stratton, 1980)

The following is a partial list of high-risk factors, derived from the
history or physical examination, that increase pregnancy risks and
may necessitate further evaluation, consultation, or referral:

Medical Problems

- Cardiovascular, renal, collagen, pulmonary, infectious, liver, and
  sexually transmitted diseases
- Chronic urinary tract infections
- Maternal viral, bacterial, and protozoan infections
- Diabetes mellitus
- Severe anemia
- Isoimmune thrombocytopenia
- Convulsive disorders

- Alcohol or other drug addiction

Obstetric Problems

- Poor obstetric history
- Maternal age under 16 or over 35 years
- Previous congenital anomalies
- Multiple gestation
- Isoimmunization
- Intrauterine growth retardation
- Third trimester bleeding
- Pregnancy-induced hypertension
- Hydramnios
- Fetal cardiac arrhythmias
- Prematurity
- Breech or transverse lie
- Rupture of the membranes for a period of time longer than 24 hours
- Chorioamnionitis
- Fetal distress

Antepartum testing for fetal well-being and fetal maturation should be available for patients when risk factors indicate the need. When the availability of these technologic resources is limited, appropriate arrangements should be made for referral to a regional center.

Gestational age is an important factor in the management of pregnancy, particularly in the presence of high-risk factors that may necessitate appropriately timed intervention. The criteria suggested for assessing fetal maturity prior to elective repeat cesarean delivery and elective induction of labor cited later in this chapter may be useful guidelines for confirming gestational age in all pregnancies.

In many instances, special obstetric problems require a multidisciplinary approach. The obstetrician should inform the pediatrician whenever there is a significant risk factor for a neonate. The pediatrician should then meet with the parents and discuss plans for the evaluation and management of the neonate's condition. Some high-risk conditions may require transport of the fetus in utero (ie, maternal-fetal transport), which in most circumstances is preferable to transport of a high-risk neonate (see Chapter 8).

Premature rupture of the membranes and premature labor are the leading causes of perinatal mortality in the United States. Despite extensive study, the causes remain unknown. Prevention is not possible; therefore, it is necessary to focus on early risk recognition, diagnosis, and treatment.

The obstetric or gynecologic history may provide some important clues to the risk of preterm delivery. A history of such deliveries, diethylstilbestrol (DES) exposure, heavy smoking, hypertension, chronic glomerulonephritis or pyelonephritis, or other chronic medical disorders has been implicated. A history of progressively earlier second trimester dilation without labor is consistent with, but not diagnostic of, cervical incompetence. Premature cervical dilation may be signaled by pelvic pressure, urinary frequency, watery vaginal discharge, cramps similar to menstrual cramps, low backache, vaginal bleeding, or uterine contractions. A high index of suspicion for premature labor, based on the history, mandates more intensive surveillance, which may lead to early diagnosis and intervention by cervical cerclage, tocolysis (see Chapter 10), or the administration of drugs that promote fetal lung maturity. Simple solutions cannot be offered for these problems, but early identification of certain risks makes it possible to anticipate needs and arrange for cooperative regional management.

For the sake of statistical reporting, postterm pregnancy is defined as a pregnancy that has extended beyond 294 days from the onset of the last menstrual period. Postterm pregnancy is a significant contributor to mortality and morbidity among infants of term size. For a small but significant number of fetuses, prolonged pregnancy increases the risk of chronic intrauterine asphyxia, meconium aspiration, long-term neurologic handicap, and, occasionally, death. Among the pathophysiologic processes that increase fetal mortality and morbidity are oligohydramnios with umbilical cord compression and uteroplacental insufficiency. Additional morbidity may result from the fact that 25% of postterm neonates weigh more than 4,000 g and their mothers may experience dystocia.

Most term-sized infants admitted to neonatal intensive care units with low Apgar scores and meconium aspiration come from postterm pregnancies. Because these infants have a high incidence of mortality and extended morbidity, postterm pregnancies require special consideration, and each hospital should develop protocols for their management. Early pregnancy dating, sizing and growth measurements, and the application of modern technology for assessment of fetal well-being can help identify those postterm fetuses who may be compromised by remaining in utero, while providing reassurance for the majority of patients whose fetuses are not at risk.

With an awareness of the conditions that increase fetal risk, the final major decision of good antepartum care can be made; namely, the selection of the health care facility that can best meet the needs of both the mother and her baby.

Patient Information

The physician and others providing antepartum care should discuss with each patient the kind of care that is provided in the office, necessary laboratory studies, the expected course of the pregnancy, signs and symptoms to be reported to the physician (such as rupture of the membranes), the timing of subsequent visits, proper diet and health habits, educational programs available, and the options for intrapartum care. At some time during the prenatal period, communication between the prospective parents and a pediatrician may be helpful. The roles of the various members of the health care team, office policies (including emergency coverage), and alternate physician coverage should also be explained. Specific information regarding costs should be provided.

Early in the third trimester, plans for hospital admission, labor, and delivery should be reviewed and information provided on what to do when labor begins, when the membranes rupture, or if bleeding occurs. Analgesic and anesthetic options should be discussed. Because a general anesthetic may be required for delivery, the patient should be advised of the hazards of ingesting food or fluid after the onset of labor. Aspects of newborn care, including the pros and cons of circumcision of male neonates, should be discussed.

Prenatal Education

The importance of prenatal education cannot be overemphasized. Health care professionals can take advantage of the pregnant woman's motivation to share in the responsibility for her own health care and to do what is best for her baby.

The physician should see that the woman is provided with information about nutrition. Smoking and alcohol consumption should be discouraged. While information relating to the risks of using psychoactive drugs during pregnancy is inconclusive, it is reasonable to caution patients to avoid their use. The patient should understand that moderate daily exercise is an important component of a healthy pregnancy; however, a sensation of fatigue suggests that activity has been excessive. Pregnancy is not the time for competitive or dangerous sports or the acquisition of new athletic skills.

A woman with an uncomplicated pregnancy and a normal fetus may continue to work until the onset of labor if her job presents no greater potential hazards than those encountered in normal daily life in the community or home. The return to work after delivery should be determined by the patient's specific circumstances and the physician's judgment.

Childbirth Education

Patients should be referred to appropriate educational literature and urged to attend childbirth education classes. Hospitals, or community agencies or groups, may offer such educational programs. The participation of physicians and hospital obstetric nurses in educational programs is desirable to ensure continuity of care and consistency of instruction.

Childbirth education classes provide an excellent opportunity for women to obtain specific information about the childbirth experience. Families should be encouraged to participate in childbirth education programs as well, because adequate preparation of family members can have a favorable and lasting effect on the mother, the neonate, and, ultimately, the family unit.

Psychosocial Support

Pregnancy is a major event in a woman's life. It is a time in which the family is "expected" to be happy. Pregnancy is a profound emotional experience, however. Conflicts may arise over the involvement of grandparents, family life, expectations, and new responsibilities. An atmosphere of acceptance allows families to communicate their feelings. Group encounters, such as childbirth classes and antepartum breast-feeding seminars, may be helpful. On occasion, referral to appropriate psychologic or psychiatric specialists may be necessary.

INTRAPARTUM CARE: LABOR AND DELIVERY

A woman should approach the unique experience of labor and delivery with a sense of confidence and trust in her antepartum preparation, in the skill and knowledge of her physician, and in the competence of the hospital staff. Childbirth is a unique family experience, and the obstetric staff should strive to make the patient and the father or other supporting persons comfortable and to keep them informed.

In large measure, the patient's and the family's perception of the intrapartum experience is determined by information provided during the antepartum period, particularly in regard to the normal physiologic processes occurring within both mother and fetus. The father or supporting person puts into practice the principles that were learned regarding the conduct of labor. Physical contact of the newborn with the parents in the delivery room may enhance future relationships, and hospital personnel should be encouraged, where feasible, to facilitate family interaction and to support the desire of the family to be together.

Intrapartum care should be both personalized and comprehensive. Because a significant proportion of patients ultimately attain high-risk status as a result of intrapartum complications, continuous surveillance of the mother and fetus is essential.

The hospital, including a birth center within the hospital complex, provides the safest setting for labor, delivery, and the postpartum period. The collection and analysis of data on the safety and outcome of deliveries in other settings, such as free-standing centers, have been problematic, as documented by a study conducted by the National Academy of Sciences. Until such data are available, the use of other settings is not encouraged. There may be exceptional, geographically isolated situations, however, that require special programs.

Any facility providing obstetric care should have at least the following services available:

- Identification of high-risk mothers and fetuses
- Equipment for continuous fetal heart rate monitoring
- Capabilities to begin a cesarean delivery within 30 minutes of a decision to do so
- Blood and fresh-frozen plasma for transfusion
- Anesthesia on a 24-hour basis
- Radiology and ultrasound examination
- Neonatal resuscitation
- Laboratory testing on a 24-hour basis
- Consultation and transfer agreement
- Nursery
- Data collection and retrieval

Admission Procedures, Medical Records, and Patient Consent Forms

It is desirable for the initial history, physical findings, and laboratory data to be transmitted to the hospital soon after the first prenatal visit. At 36 weeks of gestation, the patient's prenatal care record should be updated in the hospital's labor registration area. When the patient is admitted for labor and delivery, her prenatal care record should be reviewed; pertinent information from this record should be recorded on the admission note (eg, blood group and Rh type, presence of irregular antibodies, results of serologic and other diagnostic tests, and therapeutic measures prescribed). The nursing admission note should include the 1) reason for admission, 2) date and time of the patient's arrival and notification of the physician, and 3) time seen by the physician.

Patients in labor, with premature rupture of the membranes, or with vaginal bleeding should be admitted directly to the labor and delivery suite. Occasionally, obstetric patients who are not in labor, but require special intensive care, may also be admitted to this area. The admission of a patient in prodromal labor with no complications may be deferred, and she may be allowed to ambulate or wait in a more casual, comfortable area. Patients who have a transmissible infection, discharging skin lesions, diarrhea, or purulent vaginal discharge should be admitted to a specific labor, delivery, and recovery area where isolation techniques can be implemented according to established hospital policy (see also Chapter 6).

When a patient has had a recent examination and is not at high risk, the evaluation of her condition at admission may be restricted to an interval history and pertinent physical examination. Attention should be focused on the onset of contractions, status of the membranes, bleeding, fetal activity, history of allergies, time and content of the most recent food ingestion, and the use of any medication.

The admitting physical examination should include determination of the patient's blood pressure, pulse, and temperature. The frequency, duration, and quality of the uterine contractions should be recorded. The fetal heart rate should be determined and recorded as soon as the patient arrives in the admitting area so that a baseline measurement will be available should fetal distress be suspected later. Fetal well being should be evaluated, and the method of assessment used should be determined by departmental policy.

When there are no complications or contraindications, as established by department protocol, qualified nursing personnel may perform the initial pelvic examination. Cervical dilation, effacement, fetal presentation, and station should be documented. A urine sample should be tested to determine the presence of protein and glucose. The physician responsible for the patient's care should be informed of her status so that a decision can be made regarding present risk and further management. The timing of the physician's arrival in the labor area is determined by this information and by hospital policy. If anesthesia other than local or pudendal is likely to be needed or desired, anesthesia personnel should be informed soon after the patient's admission. After the results of the patient examination, as well as diagnostic and therapeutic orders, have been noted on the record, any necessary consent forms should be signed and attached to the record.

Departmental policies and physician preference concerning admission procedures, such as the shaving of the pubic and perineal hair, administration of enemas, taking of showers, placement of intravenous lines, use of abdominal belts or electronic fetal monitoring, and ambulatory restrictions, should take into account the patient's needs and desires. The use of drugs for analgesia and anesthesia during labor and delivery should also depend on the needs and desires of the patient and on the judgment of the attending physician.

Patients who have had no prenatal care should be considered to be at higher risk for special problems, especially infectious disease, for which routine laboratory tests are required. A patient who has not had an orientation visit to the labor and delivery area as part of a childbirth education program or who is unfamiliar with monitoring techniques that may be used during labor should be given a careful explanation of what will happen during labor.

Pain Relief During Labor and Delivery

Control of discomfort and pain during labor and delivery is more than providing personal comfort to the mother; it is a necessary part of good obstetric practice. Pain can be controlled by pharmacologic means or by techniques that the patient learned in a childbirth education and preparation program. The choice and availability of analgesic and anesthetic techniques depend on the experience and judgment of the anesthesiologist, the circumstances of labor and delivery, and the personal preferences of the obstetrician and the patient.

Of the various pharmacologic methods used for pain relief during labor and delivery, continuous lumbar epidural analgesia is the most effective and least depressant; furthermore, it allows for an alert, participating mother. Narcotics and inhalation analgesia safely provide varying degrees of pain relief, but they are potentially depressant to both mother and fetus. Barbiturates, tranquilizers, and scopolamine have no analgesic qualities and are also potentially depressant. At the time of delivery, local infiltration and pudendal block are safe techniques with or without an inhalation analgesic supplement; however, they do not provide total pain relief and, thus, are not sufficient for all vaginal births. Spinal anesthesia can provide adequate pain relief and muscle relaxation for nearly all vaginal births, but, unlike continuous lumbar epidural analgesia, spinal anesthesia is useful only at the time of birth; other measures are required for pain control during the first stage of labor. Most important, general anesthesia is rarely necessary for vaginal births and should be used only for specific indications.

Paracervical block, when used for pain relief for labor, results in bradycardia in as many as 50% of fetuses whose mothers receive the block. For this reason, close monitoring of the fetal heart rate is recommended when this method of pain relief is used. Because of adverse reactions, bupivicaine is contraindicated for use in paracervical block anesthesia.

For the uncomplicated cesarean delivery, properly administered regional or general anesthesia is effective and has little adverse effect on the newborn. Because of the risks to the mother associated with intubation and the possibility of aspiration during the induction of general anesthesia, regional analgesia may be the safer technique and should be available to all patients. The advantages and disadvantages of both techniques should be discussed with the patient as completely as possible.

If properly chosen and administered, analgesia or anesthesia during labor has little or no effect on the physiologic status of the neonate. At present, there is no evidence that the administration of analgesia or anesthesia to the woman in labor has a significant effect on the child's later mental and neurologic development.

Because the safety of obstetric anesthesia depends principally on the skill of the anesthesiologist, and because obstetric anesthesia must be considered emergency anesthesia, it demands a competence in personnel and an availability of equipment similar to or greater than those required for elective surgical procedures. Obstetricians, house officers, nurse-anesthetists, and nonphysician personnel are seldom fully competent in all forms of inhalation, intravenous, local, and regional anesthesia. It is the responsibility of the director of anesthesia services to review the qualifications and competence of each individual who is to provide analgesia or anesthesia and to determine which agents and techniques he or she may use. The director of anesthesia services, with the approval of the medical staff, should develop and enforce written policies regarding the provision of obstetric anesthesia (ie, who may do specific procedures and under what circumstances).

An obstetrician who is appropriately trained to do so may administer the anesthesia if granted privileges for these procedures. It is preferable, however, for an anesthesiologist or anesthetist to provide this care so that the obstetrician may give undivided attention to the delivery. All obstetricians should be trained in the use of infiltration anesthesia. When any type of regional anesthesia is administered, the patient should be monitored by a qualified member of the health care team.

The routine use of pain medications is not recommended. No conduction anesthesia (epidural, caudal, or spinal) or general anesthesia should be administered until the patient has been examined, the fetal status and progress of labor have been evaluated, and a qualified physician is readily available to supervise the labor and to manage any obstetric complications that may arise.

Management of Labor

Term Patients

As mentioned earlier, 20% of perinatal morbidity and mortality arise during the intrapartum period from the group of patients who have had no complications during their pregnancies. Therefore, basic standards of care should be maintained in this group of patients (ie, those without identifiable risks), in order to minimize problems of an unpredictable nature .

After the patient in labor has been admitted and her status initially evaluated, ongoing intrapartum surveillance is necessary; the degree and method of surveillance vary according to predetermined risk factors. A physician should see the patient within a reasonable period of time, as determined by her obstetric and other medical conditions, after her admission to the hospital. Each hospital should develop maximum allowable physician response times for high-risk and low-risk patients. The patient may be permitted to ambulate with the knowledge and consent of the attending physician. General care during labor should provide optimal patient comfort in addition to optimal fetal and maternal safety.

For each shift that she is in the labor and delivery area, the patient should be introduced to the nurse responsible for her care. A designated member of the obstetric team should be responsible for observing the patient, following the progress of labor, and recording the patient's vital signs and fetal heart rate on the labor record. The physician who is responsible for the patient's care should be kept informed of her progress and notified immediately of any abnormality. He or she should be readily available when the patient is in the active phase of labor. Other qualified health professionals (eg, skilled nurses and house staff) may assist in patient management.

For the patient without identifiable risks, assessment of the quality of uterine contractions, in conjunction with vaginal examinations, should be adequate to monitor the progress of labor and to detect abnormalities. The patient's temperature and pulse should be recorded every 4 hours, more often if indicated. Maternal blood pressure should be taken and recorded every hour during labor. The patient should be encouraged to void every 3 hours during labor. The amount of fluid intake should be recorded. Any new significant symptom or sign (eg, excessive vaginal bleeding or pain, or meconium-stained amniotic fluid) should be evaluated by the physician.

Patients should not take anything by mouth during labor except for small sips of water, ice chips, or preparations to moisten the mouth and lips. Hydration and nourishment during a long labor should be provided by means of the intravenous administration of fluids; this measure also minimizes acidemia and electrolyte imbalance.

Intrapartum infusion of solutions containing glucose may cause maternal hyperglycemia and hyperinsulinemia, as well as an increase in lactic acid levels in maternal and umbilical vein blood that reduces the umbilical vein pH. Because these factors can be of importance when fetal distress or fetal hypoxia is due to other perinatal events, large infusions of glucose should be avoided during the intrapartum period.

Because aspiration continues to be a leading cause of anesthetic-related maternal mortality and because the aspiration of acidic (pH less than 2.5) gastric contents is more harmful than the aspiration of less acidic gastric contents, the prophylactic administration of an antacid before the induction of a major regional or general anesthesia is appropriate. Particulate antacids may be harmful if aspirated; therefore, a clear antacid, such as 0.3 mol/L sodium citrate or a similar preparation, may be a safer choice. On rare occasions, it may be impossible to intubate an obstetric patient following induction of general anesthesia. An emergency cricothyrotomy may be lifesaving in this case, and the necessary equipment for performing this procedure should be available when general anesthesia is administered.

Vaginal examinations should be kept to a minimum and conducted with careful attention to the use of a clean technique. This is particularly important if the membranes are ruptured. Cleansing of the perineum may decrease potential contamination, and the use of a sterile lubricant reduces discomfort from the examination.

The intensity and method of fetal heart rate monitoring used during labor should be based on risk factors and delineated by department policy. It has been shown that intermittent auscultation at intervals of 15 minutes during the first stage of labor and 5 minutes during the second stage is equivalent to continuous electronic fetal heart rate monitoring. Thus, when risk factors are present during labor or when intensified monitoring is elected, the fetal heart rate should be assessed by one of these methods according to the following guidelines:

1. During the active phase of the first stage of labor, the fetal heart rate should be evaluated and recorded at least every 15 minutes, preferably following a uterine contraction, when intermittent auscultation is used. If continuous electronic fetal monitoring is used, the tracing should be evaluated at least every 15 minutes.

2. During the second stage of labor, the fetal heart rate should be evaluated and recorded at least every 5 minutes when auscultation is used and should be evaluated at least every 5 minutes when electronic fetal monitoring is used.

For low-risk patients in labor, the fetal heart rate may be monitored by auscultation. In such patients, there are no data to demonstrate optimal time intervals for intermittent auscultation. The standard practice is to evaluate and record the fetal heart rate at least every 30 minutes following a contraction in the active phase of the first stage of labor and at least every 15 minutes in the second stage of labor.

When electronic fetal heart rate monitoring is selected as the method of fetal assessment, the physician and obstetric personnel attending the patient should be qualified to identify and interpret abnormalities. It is appropriate for physicians and nurses to use the names that have been given to fetal monitoring patterns (eg, accelerations and early, late, or variable decelerations) in chart documentation and verbal communication. Consultation with qualified physicians should be sought when the staff responsible for the care of the patient cannot adequately interpret abnormal patterns. In the event of differences of interpretation among professionals involved in the care of specific patients, an established hospital policy for the resolution of such a conflict should be followed.

Internal uterine pressure monitoring can provide important information regarding the strength and frequency of contractions. This technique is not used routinely, but is reserved for those occasions when complications have developed in labor or when there is a question about the adequacy of oxytocin administration.

Notation on the monitoring strip of such items as physician or nurse presence, the patient's position in the bed, cervical status, oxygen or drug administration, hypertension or hypotension, fever, amniotomy, color of the amniotic fluid, and Valsalva efforts provides a detailed and graphic documentation of the course of events during labor. Abnormal findings should be described and interpreted. It is especially important that when a change in fetal heart rate patterns has been noted, a subsequent return to normal patterns be documented as well. Each tracing should include the patient's name, hospital number, date and time of admission and delivery, and other data required for medical records. All tracings should be stored in a way that makes them readily retrievable.

Although its exact role is controversial, determination of fetal capillary pH may be a useful adjunct to intrapartum fetal assessment.

Preterm Patients

When patients are admitted in preterm labor, fetal maturity and the possibility of fetal or maternal infection should be determined. Protocols should be developed for the use of tocolytic agents, including the indications for their use and the management of their side-effects. The pediatric service should be notified of the possibility of a preterm delivery; if necessary, transfer to a hospital with facilities for the care of these mothers and infants should be arranged. Particular attention should be given to the care of mothers and infants when delivery will occur at the early limits of viability.

Preterm, Premature Rupture of Membranes

Management of preterm, premature rupture of the membranes remains controversial. The risk of chorioamnionitis and fetal infection must often be weighed against the risks associated with the delivery of a premature infant. If amniotic fluid has pooled in the vagina, it can be examined for evidence of lung maturity. Speculum examination can permit visualization of the cervix and culturing for group B *Streptococcus* and *Neisseria gonorrhoeae*, if indicated (see Chapter 6). A digital examination should be avoided if the patient is not in labor.

In the presence of an immature fetus without signs of infection, it is reasonable to observe the patient rather than to induce labor. When infection occurs, however, it is necessary to deliver an immature fetus.

Assessment of Fetal Maturity Prior to Repeat Cesarean Delivery or Elective Induction of Labor

The assessment of fetal maturity is an important consideration in determining the timing of a repeat cesarean delivery or elective induction of labor. Fetal maturity can be assumed if at least two of the following clinical criteria for estimating gestational age are supported by at least one of the following laboratory determinations:

Clinical Criteria

1. Thirty-nine weeks have elapsed since the last menstrual period of a patient with normal menstrual cycles and no immediate antecedent use of oral contraceptives.
2. Fetal heart tones have been documented for 20 weeks by nonelectronic fetoscope.
3. Uterine size has been established by pelvic examination prior to 16 weeks of gestation.

Laboratory Determinations

1. Thirty-six weeks have elapsed since a positive serum human chorionic gonadotropin (hCG) pregnancy test
2. Ultrasound examination was used to determine gestational age through one of the following measurements:
   a. Crown rump length obtained between 6 and 14 weeks of gestation
   b. Biparietal diameter obtained before 24 weeks of gestation

If these criteria are not met, amniotic fluid analysis for lecithin:sphingomyelin (L:S) ratio or phosphatidylglycerol can provide satisfactory evidence of fetal lung maturity. When there is no evidence of fetal lung maturity, it is a reasonable option to allow a patient with no contraindications to go into labor spontaneously.

Elective repeat cesarean delivery does not necessarily constitute a high-risk situation for the neonate. Because the duties of the surgical team may preclude their caring for a distressed neonate, another qualified person skilled in neonatal resuscitation should be present in the delivery room to care for the neonate. The qualifications needed should be defined by the hospital's medical staff.

Medical Induction and Augmentation of Labor

Labor may be induced or augmented with oxytocin only after a physician who is responsible for the patient's care has evaluated the patient's condition, determined that induction or augmentation is beneficial to the mother or fetus, recorded the indication, and established a prospective plan of management. Only a physician who has privileges to perform cesarean deliveries should initiate these procedures. A physician or qualified nurse should examine the patient vaginally immediately prior to the oxytocin infusion.

Each hospital's department of obstetrics and gynecology should determine the indications for induction and augmentation of labor, and should establish a written protocol for the preparation and administration of the oxytocin solution. This protocol should delineate methods to be employed for maternal and fetal assessment. Oxytocin should be administered only intravenously, with a device that permits precise control of the flow rate.

Personnel who are familiar with the effects of oxytocin and able to identify both maternal and fetal complications should be in attendance during the administration of oxytocin. A qualified physician should be readily available to manage any complications that may arise during the infusion.

Management of Delivery

Specific preparation for delivery should be instituted at a time dictated by the patient's parity, labor progress, fetal presentation, labor complications, and anesthesia management. At least one member of the nursing staff should be present in the delivery room throughout the delivery. Under no circumstances should any attempt be made to delay the birth by physical restraint or anesthesia.

Although the lithotomy position is generally used for vaginal delivery in the United States, many physicians prefer the lateral position or partial sitting position. Regardless of the position employed, positioning of the patient must allow for the safe administration of anesthesia. If a pudendal block or local perineal block anesthesia is used, it should be administered when the patient is positioned for delivery. Obstetric forceps or vacuum extractors may be used as determined by the training and skill of the obstetrician and the obstetric conditions (see Forceps, this chapter).

Episiotomy is used to protect the perineum; it is not always necessary, however, and should not be considered routine. The presence of a short perineum, a large baby, and the need to shorten the second stage of labor are some of the current indications for its use.

The maternal blood pressure and pulse should be evaluated every 15 minutes and recorded. The fetal heart rate should be monitored at least every 5 minutes. Maternal vital signs should be evaluated upon delivery and reevaluated at 15-minute intervals (or more frequently) until the patient's condition has stabilized.

If external monitoring is being used in patients who will undergo cesarean delivery, it should be continued until the abdominal preparation is begun. If internal monitoring is being used, the scalp electrode should remain attached to the fetus and the monitoring equipment until the abdominal preparation is complete.

Emergency Cesarean Delivery

Any hospital that provides labor and delivery services should be equipped to perform an emergency cesarean delivery. The nursing, anesthesia, neonatal resuscitation, and obstetric personnel required must be either in the hospital or readily available. It should be possible to begin the operation within 30 minutes of the time that the decision is made to operate.

Vaginal Birth After Cesarean Delivery

A trial of labor after a prior cesarean birth (low transverse uterine incision) is appropriate if there are no contraindications. Recent data show that 50-80% of patients who attempt to deliver vaginally after a cesarean birth have successful vaginal births. Data also show that maternal and perinatal mortality rates associated with vaginal delivery after cesarean delivery are no higher than those for repeat cesarean delivery. Although uterine rupture can occur, it is rarely catastrophic because of the availability of modern fetal monitoring, anesthesia, and obstetric support services. A successful vaginal delivery not only eliminates operative and postoperative complications, but also shortens the patient's hospital stay.

Unless there are contraindications to vaginal delivery, women with one previous cesarean delivery should be counseled to undergo labor in their current pregnancy. The concept of routine repeat cesarean birth should be replaced by a diagnostic indication for a subsequent abdominal delivery. More specific details on vaginal birth after cesarean delivery are available from the American College of Obstetricians and Gynecologists.

Forceps

There is a place for forceps operations, applied judiciously and used within the context of the following definitions, indications, and required conditions.

DEFINITIONS

1. **Station:** The relationship of the estimated distance, in centimeters, between the leading bony portion of the fetal head and the level of the maternal ischial spines. In classifying forceps procedures, the level of engagement of the fetal head must be stated as precisely as possible. Engagement of the vertex occurs when the biparietal diameter has passed through the pelvic inlet and is clinically diagnosed when the leading bony portion of the fetal head is at or below the level of the ischial spines (station 0 or more).

2. **Outlet forceps:** The application of forceps when a) the scalp is visible at the introitus without separating the labia, b) the fetal skull has reached the pelvic floor, c) the sagittal suture is in the anterior-posterior diameter or in the right or left occiput anterior or posterior position, and d) the fetal head is at or on the perineum. According to this definition, rotation cannot exceed 45°. There is no difference in perinatal outcome when deliveries involving the use of outlet forceps are compared with similar spontaneous deliveries, and there are no data to support the concept that rotating the head on the pelvic floor 45° or less increases morbidity. Forceps delivery under these conditions may be desirable to shorten the second stage of labor.

3. **Low forceps:** The application of forceps when the leading point of the skull is at station +2 or more. Low forceps have two subdivisions: a) rotation 45° or less (eg, left occipitoanterior to occiput anterior, left occipitoposterior to occiput posterior), and b) rotation more than 45°.

4. **Midforceps:** The application of forceps when the head is engaged but the leading point of the skull is above station +2. Under very unusual circumstances, such as the sudden onset of

severe fetal or maternal compromise, application of forceps above station +2 may be attempted while simultaneously initiating preparations for a cesarean delivery in the event that the forceps maneuver is unsuccessful. Under no circumstances, however, should forceps be applied to an unengaged presenting part or when the cervix is not completely dilated.

INDICATIONS.   The indications for the forceps operation, including the position and station of the vertex at the time of application of the forceps, should be specified in a detailed operative description in the patient's medical record. These indications include the following:

1. Shortening the second stage of labor: Outlet forceps may be used to shorten the second stage of labor in the best interests of the mother or the fetus, as long as the criteria for outlet forceps are met.
2. Prolonged second stage: The following durations are approximate; when these intervals are exceeded, the risks and benefits of allowing labor to continue should be assessed and documented:
   A. Primigravida: More than 3 hours with a regional anesthetic or more than 2 hours without a regional anesthetic
   B. Multigravida: More than 2 hours with a regional anesthetic or more than 1 hour without a regional anesthetic
3. Fetal distress
4. Maternal indications (eg, cardiac, exhaustion)

REQUIRED CONDITIONS.   The following conditions are required for forceps operations:

1. An experienced person performing or supervising the procedure
2. Assessment of maternal-fetal size relationship
3. Adequate anesthesia
4. Willingness to abandon attempt if forceps procedure does not proceed easily

Assessment and Care of the Neonate in the Delivery Room

The first minutes of life may determine the quality of that life. The need for a prompt, organized, and skilled response to emergencies in this period requires institutions that provide maternal-fetal care to have written policies delineating responsibility for immediate newborn care, resuscitation, selection and maintenance of necessary equipment, and training of personnel in proper techniques.

The obstetrician is responsible for providing immediate postdelivery care of the newborn and for ascertaining that the newborn adaptations to extrauterine life are proceeding normally. The hospital rules and regulations should include protocols for the transfer of medical care of the neonate in both routine and emergency circumstances. Routine care of the healthy newborn may be delegated to appropriately trained nurses.

Recognition and immediate resuscitation of the distressed neonate require an organized plan of action and the immediate availability of qualified personnel and equipment. At least one person skilled in initiating resuscitation should be present at every delivery. Responsibility for identification and resuscitation of a distressed neonate should be assigned to a qualified individual, who may be a physician or an appropriately trained nurse-midwife, labor and delivery nurse, nurse-anesthetist, nursery nurse, or respiratory therapist. The provision of services and equipment for resuscitation should be planned jointly by the directors of the departments of obstetrics, anesthesia, and pediatrics, with the approval of the medical staff. A physician should be designated to assume primary responsibility for initiating, supervising, and reviewing the plan for management of depressed neonates in the delivery room. The following factors should be considered in this plan:

1. A list of maternal and fetal complications that require the presence in the delivery room of someone specifically qualified in newborn resuscitation should be developed (Appendix C).

2. Individuals qualified to perform neonatal resuscitation should demonstrate
   a. Skills in rapid and accurate evaluation of the newborn condition, including Apgar scoring.
   b. Knowledge of the pathogenesis and causes of a low Apgar score (eg, asphyxia, drugs, hypovolemia, trauma, anomalies, infections, and prematurity), as well as specific indications for resuscitation.
   c. Skills in airway management, laryngoscopy, endotracheal intubation, suctioning of the airway, artificial ventilation, cardiac massage, emergency administration of drugs and fluids, and maintenance of thermal stability. The ability to

recognize and decompress tension pneumothorax by needle aspiration is also a desirable skill.

3. Procedures should be developed to ensure the readiness of equipment and personnel and to provide for intermittent review and evaluation of the effectiveness of the system.

4. Contingency plans should be established for multiple births and other unusual circumstances.

5. A physician for the neonate need not be present at a delivery provided that no complications are anticipated and another skilled individual is present to care for the neonate.

6. The resuscitation steps should be documented in the records.

Apgar Score

At 1 minute and 5 minutes after the complete birth of the neonate, Apgar scores (Table 4-l) should be obtained. If the 5-minute score is less than 7, it is useful to obtain additional scores every 5 minutes until 20 minutes have passed or until two successive scores of 7 or greater are obtained.

When necessary, resuscitation should be initiated before the 1-minute Apgar score is obtained. A person (eg, a nurse) not directly involved in resuscitating the neonate should assign the Apgar score. Low scores (less than 3), especially those associated with a delay in the return of tone, are useful in identifying the neonate who is significantly depressed; the change between the one-minute score

Table 4-1. Apgar Score

Sign	0	1	2
Heart rate	Absent	Slow (<100 min)	100 beats/min
Respirations	Absent	Weak cry; hypo-ventilation	Good, strong cry
Muscle tone	Limp	Some flexion	Active motion
Reflex irritability (response to brisk slap on soles of feet)	No response	Grimace	Cough or sneeze
Color	Blue or pale	Body pink; extremities blue	Completely pink

Apgar V et al: Evaluation of the newborn infant—Second report. JAMA 168:1985,1958.
Copyright © 1958, American Medical Association

and the 5-minute score is useful in assessing the efficacy of resuscitation; and low scores at 10, 15, and 20 minutes are associated with an increased risk of neonatal and later mortality and morbidity.

If a low Apgar score is anticipated or assigned, rapid assessment of the neonate's condition is necessary in order to delineate a plan of care. Umbilical cord blood gas and pH analyses may help to distinguish metabolic acidemia secondary to hypoxia from other causes of low Apgar scores in the depressed neonate.

Maintenance of Body Temperature

Immediately following delivery, the neonate should be placed in a warm place and dried completely. Drying the neonate with prewarmed towels immediately after birth reduces evaporative heat loss. It is recommended that a radiant warmer with a servocontrol mechanism be placed in the resuscitation area, because such devices allow easy access to the neonate during resuscitation procedures.

Suctioning

The neonate's mouth may be suctioned gently to remove excess mucus or blood. Although clear mucus is suctioned from the mouth routinely in most centers, there is no evidence to support the value of this practice. Vigorous suctioning of the posterior pharynx should be avoided, as this may produce significant bradycardia.

If there is meconium in the amniotic fluid, the mouth and hypopharynx should be thoroughly suctioned with a mechanical device before delivery of the shoulders in a cephalic presentation and immediately after delivery of the head in a breech presentation. In the presence of thick or particulate meconium, the larynx should be visualized and any meconium present removed. If meconium is present, the clinician should intubate the trachea and suction to remove meconium or other aspirated material from beneath the glottis (Table 4-2; see Suctioning, Chapter 6).

Table 4-2. Guidelines for Endotracheal Tubes and Suction Catheters

Weight (kg)	Minimum Internal Diameter (mm) of Endotracheal Tube	Depth of Insertion (cm from upper lip)	Suction Catheter Size
1	2.5	7	5F
2	3.0	8	6F
3	3.5	9	8F

Resuscitation

As a part of a multiorganizational collaboration, the American Heart Association and the American Academy of Pediatrics have developed materials for teaching resuscitation skills and should be considered the primary source of more definitive information.

The need for resuscitation is determined by the condition of the neonate. The normal neonate breathes within seconds of delivery and has established regular respiration by 1 minute of age. A flaccid neonate who is not breathing spontaneously and whose heart rate is less than 80 beats/min requires immediate positive pressure ventilation. A bag and mask can often provide effective ventilation (Fig. 4-2), but it may be difficult to use this method in premature neonates with noncompliant lungs. If the neonate's heart rate does not rise promptly to more than 60-80 beats/min, endotracheal intubation is required.

Before applying positive pressure ventilation, it is important to ensure that the airway has been cleared. The head should be placed in a "sniffing" position, with care to avoid hyperextension of the neck. The middle or fourth finger should be placed behind the posterior ramus of the mandible, "thrusting" the mandible forward; no fingers (or any part of the mask) should rest on the soft tissues of

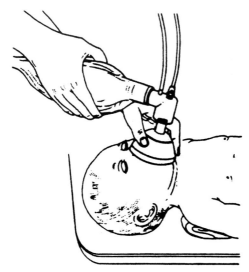

Fig. 4-2. *Artificial ventilation of the newborn with bag and mask. (American Heart Association, American Academy of Pediatrics: Textbook of Neonatal Resuscitation. Reproduced with permission, © American Heart Association, Dallas, 1987)*

the neck. Initial lung inflation may require 30-40 cm H_2O, and 15-20 cm H_2O is often adequate for succeeding breaths, which should be provided at a rate of 40/min. Preferably, oxygen should be warmed and humidified. With rare exceptions, severely asphyxiated neonates respond promptly to adequate ventilation, and this is the only resuscitation maneuver required.

Symmetric movement of the apices of the chest, equal breath sounds (heard in the axillae), and improvement in heart rate, color, and muscle tone indicate satisfactory ventilation. The response of the heart rate is the most useful and readily measurable criterion of adequate resuscitation. If the response to ventilation is not prompt, the seal between the face and the mask or the position of the endotracheal tube should be checked. If chest movement and breath sounds appear satisfactory in an intubated neonate, yet the neonate is not responding, the position of the endotracheal tube should be checked by direct visualization of the larynx with a laryngoscope.

External Cardiac Massage

If the heart rate does not rise promptly to more than 60-80 beats/min after effective ventilation with oxygen, external cardiac massage should be instituted while ventilation is continued. Two techniques are illustrated in Figure 4-3. Chest compressions should be carried out at a rate of 120 beats/min to a depth of 1/2-3/4 inch. If there is no response in the heart rate, appropriate drug therapy (and volume expansion, if indicated) should be instituted.

Drugs and Volume Expansion

The use of drugs for resuscitation of the neonate is rarely necessary in the delivery room. When drugs are needed (Table 4-3), they should not be administered until ventilation has been adequately established. The preferred route of administration is the umbilical vein. The infusion of epinephrine into the trachea via an endotracheal tube can also be an effective route of administration.

ACIDOSIS. Severely asphyxiated neonates have a combined metabolic and respiratory acidosis. The treatment of acidosis is treatment of the cause. Thus, respiratory acidosis, which is the result of hypoventilation, is treated by providing positive pressure ventilation. Metabolic acidosis is the result of hypoxemia or hypoperfusion, and the correction of these factors should correct the acidosis.

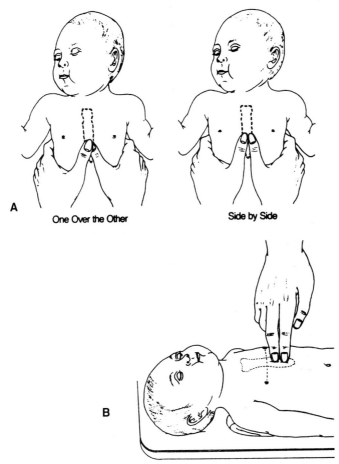

A   One Over the Other   Side by Side

B

Fig. 4-3. Techniques for external cardiac massage. **A.** The chest is encircled with both hands and the thumbs compress the sternum. **B.** The tips of the middle finger and either the index or ring finger of one hand are used for compression. (American Heart Association, American Academy of Pediatrics: Textbook of Neonatal Resuscitation. Reproduced with Permission, © American Heart Association, Dallas, 1987)

Significant acidemia is detrimental to myocardial function in the hypoxic heart. Sodium bicarbonate may be useful in a prolonged resuscitation to help correct a documented metabolic acidosis, but its use is discouraged in brief arrests or episodes of bradycardia. In the absence of adequate ventilation, sodium bicarbonate will not improve blood pH.

BRADYCARDIA. Epinephrine hydrochloride may be indicated for bradycardia that persists after adequate ventilation and cardiac massage. Dosages are given in Table 4-3.

Table 4-3. Indications for Drugs in Resuscitation of the Newborn

Indication	Drug	Dosage
Bradycardia	Epinephrine hydrochloride	0.1 ml/kg of 1:10,000 solution
Low blood volume	Albumin	10 ml/kg of 5% solution
	Ringer's lactate	10 ml/kg
Hypoglycemia	Dextrose	2 ml/kg of 10% solution
Respiratory depression secondary to narcotics	Naloxone hydrochloride	0.01-0.1 mg/kg
Metabolic acidosis with normal or low (CO_2)	Sodium bicarbonate	2 m Eq/kg slowly

HYPOVOLEMIA. It is important to recognize that most asphyxiated neonates are not hypovolemic and that there may be potential hazards (eg, intracranial hemorrhage) to rapid volume expansion. Conditions associated with hypovolemia include significant hemorrhage from the fetoplacental unit (eg, vasa praevia, fetomaternal bleeding) and compression of the umbilical cord.

If significant hypovolemia is suspected, it should be treated with repeated small infusions of volume expanders (5-10 ml/kg). The neonate's response should be assessed after each infusion. Therapy is stopped when tissue perfusion is adequate. The choice of a particular plasma expanding agent depends on the cause of the hypovolemia. For unanticipated shock, heparinized placental blood may be used; this is obtained from the umbilical cord after it has been sterilized. Blood is withdrawn into a 20-ml syringe that contains 1 ml of 50 U/ml heparin and administered through a blood set filter.

NARCOTIC-INDUCED RESPIRATORY DEPRESSION. If respiratory depression is the result of narcotics administered to the mother prior to delivery, naloxone hydrochloride, 0.01 mg/kg, may be administered to the neonate in conjunction with assisted ventilation.

POSTPARTUM AND NEWBORN CARE

Postpartum hospitalization has several purposes: to identify maternal and neonatal complications, to provide professional assistance during the time when the mother is most likely to be uncomfortable, and to allow adequate time for instruction so that the parents may return home with reasonable competence and confidence.

Emphasis in the immediate postpartum period should be placed on the initiation of positive parent-neonate relationships that can be carried over to the home environment. Adequate preparation should include provisions not only for the mother and newborn, but also for siblings and other members of the household. This preparation and introduction of other family members can begin in the hospital. In order to enhance positive interaction with the newborn, liberal visiting privileges for the immediate family are encouraged (see Visiting, this chapter).

Care of the Mother

Immediate Postpartum Care

Postpartum care begins immediately after delivery, in the recovery area or birthing room where the woman can be observed for postpartum complications, such as hemorrhage or hematoma formation. During this period of observation, maternal blood pressure and pulse should be taken and recorded every 15 minutes for the first hour, more frequently if the patient's condition warrants. The uterine fundus should be examined frequently to check for excessive bleeding and palpated to determine if it is well contracted. If the uterus has a tendency to relax or if the patient has a predisposing cause for postpartum hemorrhage (eg, an overdistended uterus) or a history of postpartum bleeding with a prior pregnancy, a dilute solution of oxytocin should be administered by intravenous drip. For postpartum hemorrhage due to uterine atony not responsive to oxytocin or ergot alkaloids, 15α-methyl prostaglandin $F_{2\alpha}$ should be available. If vaginal bleeding occurs or if the patient complains of perineal pain, the cause of the bleeding or pain should be determined by careful palpation of the uterus and by inspection and palpation of the perineum, vagina, and cervix for lacerations or hematoma formation.

The father or other supporting person may remain with the new mother during the immediate postpartum period. Parents should be encouraged to interact with the neonate unless such interaction is precluded by maternal or neonatal complications. Even though the neonate remains with the mother, the physician or nurse should make an initial assessment of the neonate's condition. Routine observation should continue during the transitional period to note any conditions, such as respiratory distress or hypothermia, that require special attention.

Following major conduction or general anesthesia for either vaginal or cesarean delivery, the patient should be observed in an appropriately staffed and equipped recovery area until she has recovered from the anesthesia. Staff assigned to the recovery area should have no other obligation. The patient should be discharged from the recovery area only at the discretion of the attending physician or the anesthesiologist in charge. A record of vital signs should be maintained and additional signs or events monitored and recorded as they occur.

Subsequent Care

The physician should sign the patient's transfer to the postpartum unit after writing the appropriate postpartum orders. When the patient is taken to her postpartum room, her vital signs, the status of the uterine fundus, and the rate of bleeding should be reassessed and recorded. This assessment should be repeated at regular intervals for the next several hours. While in the postpartum unit, the mother should be taught how to care for herself and her neonate, and problems related to her general health should be discussed. Specific postpartum policies and procedures should be established through cooperative efforts of the medical and nursing staff.

BED REST, AMBULATION, AND DIET. Bed rest is recommended for only a brief time, just long enough to allow the new mother to sleep, regain her strength, and recover from the effects of the analgesic or anesthetic agents that she may have received during labor. It may be necessary to administer fluids intravenously for hydration. Because early ambulation has been shown to decrease the incidence of subsequent thrombophlebitis, the patient should be encouraged to ambulate, with assistance, as soon as she feels able. The patient should not attempt to get out of bed initially without the help of an attendant. The mother may have a full diet as soon as she desires it, unless her physician gives other orders.

CARE OF THE VULVA. The patient should be taught to cleanse the vulva from anterior vulva to perineum and anus rather than in the reverse direction. The application of an ice bag is likely to reduce edema and pain during the first 4-6 hours after repair of episiotomy. Orally administered analgesics are commonly required and are usually sufficient for relief of discomfort from episiotomy. Pain that is not relieved by such medication suggests hematoma formation and mandates a careful examination of the vulva, vagina, and rectum. Beginning 24 hours after delivery, either dry heat with an infrared lamp or moist heat in the form of a warm sitz bath can be applied to reduce local discomfort and promote healing.

CARE OF THE BLADDER. Women often have difficulty voiding immediately after delivery, possibly because of trauma to the bladder during labor and delivery, regional anesthesia, or pain from the episiotomy site. In addition, the diuresis that sometimes follows delivery may distend the bladder before the patient is aware of it. In order to ensure adequate emptying of the bladder, the patient should be checked frequently during the first 24 hours after delivery, with particular attention to displacement of the uterine fundus and any indication of a fluid-filled bladder above the symphysis. Every effort should be made to help the patient void spontaneously; however, a single catheterization may be necessary. If the patient continues to find voiding difficult, the use of an in-dwelling catheter may be preferable to repeated catheterization.

BATHING. After the mother is able to ambulate, she may shower. She may not be comfortable with tub baths until the second postpartum day or later.

CARE OF THE BREASTS. The mother's decision about breast-feeding her newborn determines the appropriate care of the breasts. Breast care for a woman who chooses to breast-feed is outlined in Chapter 7. The woman who does not desire to breast-feed should be reassured that stopping the milk production is not a major problem. During the stage of engorgement, the breasts become painful and should be supported with a well-fitting brassiere. Ice packs or small doses of analgesics may be required to relieve discomfort during this 12- to 24-hour period. If needed, many medications are available to suppress lactation.

TEMPERATURE ELEVATION. The condition of all postpartum patients with an elevated temperature should be evaluated and appropriate cultures taken (see Chapter 6). The nursery should be notified if the mother develops a fever, especially within the first 24 hours, so that the neonate can be examined for potential infection.

POSTPARTUM STERILIZATION. Performing tubal ligation immediately after a delivery that has been conducted under major regional or general anesthesia reduces the length of the patient's hospitalization and eliminates the need for a second administration of anesthesia. If tubal sterilization necessitates the induction of anesthesia (regional or general), the anesthesiologist should carefully evaluate the patient's condition. If there is any indication of a neonatal problem, the timing of this elective procedure should be reevaluated.

IMMUNIZATION: RHIG AND RUBELLA. An unsensitized Rho(D)-negative woman who delivers an Rho(D) or Du-positive neonate should receive 300 µg RhIG postpartum, ideally within 72 hours, even when RhIG has been administered in the antepartum period. This dose may be inadequate in circumstances where there is potential fetal-maternal hemorrhage, such as abruptio placentae, placenta previa, intrauterine manipulation (as may be required for the delivery of twins), manual removal of the placenta, cesarean delivery, precipitous delivery, multifetal gestation, and polyhydramnios. In these cases, laboratory analysis should be performed to detect excessive maternal-fetal hemorrhage and thus determine the proper dosage. If indicated, additional RhIG should be administered.

A patient who has been identified as rubella-susceptible should receive the rubella vaccine in the postpartum period. Rubella vaccine can be administered after delivery prior to discharge, even if the patient is breast-feeding.

Care of the Neonate

Immediate Stabilization Period

Stabilization usually occurs during the first 12 hours after birth. Following an initial evaluation of the neonate's condition, a care plan appropriate to the individual neonate should be established and the neonate carefully observed for the next 6-12 hours. During the stabilization period, temperature, heart and respiratory rates, blood pressure, color, adequacy of peripheral circulation, type of respiration, level of consciousness, tone, and activity should be monitored and recorded at least once per hour until the neonate's condition has remained stable for 2 hours.

Neonates who appear to be healthy need not leave their mother for this stabilization period if the facilities needed for their observation are in the mother's recovery or postpartum area and there is adequate nursing personnel to observe the neonate in the manner outlined. Following these careful observations, the neonate who has no identified problem may be placed in the newborn nursery or in the mother's room for continued observation and care until discharge. After appropriate initial care in the resuscitation area, neonates who at birth are sick, small, or at high risk of becoming sick (as determined by history or physical examination) should be transferred to an intermediate or intensive care area.

NEONATE IDENTIFICATION. While the newborn is still in the delivery room, two identical bands that indicate the mother's admission number, the neonate's sex, and the date and time of birth should be placed on the wrist or ankle. The nurse in charge of the delivery room should be responsible for preparing and securely fastening these identification bands on the neonate. The birth records and identification bands should be checked before the neonate leaves the resuscitation area of the delivery room. When the neonate is taken to the nursery, both the delivery room nurse and the admitting nurse should check the identification bands and birth records, verify the sex of the neonate, and sign the neonate's record. The admitting nurse should fill out the bassinet card and attach it to the bassinet. Later, when the neonate is shown to the mother, she should be asked to verify the information on the identification bands and the sex of the neonate. It is imperative that delivery room and nursery personnel be meticulous in the preparation and placement of neonate identification bands.

Footprinting and fingerprinting have in the past been recommended for purposes of neonate identification. Newly developed techniques, such as sophisticated blood typing, appear to be more reliable means of identification, however. Individual hospitals may want to continue the practice of footprinting and fingerprinting, but universal use of this practice is no longer recommended.

ASSESSMENT OF NEONATAL RISKS. As soon as possible, no later than 2 hours after birth, admitting personnel should evaluate the neonate's status and assess risks. Necessary clinical data that were unavailable initially should be either obtained or requested at this time. Risks can be assessed through the history and physical examination.

The nurse or physician in attendance at delivery should prepare a history, including the following information:

1. History of hereditary conditions in each parent's family
2. Medical history of mother (eg, diabetes; hypertension; preeclampsia; infections; fever just prior to, during, or following delivery)
3. Past obstetric history (eg, number, duration, and outcome of previous pregnancies, with dates)
4. First day of the last menstrual period and estimated date of confinement
5. Mother's blood group and Rh type, with evidence of sensitization or immunization (eg, administration of RhIG)
6. Results of serologic test and cultures, including dates performed
7. Drugs taken during pregnancy, labor, and delivery

8. Results of measurements of fetal maturity and well-being
9. Duration of ruptured membranes and labor, including length of second stage
10. Method of delivery, including indications for operative or instrumental delivery
11. Placental abnormalities, if any
12. Estimated amount (ie, oligohydramnios, hydramnios) and description (eg, meconium staining; foul-smelling, particulate matter) of amniotic fluid
13. Apgar scores
14. Description of resuscitation, if required
15. Detailed description of abnormalities and problems occurring from birth until transfer to the admission/observation area

The admitting nurse or physician should assess the newborn's condition as soon as possible after birth, either in the recovery room or in the nursery. The neonate's physician should examine the apparently normal neonate no later than 12-18 hours after birth and within the 24 hours before discharge from the hospital. The results of these examinations should be recorded on the neonate's chart and discussed with the parents. This initial examination record should include the following information:

1. Date and time of birth
2. Date, time, and age of neonate at the time of examination
3. Sex
4. Racial origin
5. Birth weight, gestational age, length, and circumference of head
6. Vital signs, including temperature, heart rate, respiratory rate, and blood pressure
7. Complete physical examination
8. Need for isolation (see Chapter 6)
9. Anomalies (both major and minor)

BIRTH WEIGHT/GESTATIONAL AGE CLASSIFICATION. The neonate's gestational age should be calculated from the mother's menstrual history, physical examination, obstetric milestones noted during pregnancy, and the obstetrician's assessment of gestational age (Fig. 4-4). If there is a marked discrepancy between the presumed duration of pregnancy and the physical and neurologic findings in the neonate, the gestational age should be estimated on the basis of the physical examination, in conjunction with a composite of relevant obstetric information and observations.

Apgar_____1 min_____5 min
Age at exam_____(hr)
Race_____ Sex_____
B.D. _____
LMP _____
EDC _____
Gestational age
  by dates_____(wk)
Gestational age
  by exam_____(wk)
Birth weight_____(g)
  _____percentile
Length_____(cm)
  _____percentile
Head circum._____(cm)
  _____percentile
Clin. dist.____None____Mild
  ____ Mod.____Severe

Neuromuscular maturity

	0	1	2	3	4	5
Posture						
Square window (wrist)	90°	60°	45°	30°	0°	
Arm recoil	180°		100°-180°	90°-100°	<90°	
Popliteal angle	180°	160°	130°	110°	90°	<90°
Scarf sign						
Heel to ear						

Physical maturity

	0	1	2	3	4	5
Skin	gelatinous red, transparent	smooth pink, visible veins	superficial peeling &/or rash, few veins	cracking pale area, rare veins	parchment, deep cracking, no vessels	leathery, cracked, wrinkled
Lanugo	none	abundant	thinning	bald areas	mostly bald	
Plantar creases	no crease	faint red marks	anterior transverse crease only	creases ant. 2/3	creases cover entire sole	
Breast	barely percept.	flat areola, no bud	stippled areola, 1-2 mm bud	raised areola, 3-4 mm bud	full areola, 5-10 mm bud	
Ear	pinna flat, stays folded	sl. curved pinna, soft with slow recoil	well-curv. pinna, soft but ready recoil	formed & firm with instant recoil	thick cartilage, ear stiff	
Genitals ♂	scrotom empty no rugae		testes descending, few rugae	testes down, good rugae	testes pendulous, deep rugae	
Genitals ♀	prominent clitoris & labia minora		majora & minora equally prominent	majora large, minora small	clitoris & minora completely covered	

Maturity rating

Score	Weeks
5	26
10	28
15	30
20	32
25	34
30	36
35	38
40	40
45	42
50	44

Fig. 4-4. Assessment of neonatal maturity. The assessment is quickly and easily performed because the chart includes measures of physical maturity and measures of passive tone but not active tone. Items are arranged so that a neonate who scored 2 on each item would be 34 weeks. Physical maturity is most accurately assessed in the minutes or hour or so following birth. The score for each item is indicated at the top of the vertical column. However, neuromuscular maturity may be spuriously retarded in the asphyxiated neonate or the neonate obtunded by anesthetic agents or drugs. Thus, neuromuscular maturity rating should be repeated after a day or two. The sum of scores on all the items of physical and neuromuscular maturity provides a maturity in weeks (see lower right). The physical maturity score times 2 provides an approximation of maturity rating in weeks.

Data from each neonate should be plotted on a birth weight-gestational age chart that indicates whether the neonate is small, average, or large for gestational age. The determination of gestational age and its relationship to weight can be used in the identification of neonates at risk for illness. For example, neonates who are either large or small for their gestational age are at relatively increased risk for hypoglycemia and polycythemia, and appropriate tests (eg, serum glucose screen or hemoglobin determination) are indicated.

CORD BLOOD. The Rh group of the cord blood should be determined and Coombs antibody tested routinely at the time of delivery if the mother is Rho(D)-negative. Blood typing, Rh determination, and serologic tests for syphilis should be done on cord blood or on blood drawn from the neonate before discharge if the mother was not previously tested.

EYE CARE. The application of 1% silver nitrate in single-dose containers or sterile ophthalmic ointment containing tetracyline (1%) or erythromycin (0.5%) in single-use tubes is acceptable prophylaxis against gonococcal ophthalmia neonatorum. Care should be taken to ensure that the agent reaches all parts of the conjunctival sac. The eyes should not be irrigated with saline or distilled water after instillation of any of these agents; however, after 1 minute, excess solution or ointment can be wiped away. Instillation may be delayed up to 1 hour following birth (see Appendix D).

VITAMIN K. In order to prevent vitamin K-dependent hemorrhagic disease and coagulation disorders, every neonate should receive a single parenteral dose of 0.5-1 mg natural vitamin K_1 oxide (phytonadione) within 1 hour of birth. Although studies generally show that oral administration of vitamin K to the mother has some efficacy, parenteral administration to the neonate is preferred.

Subsequent Care

The condition of the neonate should be evaluated on admission to the nursery. This evaluation should include a review of the neonate's identification, the mother's health prior to pregnancy and during the prenatal and intrapartum periods, the neonate's condition at birth, and the neonate's success in adapting to extrauterine life. Based on this initial assessment, an individualized care plan should be established.

Healthy neonates born after uncomplicated pregnancies should be assigned to a care plan that includes appropriate observation for the stabilization period and the remainder of the hospital stay. Observations should be made and recorded every 8 hours until discharge; the specific times of observation should be recorded as well.

Neonates with identified problems or risk factors usually require individualized care plans. It is advisable to develop nursery guidelines to delineate those conditions (eg, low birth weight, small size for gestational age, or questionable clinical status) that require specific actions by nurses or immediate notification of the physician. Clinical conditions such as maternal drug abuse, maternal fever or infection, or low Apgar scores are associated with increased risk for neonatal illness and should prompt immediate notification of the physician. The obstetrician should be advised of the baby's status, particularly if problems arise.

OBSERVATION. The neonate should be observed for any signs of illness: 1) temperature instability; 2) change in activity, including refusal of feedings; 3) unusual skin color; 4) abnormal cardiac or respiratory rate and rhythm; or 5) delayed or abnormal stooling or voiding. The normal full-term neonate passes meconium within the first 24 hours of life. If the full-term neonate has not passed meconium by 48 hours of age, the lower gastrointestinal tract may be obstructed. Urine is normally passed within the first 12 hours. Failure to void in the first 24 hours may indicate genitourinary obstruction or abnormality, or dehydration.

SKIN AND CORD CARE. Infection is the primary concern in skin and cord care. These considerations are discussed in Chapter 6.

NURSERY ENVIRONMENT. The physical environment where care is provided to the newborn should be designed and controlled to optimize that care. Valid concerns have been expressed, however, that the newborn, especially premature or chronically ill neonates, may be adversely affected by modern nursery environments. Many nurseries are constantly illuminated at high foot-candle levels and have noise levels that are many decibels higher than desirable. While physicians and nursing personnel stay in the nursery environment for intervals of hours at most, some neonates remain there for weeks or even months.

Pending development of more specific information, prudence suggests that attempts should be made to control excessive stimulation and to correct the lack of variation in nursery environments. High-intensity noise should be avoided. (Regulations of the Occupational Safety and Health Administration (OSHA) do not permit a level of more than 80 dB for longer than 8 hours for an adult.) Light intensity of 60 foot-candles is adequate for observation and for the performance of most procedures; additional lighting can be provided when necessary. Activities of personnel and stimulation of babies for feeding or procedures can be altered to allow for diurnal cycles and rest or nap intervals.

WEIGHING. Each neonate should be weighed at least daily. The neonate must be kept warm during weighing. The scale pan should be covered with a clean paper before each neonate is weighed. The accuracy of the nursery scales should be checked once a month.

CLOTHING. Most neonates require only a cotton shirt or gown without buttons in addition to a soft diaper. They may be clothed only in a diaper during hot weather if the nursery is not air-conditioned. A supply of soft clean cotton clothing, bed pads, sheets, and blankets should be kept at the bedside.

Aniline dyes should not be used to mark clothing, blankets, or other items used in the care of newborns.

FEEDING. Under normal circumstances, newborns may nurse as soon as possible after delivery. In any case, fluid and nutrients should be administered by at least 6 hours of age. (See Chapter 7 for further details.)

BATHING. Skin care, including bathing, may be important for the health and appearance of the individual neonate and for infection control within the nursery. The medical and nursing services of each hospital should develop guidelines regarding the time of the first bath, circumstances and method of skin cleansing, and role of personnel and parents. Supervised involvement of new parents, including discussion of bathing in health education classes, is recommended.

The first bath should be postponed until thermal stability is assured. The use of special equipment, such as radiant warmers, is recommended for premature and unstable infants (see Thermal Regulation, Chapter 10).

NEONATAL SCREENING. All neonates should be entered into an adequate screening program that includes, as a minimum, tests for the persistent hyperphenylalaninemias (PHP), including phenylketonuria (PKU), and for congenital hypothyroidism in its various forms.

The program should ensure (a) participation of all neonates, (b) notification of parents, (c) reliable and prompt performance of the-screening test, (d) prompt follow-up of subjects whose tests have positive results, (e) accurate diagnosis of subjects with confirmed positive test results, and (f) appropriate counseling and treatment of patients.

A screening program should conform to the following recommendations:

1. A blood sample should be obtained from every neonate prior to discharge or transfer. Neonates whose siblings have PHP/PKU or congenital hypothyroidism merit special priority in the collection of blood samples. For PHP/PKU, an adequate sample from a full-term neonate is defined as heel blood obtained as close as possible to the time of discharge from the nursery (cord blood is not sufficient); for congenital hypothyroidism, it is cord blood at birth or heel blood at discharge. In a premature neonate, any neonate being fed parenterally, or any neonate being treated for illness, a blood sample obtained at or near 7 days of age is adequate.

2. Neonates initially screened before 24 hours of age should be rescreened for PHP/PKU, because cases may be missed by a screening test so soon after delivery. The repeat screening test should be completed no later than the third week of life.

3. Accurate analysis requires meticulous standardization of the screening method. The level considered abnormal should be defined. The specificity of the test should be monitored regularly, which requires a high volume of samples per unit of time. The analytic component in the program should be centralized to enhance ongoing evaluation of efficiency, accuracy, participation, and adequacy.

4. All patients with PHP should be investigated to rule out the tetrahydrobiopterin-deficient forms of PKU.

5. Systematic follow-up of neonates with positive results on screening tests for congenital hypothyroidism is necessary to evaluate the efficacy of efforts to ameliorate the effects of this condition and to manage premature infants with transiently low T-4 values.

In addition, many states screen for hemoglobinopathies, including sickle cell disease.

INBORN ERRORS OF METABOLISM. Although screening reveals many inborn errors of metabolism, screening is inadequate for a large group of metabolic diseases because severe signs and symptoms develop before screening results are available. Symptomatic inborn errors of metabolism of the neonate include the following disorders:

Urea Cycle Disorders
    Carbamyl phosphate synthetase deficiency
    Ornithine transcarbamylase deficiency
    Argininosuccinic acid synthetase deficiency
    Argininosuccinase deficiency

Amino Acid Disorders
    Maple syrup urine disease
    Propionic acidemia
    Methylmalonic acidemia
    Isovaleric acidemia

Carbohydrate Disorders
    Galactosemia
    Glycogen storage disease Type I
    Congenital lactic acidosis

Glutaric Acidemia Type II
    Electron transport flavoprotein deficiency
    Electron transport flavoprotein dehydrogenase deficiency

Each of these diseases is rare, but when considered as a group, they represent an important cause of morbidity among full-term infants who had no antepartum or intrapartum risk factors. Inborn errors of metabolism appear in premature and full-term infants with an approximately equal frequency; therefore, more than 90% of symptomatic inborn errors of metabolism in the neonatal period are found in full-term infants. Because effective therapy is available for many of these diseases, early diagnosis and treatment may mitigate or prevent permanent neurologic sequelae.

With few exceptions (ie, congenital lactic acidosis and glutaric acidemia Type II), neonates with inborn errors of metabolism appear normal until sometime after the first day of life. At this time, the toxic substrate has had time to accumulate to a level that produces symptoms. These symptoms are nonspecific (eg, lethargy, vomiting, respiratory distress, seizures, hypothermia) and are similar to those seen in the common diseases of premature infants.

When full-term infants become ill after 24 hours of age with no evident cause, an inborn error of metabolism should be strongly suspected. Once such a possibility is raised, it should be pursued as an emergency, because the condition of affected neonates deteriorates very rapidly. A family history should be investigated for neonatal deaths and, if the patient is a male, for an X-linked pattern of inheritance. Peculiar odors of the infant may be indicative (ie, maple syrup in maple syrup urine disease, sweaty socks in isovaleric acidemia and glutaric acidemia Type II).

A number of routine laboratory determinations are useful in suggesting an inborn error of metabolism. For example, respiratory alkalosis suggests hyperammonemia, acidosis with an anion gap suggests an organic acidemia, ketonuria suggests propionic or methylmalonic acidemia, a low level of serum urea nitrogen (less than 5 mg/dl) suggests a defect in ureagenesis, hypoglycemia suggests one of the carbohydrate disorders, and the presence of urinary reducing substance suggests galactosemia. In sick full-term infants, it is advisable to measure plasma ammonium, lactate, and pyruvate levels. These tests are available in many hospital laboratories. For a definitive laboratory diagnosis, plasma levels of amino acids measured by quantitative column chromatography and urine organic acid measured by gas chromatography-mass spectrometry usually provide sufficient information to begin disease-specific therapy. Additional studies (eg, urine orotate and tissue enzyme analyses) may be necessary, however.

When an inborn error of metabolism is suspected, it is advisable to discontinue all protein feeding and provide a high caloric intake until a diagnosis is confirmed. Progressive hyperammonemia is a serious medical emergency that demands prompt therapy; hemodialysis is the treatment of choice for neonatal hyperammonemic coma from any cause.

Because of the increasing use of DNA methodology in antenatal diagnoses of inborn errors of metabolism, it is recommended that DNA be obtained from affected infants for possible use in the assessment of their mother's subsequent pregnancies. Fibroblasts grown in culture from a skin biopsy can be a valuable source of DNA.

CIRCUMCISION. As the *Guidelines* go to press, an Academy of Pediatrics Task Force on Circumcision is reviewing current data on the effect of circumcision on cancer of the penis and cervix, sexually transmitted diseases, and urinary tract infections, as well as considerations of pain, surgical complications, and informed consent. The present policy, there is no absolute medical indication for circumcision in the neonatal period, will be modified only if data conclusively demonstrate the value of the procedure.

Parent Education

The hospital experience is to some extent a learning process; however, the reduction in the length of a patient's routine postpartum stay compromises the opportunity for parent education. Hospital resources that have traditionally been extended to parents can no longer be accommodated within the shortened hospital stay. Physicians should be willing to accept, understand, and respond to parent inquiries that arise throughout the perinatal period and make every effort to ensure that educational aspects of care are provided prior to and following hospitalization.

Closed circuit television films previewed and approved by the obstetric and pediatric staff, printed materials, and counseling by hospital personnel (eg, postpartum and nursery nurses, registered dietitians/nutritionists, and physical therapists) have been helpful to parents. Other beneficial activities are group or individual educational sessions held regularly during the postpartum period to teach and discuss patient self-care, including exercises and self-examination of the breasts; parent-infant relationships; infant care, including bathing and feeding; and child growth and development. Family planning techniques appropriate to the patient's needs and desires should be explained in detail.

The newborn undergoes rapid changes in physiology that should be explained to the parents. The neonate's cardiovascular, pulmonary, renal, and neurologic maturation should be observed by the parents with the guidance of qualified personnel. Parents should be familiar with normal and abnormal changes in wake-sleep patterns, temperature, respiration, voiding, stooling, and the appearance of the skin. They should also observe and become familiar with the behavior, temperament, and neurologic capabilities of the newborn. Some believe that parents should also learn infant cardiopulmonary resuscitation techniques.

Visiting

The father or supporting person may be with the mother as much as desired within the constraints of acceptable standards of care and hospital policy. This includes the labor, delivery (including cesarean delivery), recovery, and postpartum periods. Local policies should be developed and followed consistently. Flexible and liberal visiting policies for fathers are well accepted and should be encouraged.

Sibling visits may be desirable in the early labor and postpartum periods. Children under 6 years of age frequently experience anxiety when separated from their mother. Furthermore, contact with the mother and newborn while they are in the hospital helps prepare the siblings for the new family member. Physical contact with neonates is a topic of current concern, as such direct sibling contact may transmit viral infectious diseases to the newborn and, potentially, to other neonates if hospitalization should be prolonged. If siblings are allowed to have direct contact with the newborn, the visit may take place in the mother's private room or in a special sibling visitation area if the mother is not in a private room. Parents should share the responsibility of preventing the exposure of their newborn to a sibling with a contagious illness. Contact of the newborn with children other than siblings should be avoided.

Other family members and friends should be allowed to visit and see the newborn according to the established policy of each hospital. Special arrangements may be necessary for other persons important to the new family, such as out-of-town visitors.

Whenever possible, parents of neonates in the continuing care, intermediate care, or intensive care areas should be allowed unrestricted visits. Provisions should be made for feeding (particularly breast-feeding), handling, and holding these neonates.

No adverse effects of sibling visitation in neonatal intensive care units have been noted, but more study is needed before a general recommendation can be made. An institution that allows sibling visitation to the neonatal intensive care unit should have clearly defined written policies and procedures based on information presently available. The following guidelines may serve as the basis for policy formulation:

1. Siblings should not have been exposed to known communicable diseases (eg, chickenpox).
2. Siblings should not have fever or symptoms of acute illness, such as upper respiratory infection or gastroenteritis.
3. Children should be prepared in advance for their visit.
4. Parents are responsible for ensuring that children are properly supervised by an adult throughout their hospital visit.

Because available data are limited, there is a need for continued evaluation and reporting of the risks and benefits of sibling visitation.

This should include both psychological and infectious disease factors. Institutions that have not introduced sibling visitation should consider the opportunity to use controlled trials to study the effects of these programs.

RESOURCES AND RECOMMENDED READING

Adamsons K Jr: The role of thermal factors and neonatal life. Pediatr Clin North Am 13:599-619, 1966

American Academy of Pediatrics, Committee on Fetus and Newborn: Criteria on early infant discharge and follow-up evaluation. Pediatrics 65(3): 651, 1980

American Academy of Pediatrics, Committee on Fetus and Newborn: Postpartum Neonatal (Sibling) Visitation. Pediatrics 76(4):650, 1985

American Academy of Pediatrics, Committee on Genetics: New issues in newborn screening of phenylketonuria and congenital hypothyroidism. Pediatrics 69(1):104-106, 1982

American Academy of Pediatrics, American Thyroid Association: Newborn screening for congenital hypothyroidism: Recommended guidelines. Pediatrics 80(5):745-749, 1987

American College of Obstetricians and Gynecologists: Assessment of Maternal Nutrition. Washington DC, ACOG, 1982

American College of Obstetricians and Gynecologists: Guidelines for Vaginal Delivery after a Previous Cesarean Birth (ACOG Committee Opinion). Washington DC, ACOG, 1988

American College of Obstetricians and Gynecologists: Obstetric Anesthesia and Analgesia (ACOG Technical Bulletin 112). Washington DC, ACOG, 1988

American College of Obstetricians and Gynecologists: Obstetric Forceps (ACOG Committee Opinion). Washington DC, ACOG, 1988

American College of Obstetricians and Gynecologists: Postterm Pregnancy (ACOG Committee Opinion). Washington DC, ACOG, 1987

American College of Obstetricians and Gynecologists: Standards for Obstetric-Gynecologic Services, 6 ed. Washington DC, ACOG, 1985

American College of Obstetricians and Gynecologists, Nurses Association of the American College of Obstetricians and Gynecologists: Electronic Fetal Monitoring (Joint ACOG/NAACOG Statement). Washington DC, ACOG, 1986

American Heart Association, American Academy of Pediatrics: Textbook of Neonatal Resuscitation. Dallas, AHA, 1987

Amiel-Tison C: Neurological evaluation of the maturity of newborn infants. Arch Dis Child 43(227):89-93, 1968

Brusilow S, Horwich A: Inborn errors of urea synthesis. In: Scriver C, Beaudet A, Sly W, et al (eds): The Metabolic Basis of Inherited Disease, 5 ed. New York, McGraw-Hill, 1983

Brusilow SW, Valle D: Symptomatic inborn errors of metabolism in the neonate. In: Nelson NM (ed): Current Therapy in Neonatal-Perinatal Medicine. Philadelphia, BC Decker, 1985, pp 207-212

Caravella SJ, Clark DA, Dweck HS: Health codes for newborn care. Pediatrics 80(1):1-5, 1987

Ernhart CB, Sokol RJ, Martier S, et al: Alcohol teratogenicity in the human: A detailed assessment of specificity, critical period, and threshold. Am J Obstet Gynecol 156(1):33-39, 1987

Farr V, Mitchell RG, Neligan GA, et al: The definition of some external characteristics used in the assessment of gestational age in the newborn infant. Dev Med Child Neurol 8(5):507-511, 1966

Freeman JM (ed): Prenatal and Perinatal Factors Associated with Brain Disorders. National Institute of Child Health and Human Development and National Institute of Neurological and Communicative Disorders and Stroke, NIH Publication No. 85-1149. Washington DC, US Government Printing Office, 1985

Hudak ML, Jones MD Jr, Brusilow SW: Differentiation of transient hyperammonemia of the newborn and urea cycle enzyme defects by clinical presentation. J Pediatr 107(5):712-719, 1985

Kirkman HN: Projections of a rebound in frequency of mental retardation from phenylketonuria. Appl Res Ment Retard 3(3):319-328, 1982

Klaus MH, Fanaroff AA (eds): Care of the High Risk Neonate, 3 ed. Philadelphia, WB Saunders, 1986, p 82

Lenke RR, Levy HL: Maternal phenylketonuria and hyperphenylalaninemia. An international survey of the outcome of untreated and treated pregnancies. N Engl J Med 303(21):1202-1208, 1980

Lenke RR, Levy HL: Maternal phenylketonuria—Results of dietary therapy. Am J Obstet Gynecol 142(5):548-553, 1982

Levison H, Linsao L, Swyer PR: A comparison of infra-red and convective heating for newborn infants. Lancet 2(477):1346-1348, 1966

Lindemann R: Resuscitation of the newborn: Endotracheal administration of epinephrine. Acta Paediatr Scand 73(2):210-212, 1984

Lou HC, Lassen NA, Fris-Hansen B: Decreased cerebral blood flow after administration of sodium bicarbonate in the distressed newborn infant. Acta Neurol Scand 57(3):239-247, 1978

National Conference on Cardiopulmonary Resuscitation and Emergency Cardiac Care: Standards and guidelines for cardiopulmonary resuscitation (CPR) and emergency cardiac care (ECC). VI: Neonatal advanced life support. JAMA 255(21):2969-2973, 1986

Neurological and Communicative Disorders and Stroke (NIH Publication No. 85-1149). Washington DC, US Government Printing Office, 1985

Nurses Association of the American College of Obstetricians and Gynecologists: Standards for Obstetric, Gynecologic, and Neonatal Nursing, 3 ed. Washington DC, NAACOG, 1986

Philipson EH, Kalham SC, Riha MM, et al: Effects of maternal glucose infusion on fetal acid-base status in human pregnancy. Am J Obstet Gynecol 157(4):866-873, 1987

Press S, Tellechea C, Pregen S: Cesarean delivery of full-term infants: Identification of those at high risk for requiring resuscitation. J Pediatr 106(3):477-479, 1985

Stark AR, Thach BT: Mechanisms of airway obstruction leading to apnea in newborn infants. J Pediatr 89(6):982-985, 1976

Thompson JE, Clark DA, Salisbury B, et al: Footprinting the newborn infant: Not cost effective. J Pediatr 99(5):797-798, 1981

5
FOLLOW-UP CARE

The continuum of perinatal care that began in the antepartum period should be reinforced during hospitalization to ensure that care extends beyond discharge. A multidisciplinary, collaborative approach is frequently used to promote this continuity, as well as to ensure that care is comprehensive.

The new mother may be unsure of the normal physical changes that occur after delivery and of her ability to care for the newborn. Therefore, the postpartum hospital stay is designed to allow health care personnel not only to provide the mother with professional assistance when she is most apt to be uncomfortable and to observe the mother and infant long enough to identify early complications, but also to reinforce prenatal instructions given to prepare the family for the infant's care at home. Now that the average length of a patient's hospital stay has been reduced to 2-3 days, however, it has become more difficult for health care personnel to achieve these objectives. Special criteria once designated to accommodate early discharge now apply to the average length of stay for most patients.

Neonates who appear to be normal may have physical, metabolic, or developmental problems that cannot be recognized by the time of their discharge from the hospital. Follow-up assessments can detect such problems as congenital anomalies, hearing or visual impairment, and neurologic deficits. Nutrition is also important and should be evaluated regularly in conjunction with physical growth and development. If identified promptly, defects and problems may be ameliorated by early intervention (medical or surgical); by programs directed toward enrichment, education, or stimulation; or by suitable counseling. The aid of government or community resources should be enlisted, if appropriate.

Maternal and neonatal follow-up care should include the following components:

1. A structured discharge plan

2. An assessment of the physical and psychosocial status of both mother and neonate
3. A discussion between the physician or another health care professional and the mother (and father, if possible) about any expected perinatal problems and ways to cope with them
4. A plan for future care, both immediate and long range

DISCHARGE PLANNING

The postpartum length of stay in the hospital is based on the period required for recovery under the observation of trained personnel. When no complications are present, this period ranges from 48 hours for vaginal delivery to 96 hours for cesarean birth, excluding the day of delivery. When the mother and baby are discharged early (less than 24 hours after delivery), the baby should be examined at 2-3 days of age. Plans for continuity of care should be developed prior to delivery, reexamined during hospitalization, and reviewed at the time of the discharge.

At the time of discharge, arrangements should be made for postpartum follow-up examination of both the mother and the neonate, and specific instructions should be conveyed to the mother. The following points should be reviewed with the mother or, preferably, with both parents:

1. Condition of the neonate
2. Immediate needs of the neonate (eg, feeding methods and environmental supports)
3. Roles of the obstetrician, pediatrician, and other members of the health care team concerned with the continuous medical care of the mother and neonate
4. Availability of support systems, including psychosocial support systems
5. Instructions to follow in the event of a complication or emergency
6. Feeding techniques; skin care, including cord care; temperature assessment and measurement with the thermometer; and assessment of neonatal well-being and recognition of illness
7. Reasonable expectations for the future

Maternal Considerations

Prior to discharge, the patient should be informed of normal postpartum events, including the changes in the lochia pattern that she should expect in the first few weeks; the range of activities that she may reasonably undertake; the care of the breasts, perineum, and bladder; dietary needs, particularly if she is breast-feeding; the recommended amount of exercise; emotional responses; and observations that she should report to the physician (eg, temperature elevation, chills, leg pains, or increased vaginal bleeding). It is helpful to reinforce oral discussion with written information.

The time at which coitus may be resumed after delivery is controversial. If resumed too soon, coitus may cause vaginal laceration and pain. Risks of hemorrhage and infection are minimal after approximately 2 weeks postpartum; by this time, the uterus has involuted markedly, and the endometrium and cervix have begun to reepithelialize. After 2 weeks postpartum, therefore, patients who wish to resume coitus may do so if contraceptive issues have been resolved.

A diaphragm cannot be fitted adequately during the immediate postpartum period. If there are no contraindications, however, oral contraceptive therapy may begin approximately 3 weeks after delivery. Breast-feeding mothers may start using oral contraceptives once their milk flow is well established. Patients for whom the use of oral contraceptives is contraindicated or patients who prefer other methods of contraception, such as foam and condoms, should be instructed in the use of these other methods. At the examination, 6 weeks after delivery, methods of contraception should be fully reviewed and implemented, as appropriate.

Neonatal Considerations

Certain neonates, particularly those who have been cared for in a neonatal intensive care unit, are known to be at increased risk for mortality, medical and surgical complications, and behavioral, neurologic, developmental, and psychosocial problems. The following perinatal conditions are among those that may identify infants at risk:

1. Birth weight less than 1,500 g
2. Size that is small for the infant's gestational age (at greatest risk: those with symmetric growth retardation)
3. Perinatal asphyxia
4. Need of mechanical ventilation for longer than 24 hours
5. Central nervous system abnormalities: such as abnormal findings on a neurologic examination, seizures, and intraventricular hemorrhage; microcephaly; hydrocephaly
6. Hyperbilirubinemia that required phototherapy, exchange transfusion, or both

7. Bronchopulmonary dysplasia, tracheostomy, oxygen supplementation, or persistent apnea associated with prematurity

8. Perinatal infections as demonstrated by: positive cultures or abnormal TORCH titers

9. Specific genetic, dysmorphic, or metabolic disorders

Each hospital should develop guidelines for the discharge of high-risk infants; such guidelines may include the following:

- The infant should be physiologically stable and should be able to maintain body temperature without cold stress when the amount of clothing worn and the room temperature are appropriate.

- The infant should be able to tolerate oral feeding by breast or bottle. If the infant's clinical condition precludes normal nipple feeding, the parents or other care providers should be instructed in an alternative feeding program.

- The infant should be gaining weight steadily at the time of discharge.

- The infant should be free of apnea prior to discharge or be receiving appropriate treatment.

- The physician or discharge planner should have confirmed parental competence (eg, ability to administer medications).

- The home situation should be considered appropriate.

It is essential to have a well-coordinated plan for the discharge and follow-up care of high-risk infants:

- A complete physical examination should be performed prior to discharge in order to identify problems that require specialized monitoring (eg, heart murmur, apnea, seizures, atypical head growth pattern) and to provide data on which to base future assessments.

- Immunization against diphtheria, tetanus, and pertussis (DTP) can be initiated in medically and neurologically stable preterm infants who have attained a chronologic age of 2 months. The status of this immunization should be assessed before discharge.

- All preterm infants should be screened for anemia prior to discharge. It may be necessary to provide supplemental vitamins, iron, or blood transfusions.

- Infants with history of deafness in the family, rubella exposure in the first trimester, maxillofacial anomalies, birth weight less than 1,000 g, meningitis, hyperbilirubinemia treated with exchange transfusion, or perinatal asphyxia may require referral for audiometric evaluation.

- Because low-birth-weight infants (ie, those weighing less than 1,500 g at birth) who receive oxygen supplementation are at an increased risk for retinopathy of prematurity, they should undergo an ophthalmologic evaluation prior to discharge. They should have at least one follow-up ophthalmologic examination during the first 6 months of life.

- Parents of infants with bronchopulmonary dysplasia require specific instruction in administering medications (eg, diuretics, bronchodilators) and feeding (eg, schedules, amount, technique, problem solving, and caloric supplements). They must be adequately trained to recognize signs of acute deterioration (eg, wheezing, congestion, distress) and to carry out cardiopulmonary resuscitation (CPR). Infants who continue to be oxygen dependent may be discharged if appropriate family and community resources are available and the infant is feeding adequately, growing, and able to maintain a transcutaneous PO_2 greater than or equal to 55 torr with activity while receiving oxygen via nasal cannula at a rate no more than 1 liter/min. Initial follow-up contact every 1-2 weeks is indicated.

- Informed consent should be obtained from their parents before infants are discharged with home apnea monitors. Parents of these infants require anticipatory guidance, training in infant CPR, complete verbal and written explanation of the monitor, guidelines for home monitoring, and referral for follow-up services.

Legislation in most states mandates that infants and children from birth to 4 years of age be restrained in appropriate car seats while in motor vehicles. A recent study has indicated, however, that low-birth-weight infants are at an increased risk of oxygen desaturation- and bradycardia when placed in a standard car seat. Parents should be alerted to this risk and should be counseled regarding alternatives.

Part of the discharge plan should include an assessment of the family's strengths and weaknesses. Appropriate referrals to any of the following ancillary services can then be initiated accordingly:

- Visiting nurse
- Social service
- Women, Infants, and Children (WIC) Program
- Mental health service
- Teen support services
- Parent support groups

- Early intervention services
- Respite care services

FOLLOW-UP CARE
Maternal Follow-up Care
Postpartum Evaluation

Approximately 4-6 weeks after delivery, the woman should see her physician for postpartum review and examination. This interval should be modified according to the needs of the patient with medical, obstetric, or intercurrent complications.

Review at the first postpartum visit should include an interval history and physical examination to evaluate the patient's current status, as well as her adaptation to the newborn. Specific inquiries regarding breast feeding should be made. The examination should include an evaluation of weight, blood pressure, breast, and abdomen, as well as a pelvic examination. Family planning techniques should be reviewed. Sexual difficulties are common in the early months after childbirth, as scarring at the episiotomy site may cause the woman some discomfort during intercourse for 1-3 months. In the lactating woman, the vagina is often atrophic, and lubrication during sexual excitement may be unsatisfactory. Furthermore, the demands of infant care alter the couple's ability to find the time previously allocated to physical intimacy.

Many women experience some degree of emotional lability in the weeks postpartum. If this persists or develops into true depression, intervention may be necessary. The emotional status of women whose pregnancies had an abnormal outcome should also be reviewed. Counseling should address specific issues regarding their future health and pregnancies. For example, it may be necessary to discuss vaginal birth after a cesarean birth or the implications of diabetes, growth retardation, prematurity, hypertension, anomalies, or other conditions in which there is a risk of recurrence. Laboratory data should be obtained as indicated. This is a good time for reviewing immunizations, including immunization against rubella, for those who are susceptible and did not receive the vaccine immediately postpartum, and for discussing any special problems. The patient should be encouraged to return for subsequent periodic examinations.

Psychosocial Adaptive Factors

In the normal postpartum period, the mother's physical and psychic energies move in a predictable course. Initially, the mother's energies are focused on herself and her baby; gradually, they move to encompass others in the immediate environment and, eventually, others beyond the immediate surroundings. The new mother needs personalized care during this period to hasten the development of a healthy mother-infant relationship and a sense of maternal confidence. Support and reassurance should be provided as the mother masters infant care tasks and adapts to her maternal role. Involving the father and encouraging him to participate in the neonate's care not only provides additional support to the mother, but also can enhance the father-infant relationship.

The postpartum period is a time of developmental adjustment for the whole family. Family members now have new roles and relationships, and an effort should be made to assess the progress of the family's adaptation. If a family member—mother, father, or sibling—finds it difficult to assume the new role, the health care team should arrange for sensitive, supportive assistance. This is particularly important for the teenaged mother, and mobilization of multiple resources within the community may be indicated in these cases.

Supportive Mechanisms and Community Resources

Both in-hospital and community agencies may assist the developing family. The physician should become familiar with the many public and private groups that give assistance and with the circumstances under which these organizations may be asked for assistance:

1. The in-hospital social service department should be an integral part of the interdisciplinary effort to coordinate hospital and discharge activities, to obtain public or private assistance, and to render psychosocial support.

2. Members of the Visiting Nurses Association may be available to visit the home to assess the parents' childrearing skills, the home environment, maternal emotional stability, and infant status and development. Under the physician's direction, these nurses may administer drugs or provide other types of therapy.

3. Certain groups that lend support and provide education on special activities (eg, breast-feeding).

Normal Neonates

The frequency of follow-up visits for normal neonates varies with patient, locale, and community practices. Such visits are usually monthly in the first 3 months, bimonthly for the remainder of the first year, and trimonthly thereafter. Thus, routine visits are more frequent in the first year of life, less frequent in the second year, and still less frequent in the succeeding years of early childhood. It is important that follow-up visits be regular and that good records of development be maintained.

Assessments and Interventions at Follow-up Visits

The need for a physical examination at each visit is obvious, not only to uncover congenital anomalies that were not apparent at birth, but also to assess residual problems, such as unstable hip joints, anemia, and infection. A neurologic examination should be an integral portion of the physical examination.

Suitable screening techniques, such as the Denver Development Screening Test, allow for serial plotting of landmarks in both cognitive and physical development. Delayed development may be related to the condition known as failure to thrive, which may be due to organic causes or to parental rejection, neglect, or ignorance. Abnormal results on developmental screening tests may call for more specialized neurologic and psychologic evaluations.

Specific developmental tests are used to assess gross motor, fine motor, language, and personal social adaptive behavior in children from birth to 5 years of age. The Denver Developmental Screening Test, for example, is designed to alert pediatricians and nurses to the need for an in-depth evaluation if development is shown to be delayed in any area. The Bayley Scales of Infant Development are probably the most standardized test available for infants between 6 months and 2 years of age. Both the Stanford-Binet Intelligence Test and the McCarthy Cognitive Index are standardized tests that can be used to assess cognitive functioning in 3-year-old children, although physical handicaps may invalidate the test. For children who are 4 years of age or older, some psychologists find the Beery Visual Motor Integration (VMI) and Zimmerman Receptive Expressive Language Assessment useful in identifying visual motor and language abnormalities. Specific serial neurodevelopmental assessment is useful in identifying appropriate candidates for early intervention or preschool special education programs. The various developmental assessments are best done by a well-trained psychologist in a structured child development program.

During each follow-up visit, immunization should be considered and executed according to the recommendations of the American Academy of Pediatrics.

Hearing, speech, and language function should be screened periodically. Hearing may be roughly evaluated by the startle response during the newborn period. At 6-9 weeks of age, an infant should turn the head toward a familiar sound. At 12 months, a child should understand simple directions and a few simple words. If the child's auditory response appear abnormal, comprehensive auditory evaluation, including 1) a behavioral history, 2) behavioral observation audiometry, and 3) testing of auditory evoked potentials (if indicated), should be obtained.

Infants with any of the following characteristics are considered at risk for hearing loss:

1. Family history of childhood hearing impairment
2. Congenital perinatal infection, such as the TORCH group of infections
3. Anatomic malformations that involve the head or neck
4. Birth weight less than 1,500 g
5. Hyperbilirubinemia at a level that exceeds indications for exchange transfusion
6. Bacterial meningitis, especially that caused by *Hemophilus influenzae*
7. Severe asphyxia in the perinatal period
8. Ototoxic drugs

The hearing of infants who meet any of these risk criteria should be screened, optimally by 3 months of age, but no later than 6 months of age. It is preferable for an audiologist to supervise the screening process. The initial screening should include the observations of behavioral or electrophysiologic response to sound. If responses are consistent at appropriate sound levels, the screening process is considered complete, except when there is a possibility of progressive hearing loss. If the results of an initial screening are equivocal, the infant should be referred for diagnostic testing.

Visual acuity should be tested by at least the second year of life. Infants who have or are at risk for structural or color anomalies (eg, strabismus, amblyopia, monocular patching) should be considered for ophthalmologic referral.

Psychosocial and Behavioral Status

Assessment of the psychosocial and behavioral status of the infant and child offers a broader dimension to follow-up care. A problem-oriented questionnaire on the family background may alert the physician to nonorganic risk factors that may ultimately affect family

stability and the adequacy of child care. Such a questionnaire may
include the following information:

1. Developmental stage of the parents (eg, teenage or young adult)
2. Surrogate or foster parent care
3. Level of parental education
4. Parental attitude and behavior
5. Changes in parent-child interaction since last visit
6. Problems with siblings
7. Major stresses
8. Spousal problems and conflicts
9. Problems with agencies
10. Problems with other responsible adults
11. Low income
12. Areas in which help is needed

Additional social and behavioral questions concerning the family
and infant at risk may be used to determine whether the behavior of
family members is normal, disruptive, or developmentally incapaci-
tating. Information about social status and familial characteristics is
useful, because these factors are known to affect psychomotor
performance, especially language development. Identification of the
areas of risk in a family leads to referrals for counseling, mental health
services, parent support groups, and other resources outside the
family itself.

Physicians and others who provide follow-up care to mothers and
infants should be aware of the physical, social, and psychologic
factors associated with child abuse and its increasing occurrence. The
following factors have been associated with child abuse:

1. Prematurity
2. Illness with long periods of hospitalization, especially in neonatal intensive care units
3. Single parenthood
4. Adolescent motherhood
5. Closely spaced pregnancies
6. Infrequent family visits to hospitalized infants

Children with a history of prematurity have been shown to have a
greater incidence of irritability, hyperkinesis, and increased dependency. Prolonged hospitalization inevitably disrupts family relationships, particularly the parent-child relationship. Infants and parents

with such a history require closer follow-up than does the average family. The interaction of the parents, especially the mother, with the infant should be evaluated periodically. The infant or child who fails to thrive may be a victim of neglect, if not outright abuse, and a causal relationship between neglect and failure to thrive should always be suspected. In every state those who provide health care to children are legally obligated to report suspected child abuse.

High-Risk Neonates

The intervals of follow-up visits required by high-risk neonates should be determined by the needs of the individual infant and family. It may be necessary to examine some of these infants weekly or bimonthly at first. Neurologic, developmental, behavioral, and sensory status should be assessed more than once during the first year in high-risk infants to ensure early identification of problems and referral for remediation.

Assessments

Growth parameters should be assessed, with continued monitoring of the adequacy of weight gain, linear growth, and head growth. Growth should be plotted on standardized growth curves. Review of nutritional intake and calculation of caloric intake are helpful in case management. The physical examination should include assessment of cardiac, pulmonary, and gastrointestinal status, as well as any herniae, anomalies, or orthopedic deformities. Parents of infants who were cared for in the neonatal intensive care unit are often concerned about minor scars secondary to procedures performed in the unit, and they benefit from reassurance.

Families must be encouraged to obtain recommended follow-up vision and audiometric assessments when indicated. Audiometric assessment should include behavioral testing in a soundproof testing room and brainstem auditory evoked potential testing if behavioral results are inconclusive or if the infant is at risk for hearing loss. After the infant has reached 6 months of age, further assessment of receptive-expressive language skills, behavioral audiometry, and impedance testing are appropriate. Brainstem auditory evoked potential testing should be repeated if the results of these tests are equivocal.

Medication dosage should be reevaluated, dosages increased with weight gain and age, and blood levels monitored. Immunization status should be reviewed.

In the primary physician's office, neurologic assessment should include an appraisal of muscle tone, reflexes, and visual and auditory responses. In addition, a standard developmental screening tool, such as the Denver Developmental Screening Test, should be used. When neurologic findings are suspicious or the developmental screening suggests developmental delays, infants should be referred for more in-depth assessment, either to a neonatal follow-up program or to equivalent facilities or programs capable of providing detailed neurodevelopmental assessments. The assessment should disclose the presence of the following abnormalities:

1. Major motor deficits
2. Seizure disorders
3. Deafness, severe hearing loss
4. Retinopathy of prematurity and other visual impairment
5. Hydrocephalus, microcephalus
6. Significant developmental delay
7. Anomalies that contribute to delays (eg, cataracts, orthopedic anomalies)

In children between 1 and 5 years of age whose conditions during the perinatal period (eg, asphyxia, hypoglycemia, intracranial hemorrhage) increased the risk of neurologic defects, the following factors should be considered:

1. Fine and gross motor abnormalities
2. Visual-perceptual-motor abnormalities
3. Receptive/expressive language delay
4. Mild conductive or sensorineural hearing loss
5. Hyperkinesis, attention deficit, behavior problems

Early Intervention

Infant stimulation and enrichment programs are designed to provide developmentally appropriate activities for babies and toddlers from birth to 3 years who are at risk for a variety of conditions that may interfere with their ability to lead a full and productive life. Infants who may be considered for such a program include those with motor handicaps, visual or auditory handicaps, orthopedic anomalies, syndromes associated with developmental delay, or known developmental delay. Intervention programs offer therapeutic guidelines for families, parent support groups, respite care programs, and innovative therapy modalities. Although there are no definitive data to confirm the beneficial effects of infant stimulation programs, there are indications that early intervention may improve the social adaptation of high-risk infants and their families.

RESOURCES AND RECOMMENDED READING

American Academy of Pediatrics: Report of the Committee on Infectious Diseases, 19 ed. Evanston IL, AAP, 1986

American Academy of Pediatrics, Ad Hoc Task Force on Care of Chronically Ill Infants and Children: Guidelines for home care of infants, children, and adolescents with chronic disease. Pediatrics 74(3):434-436, 1984

American Academy of Pediatrics, Committee on Fetus and Newborn: Criteria on early infant discharge and follow-up evaluation. Pediatrics 65(3):651, 1980

American Academy of Pediatrics, Joint Committee on Infant Hearing: Position statement 1982. Pediatrics 70(3):496-497, 1982

American Heart Association, American Academy of Pediatrics: Textbook of Neonatal Resuscitation, Dallas, AHA, 1987

Hurt H (ed): Symposium on continuing care of the high-risk infant. Clin Perinatol 11(1):1-244, 1984

Willett LD, Leuschen MP, Nelson LS, et al: Risk of hypoventilation in premature infants in car seats. J Pediatr 109(2):245-248, 1986

6

CONTROL OF INFECTIONS IN OBSTETRIC AND NURSERY AREAS

Infections are relatively uncommon in healthy mothers who deliver vaginally at term and in normal newborns. Women who have had a complicated pregnancy and labor or a cesarean delivery are much more likely to develop infection, and sick or preterm neonates are infected relatively frequently. In some intensive care nurseries, 15% or more of the neonates may have one or more infections, and a high percentage may be fatal. Nosocomial infections are a constant threat.

Most infections in obstetric patients are caused by endogenous flora—microorganisms that are normally resident in the genital tract, but generally cause no disease until labor, delivery, or the puerperium. Many of these infections can be prevented through meticulous surgical and patient care techniques and appropriate use of prophylactic antibiotics. Bacterial pathogens such as group B streptococci, *Listeria monocytogenes,* or *Chlamydia,* if acquired by neonates from their mothers in the intrapartum period, occasionally cause pneumonia or septicemia during the first hours or days of postnatal life. At present, these infections are difficult to predict or prevent, although they are known to occur more frequently after prolonged rupture of the membranes or a complicated labor and delivery.

In contrast, most infections in neonates in intensive care units are caused by pathogens acquired from the hospital environment. The survival of more and more very low-birth-weight infants; the emergence of chronic disease states, such as bronchopulmonary dysplasia; and the development of new invasive procedures provide additional opportunities for infectious problems to arise. Prevention of these

113

infections requires a multifaceted approach, including meticulous patient care techniques, elimination of inappropriate antibiotic use to avoid further alteration of the balance of colonizing flora, and careful attention to all aspects of infection control.

COLONIZATION IN NEWBORN INFANTS

Most neonates emerge from a sterile intrauterine environment. During and after birth, they are exposed to numerous microorganisms that colonize their skin, nasopharynx, and gastrointestinal tract, among other areas. Ill neonates who are subjected to multiple invasive procedures are frequently colonized at multiple sites with a variety of organisms, particularly gram-negative bacteria. Many factors, some of which can be modified by medical personnel and hospital procedures, influence the type and the balance of colonizing organisms and the host response.

Full-term healthy neonates are unlikely to acquire severe infections. When such a neonate does have severe infection, it may occur secondary to group B streptococci, *Escherichia coli* (particularly strains with K1 antigen), *L . monocytogenes, Citrobacter, diversus, Salmonella, Chlamydia,* herpes simplex virus (HSV), or enteroviruses. These organisms can be transmitted to other neonates in the nursery on the hands of hospital personnel.

The skin of the newborn is a major initial site of bacterial colonization, particularly with *Staphylococcus aureus;* colonizing strains of this organism are most commonly transmitted within the nursery rather than from the mother. Any break in the integrity of the protective skin affords an opportunity for infection to develop. At birth, for example, a neonate has at least one open surgical wound (the umbilicus) that is highly susceptible to infection. A circumcision site is another area that is susceptible to infection.

The bowel flora of a neonate who is breast-fed exclusively is qualitatively and quantitatively different from that of a neonate who is formula-fed, especially if the latter is fed via continuous drip feedings administered by hospital personnel.

Nursery Admission Policies

It is not necessary to restrict nursery admission to infants born under "sterile" conditions. Those born under "unsterile" conditions (eg, after prolonged rupture of the membranes or to mothers with suspected or proved infection), those transferred from another hospital, or those readmitted after discharge may be admitted to most nurseries if precautions are taken to prevent the transmission of colonizing or infecting organisms from one neonate to another. Similarly, neonates may be moved safely from one nursery area to another under normal circumstances. Categorizing neonates as "clean" or "dirty," based on whether they were born under sterile conditions, may lead to the assumption that the "clean" neonates do not harbor organisms that can cause disease, and this may result in inappropriate care. Each neonate should be approached as if he or she were colonized with unique flora that should not be transmitted to any other neonate. Personnel need to recognize the importance of proper infant care techniques in limiting the spread of organisms.

Neonatal Intensive Care

Neonates who require intensive care undergo a variety of invasive procedures that breach normal barriers to infection, making these infants highly susceptible to colonization. Because those neonates colonized with pathogenic organisms may have no overt signs of illness, special precautions may not be exercised in their care. Thus, physicians, nurses, respiratory therapy personnel, and other person- nel who move from one neonate to another may carry these patho- genic organisms from neonates who have been colonized to those in the same nursery who have not yet been colonized. As a result, a high proportion of the neonates in a single nursery may be colonized or infected with the same strains of bacteria; respiratory tract and intestinal organisms are particularly common in such situations. In order to minimize the transmission of organisms, each individual working with these neonates and with the equipment used directly in their care should be meticulous when providing patient care. After taking care of one neonate, personnel should wash their hands before taking care of another neonate or of the same neonate at another site, and they should dispose of contaminated equipment or materials properly.

SURVEILLANCE FOR NOSOCOMIAL INFECTION

The infection control committee of each hospital should work with perinatal care personnel to establish workable definitions of nosoco- mial infection for surveillance purposes. For obstetric patients, a nosocomial infection can be broadly defined as one that is neither present nor incubating at the time the patient is admitted to the hospital. Most cases of endometritis or urinary tract infection that occur postpartum, therefore, are nosocomial, even though the causative organisms may be endogenous.

Nosocomial infection in newborns is more difficult to define. The broadest definition includes all infections that have an onset after birth, excluding only those known to have been transmitted transplacentally. Narrower definitions exclude those infections that develop within 24-72 hours of birth, because these, too, may have been caused by organisms acquired from the mother rather than from the hospital environment. The narrower, more specific definitions are probably more useful for general purposes. Definitions should include infections that become apparent within a certain period after a neonate's discharge. The definition selected should be applied consistently to allow uniform reporting and analysis of nosocomial infections.

Obstetric and nursery personnel should cooperate with hospital infection control personnel in conducting and reviewing the results of surveillance programs for nosocomial infections. This type of monitoring provides information about any unusual problems or clusters of infection, the risks associated with certain procedures or techniques, and the success of specific preventive measures. Generally, the surveillance program can be conducted most efficiently if it emphasizes the detection of infections in hospitalized patients, although most new mothers and their newborns are discharged after only a few days in the hospital.

Routine culturing of neonatal tissue for surveillance purposes is not recommended, but cultures of specimens from lesions or sites of infection can be helpful in identifying clusters of infection caused by a single strain of bacteria. As infections with organisms acquired within the nursery may not become apparent until after discharge of the newborns, it is especially important for pediatricians and others who care for the newborns to report confirmed or suspected postdischarge infections to nursery and hospital infection control personnel.

Patterns of infection are easier to recognize if the data include only those infections in which a specific site or pathogen can be identified. In neonates, however, it is frequently difficult to distinguish between the clinically insignificant presence of bacteria and disease at a site such as the lower respiratory tract. Usually, only clinically apparent infections should be recorded in the surveillance data; at times, especially during an outbreak of infection, it may be important to document organisms responsible for colonization of all neonates at certain sites. Clusters of infection that do not fit a standard definition may need to be individually investigated.

Both obstetric and nursery personnel are involved in providing perinatal care; therefore, close communication between these groups about infectious diseases is essential. In particular, nursery personnel should be notified in advance about the birth of a neonate who may have a congenital or perinatal infection, or about a mother who is known to be infected or to be a chronic carrier (eg, with *Salmonella*, hepatitis B virus (HBV), HSV, or human immunodeficiency virus (HIV)). Conversely, obstetric personnel should be informed about problems in newborns that may be associated with labor and delivery or may have a bearing on maternal health.

PREVENTION AND CONTROL OF INFECTIONS

Health Standards for Personnel

Obstetric and nursery personnel, as well as others who have significant contact with the newborn, should be free of transmissible infectious diseases. Each hospital should establish written policies and procedures for assessing the health of personnel assigned to the perinatal care services, restricting their contact with patients when necessary, maintaining their health records, and reporting any illness that they may have. These policies and procedures should address screening for tuberculosis and rubella. Routine culturing of specimens obtained from personnel is not useful, although selective culturing may be of value when a pattern of infection is suspected.

Personnel should be aware that even a mild transmissible infection may preclude contact with neonates. Ideally, individuals with a respiratory, cutaneous, mucocutaneous, hepatic, gastrointestinal, or other communicable infection have no direct contact with neonates. Personnel who have exudative skin lesions or weeping dermatitis should refrain from all direct patient care and should not handle patient care equipment until the condition resolves.

Transmission of HSV from infected personnel to infants in newborn nurseries has rarely been documented. It is not known whether personnel who have labial HSV infection ("cold sores") or who are asymptomatic oral shedders of the virus can transmit the virus to infants, but the possibility seems extremely remote. The risk of compromising patient care by excluding personnel with "cold sores" when these personnel are essential for the operation of the nursery must be weighed against the potential risk of infecting newborn infants. Personnel with "cold sores" who have direct contact with infants should cover and avoid touching their lesions, and carefully observe hand-washing policies; furthermore, they should not kiss or nuzzle newborn infants or infants with eczema. Transmission of HSV infection from personnel with genital lesions is not likely, provided that hand-washing policies are carefully observed. Personnel with herpetic hand infections (herpetic whitlow) should not participate directly in the care of patients until the lesions have healed.

Personnel in contact with neonates should report personal infections or symptoms to their immediate supervisors and be medically examined before working directly with neonates. Decisions regarding the exclusion of staff members from obstetric and nursery areas should be made on an individual basis. Exclusion is appropriate for highly contagious conditions, even if the individual feels well enough to continue working. Employee health policies should be worded and applied in a way to ensure that personnel feel free to report infectious problems without fear of income loss.

All hospital personnel, both men and women, who are susceptible to rubella should be vaccinated. Unless they are vaccinated, those working in the obstetric and nursery areas, including clinics, may contract the disease as a result of exposure to persons or neonates with rubella infection or may themselves transmit infection to pregnant women. Susceptible female personnel in the childbearing age group should be identified and offered vaccination before they become pregnant or are exposed to infected patients. Vaccine should not be administered to pregnant women. Furthermore, conception should be avoided for 3 months after vaccination; if pregnancy occurs within that time frame, however, available data do not support an assumption that the pregnancy should be terminated for that reason.

Influenza is likely to be serious or complicated in neonates, but they cannot be vaccinated against infection. Therefore, programs for immunization and chemoprophylaxis of adults who are in close contact with neonates may be an important means of protecting these infants from this disease. Annual immunization of nursery personnel against prevalent strains of influenza virus is strongly encouraged.

Personnel in neonatal units are likely to be exposed to patients who are excreting cytomegalovirus (CMV), but studies suggest that these staff members are not at greater risk for acquiring primary CMV infection. Because the majority of CMV infections are subclinical, previous infection and the current immune status of the exposed person are usually unknown. Women of childbearing age who work in neonatal units should be counseled about the relative risks of exposure should they become pregnant. A routine program of serologic testing for obstetric or nursery hospital employees is not recommended, however.

It is desirable to recruit and maintain a regular group of nurses with specialized training in obstetric and neonatal nursing to work in these specialty areas. If nurses from other areas must work in the obstetric and neonatal care areas, or if nurses from the obstetric and neonatal care areas must work on other units of the hospital, specific policies should be established for this practice. Nursing personnel should be assigned to one area for an entire shift and should not be moved back and forth indiscriminately. Ideally, nursing personnel from the perinatal care areas who work on other units should be assigned to work only with uninfected patients.

Hand-Washing

As mentioned earlier, most of the common infectious agents responsible for colonization and disease in patients, especially in the nursery, are transmitted from patient to patient on the hands of personnel. Therefore, in order to minimize this type of transmission, medical and hospital personnel must follow careful hand-washing techniques.

Agents for Hand-Washing

Antiseptic (antimicrobial) hand-washing agents have traditionally been recommended for personnel who care for neonates. Antiseptic preparations should be used for scrubbing before entering the nursery, before providing care for neonates highly susceptible to infection, before performing invasive procedures, and after providing care for infected neonates. For routine hand-washing within the nursery, however, soap and water may be sufficient.

The ideal antiseptic agent for hand-washing should kill pathogenic bacteria, be nonstaining and nonirritating to the skin, be nonsensitizing, and have persistent local action. It should also be easy to use. These requirements limit the number of useful preparations.

The antiseptics most useful for hand-washing in the nursery are chlorhexidine gluconate or iodophor (water-soluble complexes of iodine with surfactant agents) preparations; both are useful against gram-negative and gram-positive organisms. Hexachlorophene-based preparations may be especially useful during nursery outbreaks of S. aureus infection, but it is not recommended for routine hand-washing. All the antiseptic compounds are occasionally sensitizing or irritating, and some personnel may need to use plain soap or mild detergents. Liquid soap dispensers and many hand-washing agents may become contaminated; disposable brushes or pads that contain an antiseptic hand-washing agent avoid this problem.

Alcohol-containing foams kill bacteria satisfactorily when they are applied to clean hands, but they are not sufficient for cleaning physically soiled hands.

Techniques of Hand-Washing

Before handling neonates for the first time on a shift, personnel should wash their hands and arms to a point above the elbow. A small amount of antiseptic preparation should be placed in the palm of the hand and the hands, wrists, forearms, and elbows washed thoroughly; all areas should be covered, including between the fingers and the lateral surfaces of the fifth fingers. Following this initial wash, the fingernails should be cleaned with a plastic or orangewood stick and the hands washed again (a soft brush or firm pad is optional). After the hands have been washed, they should be rinsed thoroughly and dried with paper towels.

A 15-second wash—without a brush, but with soap and vigorous rubbing—is required before and after handling each neonate and after touching objects or surfaces likely to be contaminated with virulent microorganisms or hospital pathogens (eg, the hair, face, or clothing of personnel; diapers; and equipment). This type of wash usually eliminates most organisms transiently colonizing the hands, although it may not be adequate if the hands are heavily contaminated. Routine, brief activities for the care of adult patients may not require hand-washing before each contact. Hand-washing facilities and materials must be easily accessible. (See Scrub Areas, Chapter 2.)

Dress Codes

Each hospital should establish dress codes for regular and part-time personnel who enter the labor, delivery, and nursery areas.

It is preferable for physicians, nursing personnel, and others who spend most of their working day in the labor, delivery, or nursery areas to wear short-sleeved scrub gowns or short-sleeved scrub suits or dresses provided and laundered by the hospital. Fathers attending births should also be in scrub clothes.

Sterile, long-sleeved gowns should be worn by all personnel who have direct contact with the sterile field during vaginal deliveries, surgical obstetric procedures, and surgical procedures in the nursery.

Those who examine neonates should be sure that their clothing or unscrubbed portions of the body do not touch the neonates or any equipment.

Some hospitals have approved more flexible dress codes for personnel who work in birthing rooms (eg, scrub suits without gowns or masks). Little information is available about the impact of these practices on the neonates, mothers, or personnel. Because of concern about potential infection of hospital personnel with blood-borne pathogens, such as HBV and HIV, the Centers for Disease Control recommends that all health care workers who perform or assist in deliveries wear gloves, gowns, surgical masks, and goggles during the procedure. Wearing aprons or gowns made of impervious material during cesarean delivery may provide additional protection. Gloves should be worn when handling the placenta or the neonate until blood and amniotic fluid have been removed from the neonate's skin. Hands should be washed immediately after gloves are removed and/or when skin surfaces are contaminated with blood.

Personnel in nursery areas should wear a clean cover gown or other type of barrier clothing to avoid contact of the newborn with the scrub suit or clothing. In many nurseries where neonates are cared for in bassinets or open beds, physicians, nursing personnel, technicians who are not regularly assigned to the nursery, and visitors are required to wear short-sleeved gowns to cover their clothing; the need for this type of gowning as a routine infection control measure is not confirmed, however. In nurseries where all neonates are kept in forced-air, isolation type incubators, personnel who work intermittently in the nursery need not wear gowns unless they have direct contact with the infant.

If an infected or potentially infected neonate is to be handled outside the bassinet, a long-sleeved gown should be worn over the scrub suit or dress, gown, or other clothing and either discarded after use or maintained for use exclusively in the care of that neonate. If one gown is used for each neonate, the gowns should be changed every 8 hours.

When leaving the obstetric or nursery area for other hospital areas (eg, laboratories, radiology department, or cafeteria), personnel in scrub suit or dress should wear a long-sleeved gown that they discard when they reenter the obstetric or nursery area.

Although caps, beard bags, and masks are not needed during routine activities in the labor and nursery areas, they are required during deliveries and may be beneficial during surgical procedures performed in the nursery, including umbilical vessel catheterization.

Long hair should be restrained so that it does not touch the neonate or equipment during patient examination or treatments. Personnel who touch their hair, beard, mustache, or face while on duty should rewash their hands before touching a patient or the patient's equipment.

Masks have limitations; they are useful, but not usually essential, in preventing acquisition or dissemination of respiratory pathogens. High-efficiency, disposable masks should be used, but even these masks remain effective for only a few hours. Masks should be worn so that they cover both the nose and the mouth, and they should be discarded as soon as they are removed from the nose and mouth. Masks may not be effective on persons who have beards.

Sterile gloves should be used during deliveries and during all invasive procedures performed in either the obstetric (including birthing rooms) or the nursery area. Disposable, nonsterile gloves may be useful in the care of patients in isolation or in the performance of procedures that may result in heavy contamination of the hands. In such circumstances, the use of gloves may reduce the intensity of transient bacterial or viral colonization of the hands.

Personnel should remove rings, watches, and bracelets before washing their hands and entering the obstetric or nursery areas; they should not wear hand jewelry while on duty.

Suctioning

Personnel assisting in suctioning of the newborn should use mechanical devices. Equipment has been developed to allow wall suction to be used with valves that limit the amount of negative pressure generated and allow the individual to control when suctioning will occur. Direct wall suction should be avoided if possible since most wall suction outlets have negative pressure levels that may be injurious.

Traditionally, devices such as the DeLee trap have been used to avoid getting aspirated material into the mouth of personnel. When mouth suction of the airway cannot be avoided, a trap should be placed in the line. (See also Chapter 4, "Suctioning for Meconium.")

Preventive Measures on an Obstetric Service

During the past decade, the trend toward relaxation of requirements regarding attire and conduct in family-centered perinatal programs and in-hospital birthing rooms has not been associated per se with a higher risk of infection in either mother or neonate. Now, however, concern over HIV infection has resulted in stricter requirements as a safeguard to both patients and personnel. The delivery area should be considered a sterile area, especially when cesarean deliveries and tubal ligations are done in the same rooms in which vaginal deliveries are performed.

Surgical Technique

A primary principle in preventing postoperative infection is good surgical technique. Before surgery, the operative field should be prepared and draped. Shaving has been associated with a higher wound infection rate; when necessary, it should be done no earlier than 2 hours before surgery.

Vaginal Examinations

The infection rate associated with vaginal examination during labor is no higher than that associated with rectal examination; however, the greater the number of examinations, the greater the risk of maternal infection.

Sterile, water-soluble lubricants are recommended for vaginal examinations during pregnancy. Because lubricants containing antiseptics such as povidone-iodine or hexachlorophene have not been shown to decrease the frequency of infections, and because the antiseptic compounds may be absorbed through the vaginal mucosa and may be harmful to the fetus, they are not appropriate agents for vaginal antisepsis.

Intrauterine Pressure and Fetal Monitoring

Intrauterine monitoring requires rupture of the amniotic membranes. Therefore, in order to reduce the risk of infection in either the mother or the newborn, the catheter and leads should be carefully inserted by means of aseptic technique. Sterile equipment should be used for all fluid pathways in the pressure-monitoring system; the system should be closed, and extreme caution should be used to avoid contamination during procedures such as calibration.

Transducers for intravascular or intrauterine pressure monitoring have caused nosocomial infections for a variety of reasons. Contamination of equipment and subsequent infection in patients have resulted from suboptimal techniques in the assembly and use of equipment, from inadequate cleaning and sterilization of reusable equipment, and from the reuse of disposable transducer domes. In order to minimize the chance of inadvertent contamination of fluids and equipment, the components of the monitoring system should not be removed from sterile packages and set up until the system is actually needed. After use, all disposable equipment should be discarded and the transducer disinfected (if used with a disposable dome that isolates the head of the transducer from the fluid path) or cleaned and sterilized (if a reusable dome-transducer combination is used). Disposable pressure assemblies are now available and, although more expensive, may have a distinct advantage in decreasing the risk of infection.

Prophylactic Antibiotics for Obstetric Patients

In selected high-risk patients, prophylactic antibiotics decrease the frequency of infections. For cesarean delivery in patients with a high risk of infection, short courses of prophylactic antibiotics significantly decrease the incidence of operative site infections and, thus, may also decrease the length of hospital stay. Various antibiotic regimens have been effective; a 1-day or 3-dose course is as effective as a longer course. Beginning antibiotic therapy after clamping the cord has been demonstrated to be as effective as beginning it before surgery.

There are a number of objections to routine antibiotic prophylaxis for patients who have a cesarean delivery. First, if infection occurs after prophylaxis, organisms may be more resistant to therapy. Second, antibiotics administered in the intrapartum period or before the cord is clamped may alter the results of neonatal blood cultures or delay diagnosis of infection in the newborn. Third, it is not yet clear whether the prophylactic use of antibiotics for cesarean delivery prevents a high proportion of serious infection.

It is currently recommended that antibiotic prophylaxis be reserved for patients who must undergo a surgical procedure and who are at a high risk of infection or for patients in whom the consequences of infection would be life-threatening. Antibiotics are not indicated for routine use in elective cesarean deliveries. In addition, prophylactic antibiotics should be continued for no longer than 24 hours after surgery. The antibiotic chosen for prophylaxis should have a reasonable spectrum of activity against pelvic flora and should be relatively nontoxic. Finally, important therapeutic antibiotics, such as penicillin, aminoglycosides, and clindamycin, should not be used for prophylaxis.

Special Preventive Techniques and Procedures for Neonates

Invasive Procedures on Neonates

Providing care for a sick newborn demands the use of multiple invasive techniques for diagnosis, monitoring, and therapy. These procedures are relatively safe if sterile equipment and meticulous aseptic techniques are used to minimize opportunities for microorganisms to overcome the fragile host defenses of the newborn.

Like all other intravascular cannulas, arterial cannulas may become colonized and serve as a nidus of infection. Percutaneous placement of peripheral arterial cannulas is associated with a lower risk of infection than is placement by surgical cutdown, however. Ideally, cannulas should remain at one site for no longer than 4 days. They should be removed promptly if clinical signs suggest infection. A safe maximum duration of cannulation for umbilical arterial catheters has not been established; a careful assessment of risks versus benefits should be made for each neonate. Intravascular catheters should not be used or left in place unless clearly indicated for medical management of the neonate.

Although an ideal pressure-monitoring system in a closed system, arterial cannulas frequently are also used for obtaining blood samples; these samples should be obtained aseptically with precautions to avoid contamination of the system (eg, from ice used to chill syringes before obtaining the blood sample). Because some species of bacteria flourish in dextrose solutions at room temperature, this type of solution should not be used in pressure-monitoring systems unless absolutely necessary.

Total parenteral nutrition has been associated with high rates of infection, including septicemia and fungemia. When properly performed, however, parenteral feeding is safe. A cooperative team approach that involves pharmacists, nurses, and physicians is strongly recommended, as such an approach reduces the incidence of infections and other complications. Meticulous attention should be paid to aseptic insertion and maintenance of the cannula and to aseptic techniques of fluid administration. All parenteral nutrition fluids should be compounded in a central pharmacy, preferably in a laminar flow hood. Because lipid emulsions are especially susceptible to contamination with a wide variety of bacterial and fungal pathogens that can proliferate to high concentrations within hours, particular caution must be taken in the storage and administration of these emulsions. Unit-dose amounts may be delivered from the pharmacy; if bottles of emulsion are kept in the nursery refrigerator, care should be taken to prevent contamination. Opened bottles must be discarded no later than 24 hours after the seal has been broken.

Intravascular Flush Solutions

The uniqueness of caring for neonates, especially those of low birth weight, was dramatically illustrated by the clinical problems caused by the use of benzyl alcohol as a preservative in intravascular flush solutions. When administered to neonates, solutions with benzyl alcohol may lead to severe metabolic acidosis, encephalopathy, and even death. Intravascular flush solutions that are available in multi-dose vials usually contain benzyl alcohol or some other preservative, necessitating the use of alternatives in the care of neonates. Although numerous medications used for neonates are also preserved with benzyl alcohol or other agents, the volume of preservative received in medication does not appear to be toxic if the intravascular flush solutions do not contain preservatives.

The hospital pharmacy should establish a system to ensure a satisfactory and safe means of providing sterile, unpreserved fluids to the nursery areas. If the fluid administered is to contain heparin, it should be added to the fluid in the hospital pharmacy whenever possible. Refrigeration retards the growth of most bacteria that may contaminate solutions during preparation; therefore, once the seal of a container has been broken for admixture or unit-dose dispensing, the remaining fluid should be refrigerated in the pharmacy. Cold fluids should not be administered to neonates, but flush solutions should be kept at room temperature no longer than 8 hours before being used or discarded.

Antibiotics for Neonates

Antibiotics, usually in combination, are commonly used in intensive care nurseries to treat presumed infections and to prevent infections in high-risk neonates who are undergoing multiple invasive proce-dures. The efficacy of antibiotics used for prophylaxis has not been documented, however, and such use should be strongly discouraged. Topical antibiotics should be used only for very specific indications and only on the order of a physician. The indiscriminate and inappropriate use of either systemic or topical antibiotics may alter the established flora of the neonate and may result in the emergence of resistant strains of bacteria, making subsequent therapy for clinical infections more difficult and dangerous. In addition, systemic pro-phylactic therapy may alter the clinical expression of infection, making diagnosis more difficult and delaying appropriate antimicrobial therapy.

A specimen for appropriate cultures should be obtained before antibiotics are administered. Broad-spectrum coverage, such as that obtained with a penicillin and an aminoglycoside, is necessary. The newer broad-spectrum drugs should be reserved for later therapy, if required, although recommendations for use may change as these new drugs are further evaluated for treatment of neonatal sepsis, meningitis, and other specific infections. If the neonate's condition improves and the results of cultures are not positive within 2-4 days, the discontinuation of antibiotic therapy should be strongly considered. If infection is documented and continued treatment is indicated, the antibiotic should be changed, if necessary, to the drug or drugs most appropriate for the specific organism, its susceptibility, and the site of infection.

The relative frequencies of documented infection with different bacteria in neonates, along with patterns of antimicrobial susceptibility, should be monitored by the infection control committee. The most innocuous and specific antibiotic regimens should be selected after analysis of these data. For example, if kanamycin-resistant, gram-negative bacteria only rarely cause infections during the first week of postnatal life, but cause infections more frequently in older infants, kanamycin can be used selectively in the younger group.

Skin Care of the Newborn

The risks and benefits of different skin care techniques for newborns should be considered, such as what effect each technique has on the skin itself, whether the agent used is absorbed and may be toxic, and whether the agent changes skin flora and may give rise to infectious problems.

Cleansing should be delayed until the neonate's temperature has stabilized. Whole-body bathing of the infant may not be necessary. Localized skin care or techniques that minimize exposure to water may reduce the neonate's heat loss. Sterile cotton sponges (not gauze) soaked with warm water may be used to remove blood and meconium from the neonate's face, head, and body. Alternatively, a mild, nonmedicated soap, preferably in a single-use container or in a small bar reserved for a single neonate, can be used with careful water rinsing. Careful drying of the neonate's skin and removal of blood after birth may minimize the risk of infection with potentially contaminating microorganisms, such as HBV, HSV, and HIV. If the neonate's skin is not grossly soiled, it may not require much cleansing. The vernix caseosa may have a protective function, although some believe it does not; there is no evidence to indicate that it is harmful, however.

For the remainder of the neonate's stay in the hospital nursery, the buttocks and perianal regions should be cleansed with fresh water and cotton, with a mild soap and water at diaper changes, or as often as required.

Various antiseptic compounds for skin care have been studied to determine their safety and effectiveness in preventing colonization and infection in neonates. Hexachlorophene, which was widely used during the 1950s and 1960s, is relatively effective against gram-positive bacteria, particularly *S. aureus;* it should not be used routinely for bathing neonates, however, because it may be absorbed through intact skin and is potentially neurotoxic for neonates. Although good antiseptics, iodophors have not been proved both safe and effective for routine skin care to prevent colonization and disease in newborns. Chlorhexidine gluconate, a compound that is poorly absorbed through intact skin, is useful for bathing or localized skin care.

No single method of cord care has proved superior in preventing colonization and disease. Current methods include the local application of antimicrobial agents, such as bacitracin, or of triple dye. The skin absorption and toxicity of the triple dye agents in newborns have not been carefully studied. Alcohol hastens the drying of the cord, but, although frequently used as an antiseptic, is probably not effective in preventing cord colonization and omphalitis.

Ideally, agents used on the newborn's skin should be dispensed in single-use containers or each patient should have a personal dispenser.

Immunization of Premature Neonates and Long-Term Nursery Residents

With improved neonatal care, more prematurely born infants are surviving the neonatal period (28 days), with and without complications. As a result, the number of infants who have been hospitalized continually since birth and whose length of stay exceeds 2 months has been increasing. Yet a recent survey of 25 neonatal intensive care units in the United States and Canada showed that 40% of the units had no immunization policy, there was no uniformity in the plans of those units with a stated policy, and the policy was not always enforced.

Pertussis, a serious disease in infancy, is being reported with increasing frequency in infants born prematurely. In one recent report, 11 of 29 infants hospitalized with pertussis had been born prematurely. There have been relatively few studies on the immunization of preterm infants, however. The few studies reported have shown an adequate antibody response with a low incidence of side-effects. For example, the response of premature infants to diphtheria toxoid immunization at birth is not significantly different from the response of full-term infants. Premature infants immunized at their expected birth day (ie, 1-3 months after their birth) developed higher antibody rates than did full-term infants immunized at birth. One study indicated a similar response to oral polio vaccine (OPV) given to premature and full-term infants at ages 2 and 4 months. No data are available on the efficacy of immunization of premature infants with hepatitis B vaccine (see Hepatitis Infection, this chapter).

The following immunization guidelines are based on the premise that premature infants do not have significant antibody that will interfere with immunization and that most of these infants have the ability to produce IgM and IgG when stimulated with a variety of antigens:

1. All neonatal intensive care nurseries should implement a policy for immunization of premature infants.

2. Prematurely born infants can be given diphtheria, tetanus, and pertussis (DTP) vaccine and OPV at the appropriate chronologic age (ie, 2 months).

3. If the infant remains in the hospital, only DTP should be given to avoid cross-infection with OPV in the nursery; the OPV series can be initiated on discharge.

4. If the infant leaves the hospital at 2 months of age, both DTP and OPV can be given on discharge.

In addition, consideration of a policy for priority immunization against influenza to personnel is recommended. (See Health Standards for Personnel, this chapter.)

Precautions to Prevent Transmission of Blood-Borne Pathogens

Medical history and examination do not reliably identify all patients infected with the blood-borne pathogens, such as HBV or HIV, that are of concern to health care personnel. For this reason, the Centers for Disease Control recommends that blood and body fluid precautions be used consistently for all patients. This approach, referred to as universal precautions, is particularly important when the risk of blood exposure is high and the potential infectious status of the patient is not known.

The primary element of universal precautions is the use of appropriate barrier precautions by all health care personnel to prevent the exposure of their skin and mucous membranes to the blood or other body fluids of any patient. Gloves should be worn when it is necessary to have direct contact with blood and potentially infectious body fluids, mucous membranes, or nonintact skin of any patient; to handle items or surfaces soiled with blood or potentially infectious body fluids; and to perform venipuncture and other vascular access procedures. Hands should be washed immediately after the gloves are removed, and skin surfaces contaminated with blood or other potentially infectious material should be washed immediately and thoroughly.

Masks and protective eye wear or face shields should be worn during procedures that are likely to disperse droplets of blood or other body fluids, and gowns or aprons should be worn during procedures that are likely to generate splashes of these fluids (see Dress Codes, this chapter).

All health care personnel should take precautions with needles, scalpels, and other sharp instruments in order to prevent injuries. Hospital infection control policies for handling and disposing of needles and other sharp objects should be clearly understood and followed by all personnel.

In order avoid the need for emergency mouth-to-mouth resuscitation of patients, mouth pieces, endotracheal tubes, resuscitation bags and other ventilation devices, and suction equipment should be available for use in all areas where the need for resuscitation may arise.

Isolation of Mothers and Neonates with Infections

Isolation procedures for patients with infectious diseases are intended to minimize or prevent the spread of microorganisms among patients, hospital personnel, and visitors. The current system of patient isolation recommended for most hospitals in the United States is designed around seven basic categories:

1. Strict isolation
2. Respiratory isolation
3. Contact isolation
4. Drainage/secretion precautions
5. Enteric precautions
6. Blood/body fluid precautions
7. Tuberculosis isolation

The appropriate management of patients with infectious diseases depends on the isolation category and the disease. Contact isolation is useful for patients with highly transmissible or epidemiologically important infections (eg, patients colonized or infected with highly resistant bacteria) who do not require strict isolation. Drainage/secretion precautions are useful in managing patients with infectious discharge from wounds, lesions, and mucosal surfaces. Blood/body fluid precautions are intended for patients with infectious blood or body fluids, such as those with HBV infections. Detailed descriptions of the isolation categories and requirements are provided in *Guidelines for Isolation Precautions in Hospitals*. The isolation categories were not designed for the special needs of neonates and nurseries, however, so specific procedures used within each category may need modification for neonates.

Obstetric patients with infections that may be transmitted to other patients or to medical or hospital personnel must be appropriately isolated. Frequently, this can be accomplished without moving the patient to a private room or away from the obstetric floor. It can be accomplished, for example, by ensuring that drainage or discharge from infectious lesions is adequately contained; that persons having contact with the infectious lesions use careful techniques (including, when appropriate, gown, gloves, and "no-touch" dressing change techniques); and that contaminated dressings, instruments, and other materials are appropriately discarded or wrapped before being sent for cleaning and disinfection or sterilization.

Isolation of Infected Postpartum Patients

Patients with group A streptococcal puerperal endometritis should be managed with contact isolation until 24 hours after the initiation of adequate antimicrobial therapy; a private room is desirable, particularly if patient hygiene is poor. A gown and gloves should be used for direct contact with the infected area or drainage. Patients with abscesses or draining infections of the perineum or of abdominal wounds should be managed with drainage/secretion precautions or, if necessary, contact isolation; a private room may be desirable.

Control measures needed in the care of febrile puerperal patients are similar to those for patients with minor infections. A private room is not essential, but patients should be placed on drainage/secretion precautions. Careful attention to aseptic patient care techniques and meticulous hand-washing after contact with patients, especially after direct contact with infected areas, are essential. Gowns should be worn during direct patient contact and gloves used for contact with potentially infected areas or for changing dressings. Perineal pads, sanitary napkins, and dressings contaminated with potentially infectious drainage should be handled with instruments, promptly placed in double plastic bags, sealed, and incinerated. Contaminated instruments should be sealed in a plastic bag, labeled as contaminated, and sent for decontamination, cleaning, and sterilizing. Contaminated or potentially contaminated linen should be bagged, labeled, and handled appropriately.

Postpartum patients with communicable diseases that are not unique to obstetric patients should be managed with appropriate precautions or isolation. If there is a significant risk that such a disease will be transmitted to other patients or if the necessary procedures cannot be performed adequately on the obstetric unit, such patients should be transferred to another nursing unit that can provide proper care.

Contact of Neonates with Their Infected Mothers

Most maternal genital infections, with the exception of group A streptococcal disease, are caused by endogenous microorganisms that ascend into the uterus from the lower genital tract; postnatal spread of infection from this site to neonates is rare. Consequently, a febrile postpartum woman without a specifically identified site of infection usually may be allowed to handle and feed her newborn if she 1) is feeling well enough; 2) washes her hands thoroughly, under supervision; and 3) wears a clean hospital cover gown to prevent contact of the neonate with contaminated items, such as bedclothes, pads, and linen. A woman with a communicable disease that is likely to be transmitted to her newborn should be separated from the newborn until the infection is no longer communicable.

A mother with a respiratory tract infection should be fully informed that such infections are easily transmitted on hands or by fomites, and she should be instructed in careful hand-washing techniques and appropriate handling of tissues or other items contaminated with infectious secretions. It may be wise for her to use a surgical mask when she is with her newborn to reduce the chance of droplet spread of infection.

Breast-feeding is usually possible even if the mother has an overt infection or if she is receiving antibiotics. Although antibiotics are secreted in breast milk in small amounts, this is usually not a contraindication to the continuation of breast-feeding (see Chapter 7).

Use of Cohorts for Infection Control

In large nurseries, cohorts of neonates may be established to minimize transmission of microorganisms or infectious diseases among different groups of neonates. A cohort usually consists of well neonates born during the same 24- or 48-hour period; these neonates are kept in a single nursery room and, ideally, are cared for by a single group of personnel who do not care for any other cohort during a given shift. After the neonates in a cohort have been discharged, the room should be thoroughly cleaned and prepared to accept the next cohort.

The use of cohorts is not usually practical for small hospitals or for those facilities with intensive care and graded care units. Even in these facilities, however, this approach can be useful in efforts to control epidemics or in the management of a group of neonates colonized or infected with a specific microbial strain. Although separate rooms for these cohorts are ideal, they are not mandatory if there is a means to demarcate cohort lines within a single large room and if personnel assigned to a cohort provide care only for neonates in that cohort.

During an epidemic, neonates with overt infection and those who are colonized should be identified rapidly and placed in cohorts. If rapid identification of these neonates is not possible, separate cohorts should be established for neonates with disease, those who have been exposed, those who have not been exposed, and those who are newly admitted. The success of cohort programs depends largely on the willingness and ability of nursery and ancillary personnel to adhere strictly to the cohort system and to follow established practices.

Neonates with Suspected or Proved Infections

The housing of an infected neonate depends on the overall condition of the neonate and the type of care required, the available space and facilities, the nurse:patient ratio, and the size and type of the neonatal care service. Other factors to be considered include the type of infection (ie, specific viral or bacterial pathogen), the clinical manifestations, the infection's source and the possible modes of its transmission, and the number of colonized or infected neonates.

In many instances, isolation rooms are unnecessary for infected neonates if 1) sufficient nursing and medical staff are on duty to provide comprehensive care, 2) there is sufficient space for a 4- to 6-ft aisle or area between neonatal stations, 3) two or more sinks for hand-washing are available in each nursery room or area, and 4) continuing instruction is provided about the ways in which infections spread. If these criteria are not met, an isolation room with separate scrub facilities is necessary.

It has often been assumed that forced-air incubators provide adequate isolation for infected neonates. While these incubators filter incoming air, they do not filter the air that is discharged into the nursery. They are satisfactory, therefore, for limited protective isolation of neonates; they should not be relied upon to prevent transmission of microorganisms from infected neonates to others, however, because the surfaces of incubators are readily contaminated with the microorganisms that have infected or colonized the neonates. Furthermore, the hands and forearms of personnel working with the neonates through portholes may be contaminated.

Specific management of neonates with suspected or definite infections varies somewhat from nursery to nursery. For optimal management, hospitals should have written procedures appropriate to the facilities and staff that are available. Each instance of infectious disease should be investigated to determine its etiology, probable source of infection, and mode of spread. Neonates that are at risk of developing an infection should be cared for in a way that prevents transmission of infection (or colonizing microorganisms) to other neonates.

It may be necessary to investigate the possibility of sepsis in neonates delivered after prolonged rupture of the membranes if their mothers have had clinical chorioamnionitis or if the neonates' own history (including the need for special resuscitative procedures) or condition suggests the presence of infection. Cultures from skin and mucosal surfaces, or urine or gastric aspirates, are not recommended routinely in such cases, because positive cultures from these sites do not necessarily indicate those pathogens that are causing systemic disease. Specific specimens required for culture should be determined by the clinical condition of the neonate. Those who were delivered after prolonged rupture of the membranes, but who have no signs that suggest infection and whose mothers have no signs or symptoms that suggest infection, should be observed carefully and cultures obtained if appropriate.

NEONATES WITH SEVERE BACTERIAL INFECTIONS.   Given satisfactory conditions in the nursery, neonates with severe bacterial infections may be cared for in the admission/observation area or in the regular newborn care area. Under ideal conditions, neonates with septicemia, bacterial meningitis, or pneumonia present little additional risk of infection to other neonates. In order to receive satisfactory care, these neonates should be treated in the intensive care unit.

NEONATES WITH GASTROENTERITIS OR DRAINING LESIONS. It is easiest to isolate neonates with gastroenteritis (diarrhea), draining lesions (eg, caused by *S. aureus*), or purulent conjunctivitis by placing them in a separate or isolation room. They may be treated in the general newborn, intermediate, or intensive care areas, provided that these areas are adequately staffed and have sufficient space and equipment to allow isolation and proper care. The most important factor in preventing the spread of infection is the presence of sufficient nursing personnel. If more than one neonate is infected, a cohort approach should be taken.

Enteric precautions or drainage/secretion precautions should be observed. All personnel should use a gown and disposable gloves when providing direct patient care. Contaminated items should be discarded properly. The environment may be heavily contaminated with the infecting microorganism and transmission of these organisms to other neonates often occurs on the hands of personnel.

NEONATES WITH CONGENITAL INFECTIONS. Neonates who have congenital infections such as cytomegalovirus, rubella, and syphilis may be highly infectious. Depending on the infection, they may excrete high titers of the infectious agent in urine, from the nasopharynx, and from mucous membrane or cutaneous lesions—even if they themselves are asymptomatic or have only mild infections. The length of time for which they excrete the infecting microorganism is variable, but it may be months.

Neonates with these congenital infections should be physically segregated (if available, a private room may be desirable) and managed with drainage/secretion precautions. Hand-washing, particularly after a diaper change, should be thorough; gowns and disposable gloves may be desirable for direct patient contact. Neonates with congenital toxoplasmosis need not be isolated.

NEONATES WITH VIRAL INFECTIONS. Many viruses, such as respiratory syncytial virus, coxsackieviruses, or echoviruses, spread rapidly among neonates and personnel in a nursery; such viral infections can be serious in neonates, sometimes resulting in death. As neonates may shed selected viruses after their clinical illness has been resolved, they become reservoirs of infection. It is believed that the viruses are transmitted predominantly by direct or indirect contact with the contaminated hands of personnel or with contaminated environmental surfaces or fomites. Contact isolation may be required to prevent this type of spread, but specific requirements vary with the infecting virus. For example, respiratory syncytial virus is shed primarily from the respiratory tract, while coxsackieviruses or echoviruses can be shed from the throat or in the stool.

Airborne Transmission of Infection

Neonates are usually ineffective disseminators of infectious bacterial or viral aerosols. Neonates with confirmed or possible infections caused by a viral agent that could be transmitted by the airborne route should be separated from other neonates 1) by transfer from the nursery area, 2) by rooming-in with the mother, or 3) by enclosure of all other neonates in the area in incubators (ie, reverse isolation).

SPECIFIC INFECTIOUS PROBLEMS

Certain infections that occur antepartum or intrapartum may have a significant effect on the fetus and newborn; proper management of the mother during pregnancy and at delivery and of the newborn postnatally can prevent or modify many serious problems and can minimize the risk of subsequent transmission of infection in the nursery. Close communication and cooperation among all perinatal care personnel are essential to obtain the best results.

Cytomegalovirus Infections

A ubiquitous virus, CMV causes chronic (usually latent) infection of little direct concern to healthy adults. The incidence of neonatal infection ranges from 0.2-2.2% of live births. Although the epidemiology of infection is not completely known, it is known that the virus can be transmitted from person to person by saliva and possibly urine, as well as by sexual contact. A fetus or newborn can acquire CMV from an infected mother transplacentally, during passage through the genital tract, and by ingestion of CMV-positive human milk.

The prevalence of CMV seropositivity in pregnant women in the United States varies by socioeconomic class, ranging from approximately 50-85%. Maternal antibody does not prevent reactivation of latent infection during pregnancy, but the great majority of these recurrent maternal infections do not result in congenital infection of the neonate; it has been estimated that 0.15% to approximately 1% of the neonates of mothers with latent CMV are congenitally infected. No more than 1% of these infected neonates are believed to have clinically apparent disease or sequelae.

Of women susceptible to CMV, the risk of primary infection during pregnancy is approximately 2% (range of 1-4%); the risk is higher for women in lower socioeconomic groups. Primary CMV infections during pregnancy are usually asymptomatic, but the probability of intrauterine transmission of infection to the fetus is approximately 40%. Only 10-15% of these congenitally infected infants have clinically apparent disease; of those who do, however, the mortality ranges from 20-30%, and more than 90% of survivors develop significant sequelae. Of the congenitally infected infants who do not have clinically apparent infection as newborns, 5-15% develop late complications or sequelae, with sensorineural hearing loss being the most common. In general, the risk of neonatal disease with subsequent complications is higher if the mother has a primary CMV infection during the first half of pregnancy.

No specific recommendations can be made to prevent primary CMV infections of pregnant women. It may be useful to avoid intimate contact with persons known to be infected. Good personal hygiene is probably important in preventing infection. Serologic testing can be used to identify susceptible individuals; although there is no prophylactic treatment, subsequent serologic testing will establish if infection has occurred. Routine serologic screening of pregnant women is of limited value, because there is no reliable way to determine if intrauterine infection or fetal disease has occurred and the incidence is very low.

Up to 3% of neonates in nurseries may be excreting CMV in urine and respiratory secretions, even though they have no clinical manifestations of infection. Drainage/secretion precautions may be indicated in the management of neonates with known or suspected infection. Personnel should wash their hands carefully after providing care for these neonates or handling contaminated objects, particularly diapers.

Neonates of seronegative mothers are at risk of severe morbidity or death if they acquire CMV infection. These infections can be transmitted to neonates by transfusion of blood from seropositive donors or by ingestion of CMV-contaminated milk from human milk banks. Transmission of CMV by these routes can be virtually eliminated by the use of blood or milk from CMV-negative donors or of frozen deglycerolized red cells. The use of CMV hyperimmune globulin is under investigation.

Hepatitis Infections

Management of Maternal Hepatitis Type B Infection

In a pregnant woman, HBV infection may result in severe disease for the mother and chronic infection for the newborn, including chronic hepatitis, cirrhosis, and primary hepatocellular carcinoma (see nomenclature in Table 6-1). Transmission of HBV from mother to neonate apparently occurs most often during delivery. Neonates born to mothers who have HBV during the last trimester of pregnancy or during the postpartum period are at high risk of acquiring infection.

Neonates born to mothers who are chronic carriers of hepatitis B antigen (HBsAg) are at risk of developing infection. Factors that increase the risk of transmission from mothers to neonates are a high maternal titer of HBsAg and the presence of e antigen (HBeAg). In fact, HBeAg is a useful marker in determining the degree of contagiousness of a chronic HBsAg carrier. Approximately 80% of neonates born to HBeAg-positive mothers become infected, and most become chronic carriers. Mothers with antibody against HBeAg are unlikely to transmit infection to their newborns.

Although the prevalence of HBV infection in the general population in the United States is low (the HBsAg carrier rate in low-risk populations is approximately 0.1%), chronic infection with HBV is

Table 6-1. Hepatitis Type B Nomenclature

Abbreviation	Term	Comments
HBV	Hepatitis B virus	Etiologic agent of hepatitis type B (previously "serum" or "long incubation" hepatitis); also known as Dane particle.
HBsAg	Hepatitis B surface antigen	Surface antigen(s) of HBV, detectable in large quantity in serum; several subtypes identified.
HBeAg	Hepatitis B e antigen	Soluble antigen; correlates with HBV replication, high titer HBV in serum, and infectivity of serum.
HBcAg	Hepatitis B core antigen	No commercial test available.
Anti-HBs	Antibody to HBsAg	Indicates past infection with and immunity to HBV, passive antibody from HBIG, or immune response from HBV vaccine.
Anti-HBe	Antibody to HBeAg	Presence in serum of HBsAg carrier suggests low titer of HBV.
Anti-HBc	Antibody to HBcAg	Indicates past infection with HBV at some undefined time.
HBIG	Hepatitis B immune globulin	

much higher in selected subpopulations (see Vaccination Against Hepatitis B, this chapter). Because of the susceptibility of neonates to HBV infection and the high probability that those infected will develop chronic disease, it is important to identify pregnant women who are chronic HBsAg carriers. Studies have shown that historical information about risk factors reveals only a portion of women who are chronic carriers. A strong argument can be made, therefore, for routinely screening all pregnant women for HBsAg rather than only those considered to be at high risk. Physicians and hospitals should consider this approach. Once pregnant women who are chronic HBsAg carriers have been identified, prophylactic treatment with hepatitis B immune globulin (HBIG) and vaccine can be provided for their newborns. Prophylaxis for exposed newborns can significantly reduce the frequency of neonatal infection and, probably, the frequency of the potentially life-threatening sequelae. The efficacy of newborn hepatitis B prophylaxis depends on the administration of HBIG as soon as possible after delivery.

Chronic carriers of HBsAg should be managed in the office or clinic and hospital with blood/body fluid precautions. Labor, delivery, and nursery personnel should be notified in advance of the anticipated delivery, and arrangements should be made to have HBIG available at delivery. Precautions should be taken to prevent transmission of HBV infection to hospital personnel during the labor, delivery, and the postpartum period.

Vaccination Against Hepatitis B

Two types of hepatitis B vaccines, one derived from human plasma and one derived from recombinant antigen, are available in the United States. The plasma-derived vaccine has been highly purified and processed in a multistep procedure that inactivates representatives of all classes of virus found in human blood, including HIV, which causes acquired immune deficiency syndrome (AIDS).

Field trials of the vaccine manufactured in the United States have shown an 80-95% efficacy in preventing infection or hepatitis among susceptible groups. Because of its cost, the vaccine is indicated only for those at high risk of HBV infection, however. Women in the United States at highest risk of HBV infection include

- Women of Asian, Pacific Island, or Alaskan Eskimo descent, whether immigrant or born in the United States
- Women born in Haiti or sub-Saharan Africa

- Women with histories of
  - Acute or chronic liver disease
  - Work or treatment in a hemodialysis unit
  - Work or residence in an institution for the mentally retarded
  - Rejection as a blood donor
  - Repeated blood transfusions
  - Frequent occupational exposure to blood in medical-dental settings
  - Household contact with an HBV carrier or hemodialysis patient
  - Multiple episodes of sexually transmitted diseases
  - Prostitution
  - Percutaneous use of illicit drugs
  - Sexual partners of men in aforementioned groups

Women who are HBsAg-negative, but have a history placing them at continuing high risk of HBV infection, should be counseled about the advisability of vaccination. The cost-effectiveness of testing for hepatitis B surface antibody (HBsAb) or core antibody (HBcAb) prior to vaccination in order to avoid vaccination of those who have already been infected has not been determined. The adult dosage is 1 ml injected in the deltoid muscle; intramuscular injection in the buttocks is not as effective. A series of three doses is required; the second and third doses are given 1 and 6 months, respectively, after the first. Pregnancy is not a contraindication to vaccination.

Management of Newborns Exposed to HBV

Because neonates infected at birth with HBV frequently become chronic carriers of HBsAg and have a high frequency of serious chronic sequelae, every effort should be made to prevent infection. Neonates born to mothers who are HBsAg-positive should be bathed carefully as soon as possible to remove the maternal blood and secretions that contaminated their skin during birth. Personnel who handle the blood-contaminated neonates should wear gloves to protect themselves. After being bathed, the neonates may be managed without special precautions for the remainder of their stay in the nursery. Neonates and mothers may have normal contact, or they may room-in (see Chapter 7 for recommendations on breast-feeding).

Neonates born to mothers who have acute hepatitis B or those who are HBsAg-positive (regardless of HBeAg status) should be given an injection of HBIG, 0.5 ml intramuscularly, as soon as possible after birth to reduce the risk of infection. In order to avoid inoculation of virus contaminating the skin, the injection site should be thoroughly cleaned before the administration of HBIG (or other agents). The need to administer HBIG promptly after birth, preferably within 48 hours of birth, cannot be overemphasized. If a mother is found to be HBsAg-positive after this time, however, the administration of HBIG may still be of some value to the neonate.

Newborn infants of HBsAg-positive mothers should receive, in addition to HBIG, 3 doses of hepatitis B vaccine (0.5 ml, or half the adult dose). The first dose can be administered at the same time that HBIG is given if separate syringes and different sites are used. The second and third doses are given 1 and 6 months, respectively, after the first. Administration of the first dose within 7 days of birth and prior to discharge from the hospital is encouraged to increase the likelihood that vaccination will be successful and to reduce the number of visits required after discharge. Data on the effectiveness of hepatitis B vaccine for neonates who weighed less than 2,000 g at birth are not available. If necessary, the administration of the vaccine (but not that of HBIG) may be delayed, but it should be given within 1 month, if possible. If vaccination is delayed for as long as 3 months, a second dose of HBIG (0.5 ml) should be given.

Hepatitis B vaccine can be given at the same time that DTP vaccine is given (see Immunization of Premature Neonates and Long-Term Nursery Residents, this chapter), but it should be given at a separate site and with a different syringe. Infants should be tested at 9 months of age or later (1 month or more after the third vaccine dose) for HBsAg and antibodies to hepatitis B in order to determine the outcome of immunoprophylaxis. All HBsAg-positive infants should have follow-up testing to determine if they have become chronic carriers.

Management of Newborns Exposed to Hepatitis A Virus

Neonates of mothers who have hepatitis A infection during pregnancy should not receive immune globulin, as they will have passively transferred antibody. Neonates born to mothers with hepatitis A infection (jaundice) at delivery or during the postpartum period may be given 0.02 ml/kg immune globulin intramuscularly at birth or as soon as maternal infection is diagnosed, although its efficacy in this circumstance has not been established. In the nursery, the neonates of these mothers should be bathed carefully, but no other special precautions are necessary. Breast-feeding may be permitted if the mother desires. The importance of proper hygiene, especially hand-washing, should be emphasized to the mother.

Herpes Simplex Infections

Maternal Infection and Management of Delivery

CLINICAL AND EPIDEMIOLOGIC CONSIDERATIONS. Symptomatic genital infection with HSV is characterized by multiple, painful vesicles and ulcers in various stages of development. Many HSV infections, particularly recurrent infections, are subclinical or asymptomatic, however. Most genital herpes infections are caused by HSV type 2 (HSV-2), although the frequency of genital infections caused by HSV type 1 (HSV-1), the type that most often causes perioral infection and gingivostomatitis, is increasing in some populations.

Primary HSV infection occurs in a person never previously infected with HSV at any site. Nonprimary, first-episode genital infection is a new infection in a person who has serologic evidence of previous infection with HSV; most commonly, this is a new genital HSV-2 infection in a person who had primary HSV-1 infection as a child (most often asymptomatic infection or gingivostomatitis). Clinically, primary infection produces the most severe local symptoms; furthermore, the lesions persist and shed virus for the longest period of time. Approximately 80% of persons with primary genital HSV-2 infection have recurrences during the first year; recurrences after primary genital HSV-1 infection may be less frequent. Intermittent, asymptomatic shedding of HSV in saliva, as well as in cervical and seminal secretions, also occurs. The virus can be transmitted to others during periods of both symptomatic and asymptomatic excretion of virus.

LABORATORY DIAGNOSIS OF GENITAL HERPES INFECTION. The most reliable and sensitive technique for diagnosis of HSV infection is virus culture of labial or cervical lesions or, in the absence of lesions, of secretions from the cervix and vulva. Because a positive culture has been used as the diagnostic standard, the sensitivity of this test cannot be determined. Cultures of fluid obtained from vesicles are more likely to be positive than are those of scrapings obtained from ulcers or crusted lesions. It is usually 1-3 days after inoculation of cell cultures before HSV can be isolated. Special transport media should be used for specimens that cannot be inoculated immediately.

Cytologic tests, such as Papanicolaou smears of the cervix and Tzanck preparations, can be examined for multinucleated giant cells and intranuclear inclusions, which are suggestive of HSV infection. These tests have a sensitivity of approximately 75% compared with that of cultures, but they are less expensive and the results are available more rapidly. In contrast to cultures, cytologic tests are more likely to be positive during the later stages of lesion development (ie, ulceration and crusting). Neither a negative culture nor a negative cytologic test excludes a diagnosis of HSV infection.

Other diagnostic techniques, such as enzyme-linked immunosorbent assays or direct fluorescent antibody staining of vesicle scrapings, are still under investigation; the sensitivity and specificity vary widely, depending on the exact procedure and reagents used. Antigen detection assays in which these techniques are used with monoclonal antibodies may improve rapid diagnostic capabilities in the future.

Serologic tests are useful only for establishing a diagnosis of primary HSV infection. Routine serologic screening of pregnant women is not recommended.

HERPES INFECTIONS DURING PREGNANCY. Two patterns of HSV infection are associated with significant consequences during pregnancy. First, disseminated infection with extension of infection beyond the usual sites (ie, oropharynx and genitals) occurs rarely. Disseminated cutaneous or visceral involvement, however, may be associated with maternal fatality and a fetal loss rate of approximately 50%. Second, maternal genital infection can be transmitted to the fetus or newborn and cause neonatal HSV disease. Primary maternal genital HSV infection poses the greatest risk to the fetus. In early pregnancy, primary infection is associated with an increased risk of spontaneous abortion and stillbirth. Women with primary infection at delivery have an approximately 50% risk of transmitting infection to infants born vaginally; women with recurrent infection have an approximately 3-5% risk of transmitting infection to their infants. Maternal genital HSV infection is also associated with the preterm onset of labor and, rarely, congenital anomalies.

Recurrent genital infection is the most common type of HSV infection during pregnancy. The probability of HSV infection in the newborn whose mother has recurrent genital infection appears to depend on multiple factors, such as viral shedding at the time of delivery, the presence of cervical lesions, and the fetus' lack of transplacentally acquired neutralizing antibody. Viral shedding during pregnancy and at delivery is infrequent. In one large study, pregnant women with a history of recurrent genital infection were monitored by means of serial cultures; only 4.1% of women had even a single positive culture during asymptomatic periods. In only 0.6% of specimens obtained during the asymptomatic periods was HSV detected. At delivery, HSV was isolated from 1% of the women who were asymptomatic at the onset of labor; each of the women who was HSV-positive had had multiple cultures obtained during the 4 weeks before delivery, and none had been positive. In other studies involving unselected patient populations, HSV shedding was documented in only 0.1-0.4% of women at delivery. The incidence of neonatal HSV disease is many times lower (0.01-0.04%).

OBSTETRIC MANAGEMENT OF WOMEN WITH GENITAL HERPES INFECTION. Expert opinion has varied widely on the best way to manage pregnant women with genital herpes infection to minimize the risk of neonatal HSV infection. Women with a history of genital herpes, with signs or symptoms of genital herpes during pregnancy, or whose sexual partner has genital herpes are at an increased risk of transmitting HSV to their neonates; however, several studies have shown that the majority of neonates infected with HSV were born to women who had none of these risk factors.

During the early 1980s, most experts recommended that all pregnant women with a history of HSV infection before or during pregnancy be monitored weekly during the last several months of pregnancy for evidence of HSV infection; those who were found to be virus-positive or to have clinical lesions underwent a cesarean delivery. Experience during the past several years has shown that this management plan is not totally satisfactory, however: 1) it does not prevent all neonatal HSV infection, because many infected infants are born to women who do not fulfill the criteria for monitoring; 2) there is little correlation between antepartum HSV infection and viral shedding at delivery; 3) cesarean delivery, even over intact membranes, does not provide complete protection against neonatal HSV infection (as indicated by a recent multicenter study in which it was found that 12% of reported neonatal herpes cases had been delivered by cesarean section over intact membranes); 4) the incidence of neonatal HSV infection is low compared with the incidence of known HSV infection in pregnant women; and 5) the cost of screening and possibly unnecessary cesarean deliveries is high in relation to the number of neonatal infections potentially averted.

Because the results of cultures of women with recurrent HSV infections during pregnancy correlate poorly with viral shedding during labor, this type of monitoring has little impact on the incidence of neonatal infection. The recommendations for HSV screening cultures in women at high risk of infections have continued to evolve as new information becomes available. The data currently available do not support the routine use of antepartum cultures to determine the route of delivery.

During the initial prenatal visit, all pregnant women should be questioned about a history of HSV infection in themselves and in their sexual partner. In addition, signs and symptoms of current infection should be sought during prenatal examination and upon admission for delivery. The management of pregnant women with a history of HSV infection in themselves or in their sexual partner should be determined on an individual basis. Decisions regarding the need for cultures or other laboratory procedures for women at risk of active infection during late pregnancy should be based on the timing and frequency of recurrent HSV lesions during pregnancy and the laboratory facilities available.

Although no single management plan can be recommended for all pregnant women with genital herpes infection, current recommendations include the following:

1. In the absence of active lesions, it is not necessary to obtain cultures from pregnant women with a history of HSV infection, and vaginal delivery is acceptable.

2. When a woman has active HSV lesions during pregnancy, culture should be obtained to confirm the diagnosis. If there are no active lesions at term, vaginal delivery is acceptable.

3. Patients who have active lesions near or at term and who are in labor, or who have ruptured membranes, should undergo expeditious cesarean delivery.

Because fetal scalp electrodes may inoculate the fetus with HSV if the mother is infected, even if the mother's infection is asymptomatic, the need for internal monitoring by fetal scalp electrode should be assessed carefully and avoided, if possible. If the mother has a history of recurrent HSV infection, cultures from the cervix and vulva at the time of admission for labor and delivery may be helpful in making decisions on neonatal management.

Women in labor who have nongenital HSV infections, but no history or evidence of genital infection, should be delivered vaginally. The lesions should be covered to prevent direct neonatal contact during the intrapartum and postpartum periods, and the mother should be taught how to prevent infection of her newborn from these lesions.

TREATMENT AND COUNSELING OF PREGNANT WOMEN WITH HERPES INFECTIONS. Couples should be educated about the natural history of genital HSV infection and should be advised that, if only one partner is infected, they should abstain from sexual contact while lesions are present. Some consultants also recommend that asymptomatic HSV-infected persons use condoms in an attempt to minimize the risk of transmitting the infection to their partners. Pregnant women should be advised that it is particularly important to avoid sexual contact during the last several months of gestation if their partners have genital HSV infection.

The safety of administering acyclovir systemically for the treatment of HSV-infected pregnant women has not been established. Prophylactic administration of antiviral drugs to women with genital HSV infection at delivery is not indicated.

POSTPARTUM MANAGEMENT OF WOMEN WITH HERPES INFECTION. Women with either genital or nongenital HSV infection can be managed safely with drainage/secretion precautions in the labor, delivery, and postpartum care areas. Those with severe primary lesions should be managed with contact isolation in private rooms. Health care personnel and the patient herself should use gloves for direct contact with the infected area or with contaminated dressings, and meticulous hand-washing is essential. Labor and delivery rooms require only routine, careful cleaning and disinfection before being used by another patient.

Management of Exposed Newborns

EPIDEMIOLOGY AND PATTERN OF INFECTIONS. The incidence of neonatal HSV infection is low; estimates range from 1/3,000 to 1/20,000 live births. Most infants who develop HSV infection acquire their infection perinatally from their mothers. Most frequently, HSV infects a neonate during passage through the infected maternal lower genital tract, or it ascends to the fetus, sometimes even though membranes are apparently intact. Less common sources of neonatal infection include 1) postnatal transmission from the mother or father, most often from a nongenital infection (eg, mouth, hands, or around the breasts), or 2) postnatal transmission in the nursery from another infected neonate, probably on the hands of personnel attending the infants. Postnatal transmission from personnel with fever blisters to neonates appears to occur extremely rarely, if at all. Congenital infection also occurs rarely.

Patterns of HSV infection in newborns include a generalized, systemic infection that involves the liver and other organs, including the central nervous system; localized central nervous system disease; or localized infection of the skin, eyes, or mouth. Clinical onset of disease may occur at any time during the first month. Disseminated disease usually occurs during the first 1-2 weeks of life; disease localized to the central nervous system or to the skin, eyes, or mouth more often occurs during the second or third week. Approximately one-third of neonates with HSV infection develop lesions of the skin, eyes, or mouth as an early manifestation; in another one-third, there may be other evidence of systemic or central nervous system disease before the mucocutaneous lesions appear; and in one-third, there are no visible lesions. Asymptomatic HSV infection of newborns occurs rarely, if at all.

NURSERY MANAGEMENT OF INFANTS EXPOSED TO OR INFECTED WITH HSV. Because HSV infection has occasionally been transmitted among neonates in nurseries and because this infection is potentially severe in newborns, precautions should be taken to minimize the risk of transmission within the nursery. Neonates with documented perinatal exposure to HSV may be in the incubation phase of infection and should be handled expectantly. Neonates born vaginally (or by cesarean delivery if the membranes had been ruptured for longer than 4-6 hours) to a mother with active HSV lesions should be physically separated from other neonates and managed with contact isolation if they remain in the nursery during the incubation period; an isolation room is not essential. An alternative approach is to have the neonate room continuously with the mother in a private mother-infant room. Personnel working with these potentially infected neonates should wash their hands meticulously after caring for the neonates and should use techniques established to prevent the transmission of any virus that may be shed during the incubation or clinical stages of infection.

The risk of HSV infection in possibly exposed neonates (eg, those born to a mother with a history of recurrent genital herpes or by cesarean delivery before rupture of the membranes) is low; although expert opinion varies, special isolation precautions are probably not needed for most of these neonates. They should be observed for several days and followed closely after discharge, however, and their parents should be instructed to observe them carefully for early signs of infection.

EARLY DIAGNOSIS AND MANAGEMENT OF SUSPECTED HSV DISEASE. Early signs of HSV infection in newborns are frequently nonspecific and subtle. A neonate known to have been exposed to HSV should be observed carefully for vesicular lesions or for unexplained illnesses, including respiratory distress, convulsions, or signs of sepsis. If any of these occur, the possibility of HSV infection should be investigated. Skin lesions and other sites, as appropriate, should be cultured for HSV. The neonate should be physically segregated and managed with contact isolation; an isolation room is desirable. Personnel having contact with skin lesions or potentially infectious secretions should use gowns and gloves. Antiviral therapy should be initiated if HSV is strongly suspected; expert consultation about recommended antiviral drug therapy should be sought. Neonates with HSV disease should be managed in a facility that provides level III care.

As suggested earlier, decisions about the management of neonates who may have been exposed to HSV may be easier if cultures are done on specimens obtained from the mother's cervix and vulva during labor. Similarly, if laboratory facilities are available, cultures obtained from the nasopharynx or mouth and the conjunctivae of neonates born to mothers known or strongly suspected of being infected with HSV can assist in management decisions. Cultures obtained from the neonate shortly after birth are helpful in identifying exposed neonates, but they do not indicate HSV infection. Furthermore, the sensitivity of these cultures in predicting infection is unknown. A positive culture obtained 24-48 hours or longer after birth suggests HSV infection and is an indication for immediate institution of antiviral therapy, even in the absence of symptoms.

Although HSV infection is more likely to occur at a site of skin trauma, there are no data to indicate that the circumcision of male neonates who may have been exposed at birth should be postponed. Delay of circumcision for approximately 1 month for those neonates at highest risk of disease (eg, those born vaginally to mothers with active genital lesions) may be prudent, however.

Contact of Neonates with Their HSV-Infected Mothers

A mother with HSV infection should be instructed about her infection and taught hygienic measures to prevent the postnatal transmission of the infection to her neonate. Before touching her newborn, the mother should wash her hands carefully and don a clean gown or use a clean barrier to ensure that the neonate does not come into contact with lesions or potentially infectious material. If the mother has genital herpes infection, her newborn may room-in with her after she has been taught protective measures. Breast-feeding is permissible if the mother has no vesicular herpetic lesions in the breast area and all active cutaneous lesions are covered.

A mother with herpes labialis (cold sore) or stomatitis should wear a disposable surgical mask when she touches her newborn until the lesions have crusted and dried; she should not kiss or nuzzle her newborn until the lesions have cleared. Herpetic lesions on other skin sites should be covered. Direct contact of a newborn with other family members or friends who have active HSV infection should be avoided.

HIV Infection

Infection with HIV, the virus that causes acquired immune deficiency syndrome (AIDS), has become a significant medical problem during the 1980s. Although fewer than 10% of persons with AIDS in the United States have been women and children, this percentage represents hundreds of cases in infants and thousands of cases in women. It is probable that thousands more women are infected with HIV and, thus, at risk of AIDS and capable of transmitting the virus to their sex partners or to their offspring if they become pregnant.

Clinical Features of AIDS and HIV Infection in Women and Infants

Acquired immune deficiency syndrome is the end stage of infection with HIV. This human retrovirus infects predominantly T-helper lymphocytes, the primary regulatory cell of the immune system, but it can also infect other cells in the immune system, the central nervous system, and perhaps other tissues. Once established, infection is chronic and persists for the life of most of those who are infected. Virus is most likely to be isolated from specimens obtained from peripheral blood lymphocytes, although HIV has been isolated from a variety of human tissues, secretions, and other body fluids.

Acute infection with HIV may be asymptomatic, or it may result in a mononucleosis-like illness with fever, rash, and lymphadenopathy. Acute infection is followed by a period of asymptomatic infection that ranges in duration from months to years. During this period, the person with HIV is potentially infectious to other people through sexual or parenteral (eg, through blood) contact and to a fetus or newborn transplacentally or intrapartally. As infection persists, the person typically develops laboratory evidence of cellular immune dysfunction, followed by the occurrence of clinical conditions that may include fever, weight loss, malaise, lethargy, central nervous system dysfunction, and opportunistic infections caused by pathogens such as HSV or *Candida*. Usually progressive, these nonspecific conditions and less severe infections may eventually result in significant disability, or they may be a prelude to a major opportunistic disease, such as *Pneumocystis carinii* pneumonia, that is diagnostic of AIDS. Classification systems have been developed to categorize the range of HIV infection in both adults and children.

At any given time, there are likely to be many more people who are asymptomatically infected with HIV than there are those who have AIDS or other associated conditions. The risk of AIDS or associated conditions in an infected person depends on multiple factors, many of which are not yet understood. One of the most important is the duration of infection; the longer that a person has been infected with HIV, the higher the probability that he or she will experience immune dysfunction and clinical illness secondary to the infection. The ultimate risk of AIDS or associated conditions in a population of infected persons is unknown. Studies in selected populations show that, after 7 years of HIV infection, more than 30% have AIDS and an additional 30-50% have other clinical manifestations of HIV infection. In adults, AIDS is seldom diagnosed during the first 2 years after infection; some adults have remained well for 8 or 9 years after documented HIV infection. One study has suggested that pregnancy may increase the risk of AIDS or other associated conditions in women infected with HIV, but this finding has not been confirmed.

Clinical findings in infants and children with AIDS are frequently similar to those in adults. Infants with congenital or perinatal HIV infection often become symptomatic during the first year or two of life. Early manifestations of HIV infection include lymphocytic interstitial pneumonitis, weight loss and failure to thrive, hepatomegaly or splenomegaly, generalized lymphadenopathy, and chronic diarrhea; parotid swelling has also been reported. Oral candidiasis is often present and may progress to esophageal or disseminated candidiasis. Opportunistic infections, particularly *P. carinii* pneumonia, are common later in the disease process. Recurrent severe bacterial infections and sepsis are more common in pediatric patients with HIV infection than in adults with HIV infection. Neurologic problems, including encephalopathy and dementia, have been reported; developmental regression is common. Malignancies are unusual, but do occur. Dysmorphic features have been reported in a small number of infants with congenital HIV infection, but it is not clear whether they are due only to HIV or to other factors. Reported mortality for children with AIDS is high; more than 65% have died.

Epidemiologic Features of AIDS and HIV Infection in Women and Infants

Human immunodeficiency virus may be present in the blood and semen or vaginal and cervical secretions of infected persons. The primary means of transmission have been sexual contact (male to female, female to male, and male to male) and shared use of blood-contaminated needles and syringes in intravenous drug abuse.

The reported cases of AIDS in women indicate that women are most likely to be infected through intravenous drug abuse (49%), sexual contact with a man known to be at risk of HIV infection (30%), and blood transfusions or clotting factor therapy given before mid-1985 when programs to screen blood for HIV began (11%). The significance of intravenous drug abuse in the transmission of HIV to women is magnified by the fact that most of the heterosexually transmitted infections occurred from sexual contact with a man infected through drug abuse. Most cases (78%) occur in women of childbearing age. Although most states have reported at least one woman with AIDS, 76% of the cases in women have been reported from only four states: New York (47%), New Jersey (13%), Florida (10%), and California (6%). The racial distribution of AIDS cases in women in the United States is quite different from that of AIDS cases in men. More than one-half the cases are in blacks (53%). Whites account for 27% of cases; Hispanics, 19%; and other races, 1%.

Although the first cases of intrauterine/perinatal HIV transmission occurred during the late 1970s, most infants with HIV infection and AIDS have been born in the middle to late 1980s. In 78% of cases reported in children, the mother has been found to be infected or at risk of HIV infection; of these, drug abuse (66%) and heterosexual transmission (22%) are the most common risk factors. In another 5% of cases, the mother has AIDS, but a specific risk factor is not known. Blood transfusion, use of clotting-factor concentrates, and unknown risk factors account for the balance of infection in the mothers.

The states that have reported the majority of cases in women have also reported the largest number of cases in infants. The racial distribution of pediatric AIDS cases is highly skewed. The majority (54%) occur in blacks, with smaller percentages being reported in Hispanics (24%), whites (21%), and other racial groups (1%). The cumulative incidence rate of AIDS in black and Hispanic children in the United States is many times that of white children. The sex distribution of pediatric AIDS cases is relatively even (54% male, 46% female), in marked contrast to that of all AIDS cases (93% of cases in males).

Risk and Means of Fetal/Neonatal HIV Infection

The risk of congenital (intrauterine, presumably transplacental) or intrapartum transmission of HIV from an infected woman to her fetus or newborn depends on multiple factors that are not yet clearly defined. In one study of infants born to infected mothers who already had one child with AIDS, 50% had serologic or clinical evidence of infection with HIV. Other studies of infected women and their children suggest a lower risk of transmission. The best estimates of the risk of congenital or perinatal transmission of HIV from an infected woman range from 30-50%; additional studies are necessary to define more precisely the risk and variables associated with this type of HIV transmission.

The relative frequency of intrauterine, intrapartum, and postpartum transmission of HIV from an infected woman to her fetus or newborn is unknown. Similarly, the effects of the onset and duration of maternal infection and other variables that may influence intrauterine transmission and infection in the fetus are not known. Intrapartum transmission of HIV appears to occur considerably less frequently than does intrapartum transmission of an infection such as maternal hepatitis type B. Preliminary studies suggest that cesarean delivery does not protect the neonate from HIV infection, but further information is necessary to confirm this finding.

A few case reports suggest that women who were infected with HIV postpartum (through blood transfusion) transmitted the infection to their infants through breast-feeding. Others have shown that infants breast-fed for up to 7 months after birth by mothers infected antepartum with HIV did not become infected with HIV, suggesting that the risk of HIV transmission through breast-feeding is low compared with the risk of intrauterine transmission. Other types of postpartum transmission from a mother to her newborn (eg, through routine care and affection for the infant) have not been documented; the relative risk of this type of transmission appears to be very low.

Diagnosis of AIDS and HIV Infection

Acquired immune deficiency syndrome is a clinical diagnosis based on clinical findings and the results of appropriate microbiologic, histologic, immunologic, radiologic, and serologic procedures for the suspected conditions, opportunistic infections, and cancers. In infants, primary immunodeficiency diseases must be excluded (eg, severe combined immunodeficiency, DiGeorge syndrome, Wiskott-Aldrich syndrome). Serologic confirmation of HIV infection is often useful.

DIAGNOSIS OF HIV INFECTION IN ADULTS AND CHILDREN. Because persons infected with HIV usually develop antibody within 6-12 weeks of infection, the diagnosis of HIV infection in adults and older children is most easily established through a validated serologic test for antibody. Screening tests based on enzyme immunoassay (EIA or ELISA) are highly sensitive and specific when a serum specimen is found to give consistently reactive results. Because of the low prevalence of HIV infection in many populations, however, and because of the extraordinary social and medical implications of positive test results, the serum specimen from a person with a repeatedly reactive EIA should also be tested by a supplemental or validation test. Currently, this is most often a Western blot test, although radioimmunoprecipitation assays and fluorescent antibody assays are also used by some laboratories.

Only one manufacturer is currently licensed to market Western blot test kits in the United States to validate HIV antibody screening tests; other test kits will probably be licensed in the future, and many laboratories produce their own reagents and materials for Western blot tests. When the manufacturer's strict criteria are used for interpreting results of the licensed test, the probability of a false-positive test is almost negligible. Some people with reactive EIA tests who are tested with this Western blot have a nonspecific pattern on the blot that is interpreted as equivocal, however. For example, a person recently infected with HIV may show an equivocal Western blot pattern. Repeating the test on a second specimen obtained 3-6 months after the initial specimen was obtained usually shows progression of the blot pattern to one that is positive if the person has been infected with HIV. The equivocal blot pattern generally persists when a second specimen is tested 3-6 months later if the person has not been infected. Because of the potential problems in performing and interpreting validation tests for HIV infection, physicians who request these tests should use only the best laboratories and should seek confirmation of the laboratory's performance on HIV antibody tests.

It is possible to isolate HIV from lymphocytes and selected other human fluids and tissues in laboratories equipped for retroviral culture. A confirmed positive culture indicates infection with HIV. Because the sensitivity of culture varies widely, however, a negative culture does not indicate the absence of infection.

Additional types of laboratory procedures for diagnosis of HIV infection will be available in the future. Tests for HIV antigen are currently being evaluated; they are useful for confirming cultures of HIV in the laboratory and possibly for evaluation of patient status in experimental studies. Because HIV antigen is not always detectable in serum once specific antibody develops, the HIV antigen tests will not replace antibody tests for screening donated blood or for determining reliably which patients are infected with HIV. Tests for viral nucleic acids in infected cells are being evaluated and may be a practical clinical test in the future.

DIAGNOSIS OF HIV INFECTION IN INFANTS. Because of the transplacental passage of maternal HIV antibody to virtually all infants born to mothers who are infected, the diagnosis of HIV infection in newborns is extremely difficult with the laboratory methods currently available. The presence of HIV antibody as detected by EIA, Western blot tests, or other methods should be expected in the serum of an infant born to a seropositive mother. An infant who is not infected should remain healthy, and the titer of antibody should decline during the first year; a few infants have not seroreverted until 15 months after birth. The loss of HIV antibody is not unequivocal evidence that the infant is free of infection, however, because a percentage of infants who serorevert are HIV infected, but appear to be immune tolerant. Infection of the infant is suggested when serial specimens assayed at one time by the same technique show persistent or rising titers of HIV antibody or when new HIV-specific antibody bands not present in the mother's serum appear on diagnostic tests such as Western blot or radioimmunoprecipitation assay.

Assays for HIV-specific IgM have been developed and are being evaluated; results to date are mixed because of technical difficulties with the tests and transient IgM production. Also, the effects of the time and means of infection of the fetus or infant on IgM production are not known.

Currently, definitive evidence of HIV infection in infants must be based on 1) a diagnosis of AIDS, 2) a combination of HIV antibody and a compatible immunologic profile and clinical course, or 3) detection of HIV in blood or tissues. Methods for detection of HIV in blood include virus culture, which is definitive if positive, but is not highly sensitive; tests for HIV antigen, which will be widely available in the near future, but do not yet have documented sensitivity and specificity in infants; and assay for viral nucleic acids, which is likely to be sensitive and specific, but is still experimental.

Prevention of AIDS and HIV Infection

PREVALENCE OF HIV INFECTION IN WOMEN OF CHILDBEARING AGE. In the United States, the prevalence of HIV infection in women of childbear ing age is highly variable, ranging from approximately 0.01% (1/ 10,000) in women who donate blood to 50% or higher in women who are chronic intravenous drug users or who are steady sexual partners of men infected with HIV. During 1986-1987, in several cities in the United States, serosurveys of blood obtained from unselected pregnant women (or of cord blood) revealed a prevalence of HIV infection as high as 1-2%; in one study, as many as 40% of the seropositive women had no specific risk factor for HIV infection. Women in the following groups have a significant risk of HIV infection:

- Those who use (or have used) drugs intravenously for nonmedical purposes
- Those whose sexual partners have clinical or serologic evidence of HIV infection or who themselves are at significant risk of infection (eg, because of male homosexual contact, intravenous drug abuse, or hemophilia)
- Those who are living in communities in the United States or who were born in countries where there is a known or suspected high prevalence of infection among women
- Those who have engaged in prostitution (often associated with drug dependency), who have had multiple sexual partners, or who are being treated for a sexually transmitted disease
- Those who received a transfusion before blood was screened for HIV antibody, but after HIV infection occurred (eg, between 1978 and 1985)

In most areas of the United States, the current probability of HIV infection is relatively low for a woman whose only risk factor is the fact that she has had multiple heterosexual partners, but the risk increases with the number of partners she has had, the prevalence of HIV infection in the area, and the possibility that one or more of her partners is bisexual or has used drugs intravenously.

PREVENTION THROUGH COUNSELING AND HIV ANTIBODY TESTING. The purpose of counseling and HIV antibody testing is to provide women who are HIV infected, or who are or have been at risk of HIV infection—particularly those of childbearing age—with information about their own status, about the means of preventing infection in themselves if they are not infected, and about the means of preventing transmission from themselves to others if they are already infected. Counseling and testing are recommended in any medical care setting in which women at risk of infection are encountered, including private obstetric and gynecologic practices, clinics for those with sexually transmitted disease, family planning and fertility services, prenatal and obstetric clinics, clinics or services for drug users or prostitutes, and comprehensive or family-oriented hemophilia treatment services. In particular, all pregnant women believed to be at increased risk of HIV infection should routinely be counseled and strongly urged to undergo testing for HIV antibody. The identification of HIV-infected pregnant women as early in pregnancy as possible is important to ensure appropriate medical care for them; to plan medical care for their infants, and to provide counseling about family planning, future pregnancies, and the risk of sexual transmission of HIV to others.

Women with clinical, virologic, or serologic evidence of HIV infection should be educated about the significance of the infection and the means to prevent transmission to others. An important aspect of counseling is supporting the patient in informing her sexual partners of her infection. If patients prefer, health department personnel may be able to notify their patients anonymously and counsel them regarding testing and the significance of infections. Because antibody to HIV may not be detectable for several months after infection, women who have been exposed recently or who continue to be exposed may need to be tested periodically to determine if infection has occurred. Women who are at risk of HIV infection, but are not infected (ie, clinically well and serologically negative) should be counseled about the need to take appropriate precautions to avoid becoming infected.

It is assumed that sexual transmission of HIV can be prevented by barriers that markedly decrease or eliminate contact of an uninfected person with infectious semen or vaginal and cervical secretions. Educating sexual partners about the HIV infection, conscientiously using condoms during sexual foreplay and intercourse, and avoiding deep (tongue) kissing should significantly reduce the possibility of sexual transmission of HIV. Laboratory experiments have shown that some spermicides kill the virus, and use of spermicides in conjunction with a condom may provide a greater margin of safety. There have been no studies that document the efficacy of specific means of preventing interpersonal transmission of HIV, however. Information and materials for counseling can be obtained from most state and local health departments.

CONFIDENTIALITY AND ETHICAL ISSUES OF HIV INFECTION.   A plethora of social and ethical concerns attend AIDS and HIV infection. Physicians who treat and counsel patients with AIDS or HIV infection should be aware of all applicable state laws and regulations. For example, it is illegal in some areas to document the results of HIV antibody tests on a medical record; in other areas, it is illegal to tell any other person about the patient's clinical condition or about the results of the patient's antibody test without the specific informed consent of the patient. Apart from these issues, it is important for physicians to be aware that people found to be infected with the virus may face social or employment discrimination or may be unable to obtain life or medical insurance coverage.

Because of their extreme significance to the patient and her family, it is important to ensure that the patient understands the potential implications of HIV antibody testing before she undergoes the test and that she agrees to be tested and to receive the counseling necessary after the test results are available. It is also important to protect all medical records, reports, and information pertaining to the test results from unauthorized disclosure. This often requires special training or instruction for employees and others who work in the office or medical care setting.

Hospital Obstetric Management of an HIV-Infected Mother and Her Infant

MANAGEMENT OF DELIVERY AND THE POSTPARTUM PERIOD. Because HIV may be present in blood, vaginal secretions, and perhaps other fluids (eg, amniotic fluid) special precautions should be followed for vaginal and cesarean deliveries and other invasive procedures performed on HIV-infected women during which personnel may be exposed to blood and other potentially infectious fluids. Gloves should be used when handling the placenta or the neonate until blood and amniotic fluid have been removed from the neonate's skin. Recommended precautions have been discussed earlier in this chapter.

After delivery, women infected with HIV can be managed in the postpartum care unit with blood/body fluid precautions. Special care should be taken to protect the confidentiality of sensitive information. Appropriate medical follow-up for the mother should be arranged to minimize complications from her HIV infection.

MANAGEMENT OF THE INFANT OF A MOTHER WITH HIV INFECTION. Few infants with HIV infection show clinical evidence of infection in the first weeks after birth. In order to minimize the risk to health care personnel, all infants should be managed with universal precautions. Prompt and careful removal of blood from a neonate's skin is important. There is no need for other special precautions or for isolation of the neonate with an HIV-infected mother; rooming in is an acceptable alternative to isolation. Gloves should be worn for contact with blood or blood-containing fluids and for procedures that involve exposure to blood. Gloves are not required for prevention of HIV transmission while changing diapers in usual circumstances.

In the United States and other countries where a safe alternative is available, the HIV-infected mother should be advised against breast-feeding her infant to avoid the possibility of transmitting the infection to her infant by that route.

The potential for HIV infection in neonates whose mothers are infected should be kept in mind and diagnostic procedures requested as appropriate and available. Because potentially HIV-infected infants may have special diagnostic and care needs in the future, arrangements for appropriate pediatric care should be made before these infants are discharged from the hospital.

Human Papillomavirus Infections

Genital warts caused by human papillomavirus (HPV) are becoming more common in clinical obstetric practice. Infections with HPV, which account for a large proportion of abnormal Papanicolaou smears, may be related to the subsequent development of genital neoplasms. Cervical or vaginal HPV infections are usually asymptomatic, and Papanicolaou smears are useful for the diagnosis of cervical infection. Most genital HPV infections are sexually transmitted. Recurrence of the warts and associated symptoms may be caused by reinfection or by activation of latent virus. Because nosocomial transmission of HPV via vaginal speculums has been documented, disposable or sterile instruments should be used.

Genital HPV infections may be more difficult to manage during pregnancy. The papillary lesions may proliferate on the vulva and in the vagina, sometimes necessitating cesarean delivery to prevent extensive vaginal damage. Lesions may become increasingly friable during pregnancy, causing additional problems. No randomized studies of the treatment of genital HPV infection in pregnancy have been reported, but many clinicians have suggested that cryotherapy may be the safest treatment of external lesions during pregnancy. Podophyllin, 5-fluorouracil, and immunotherapy should be avoided for treatment of genital warts during pregnancy.

There is some risk that an infant whose mother has a genital HPV infection will be infected during birth, leading to the later development of laryngeal papillomata. These lesions are now known to be caused by HPV types 6 and 11. Possible modes of transmission include contact between the fetus and the infected genital tract of the mother, transplacental passage of maternal infection, or postnatal contact with an infected individual.

There is usually a latent period of years before HPV lesions become clinically signficant in children. On the basis of the number of abnormal Papanicolaou smears in the general female population, it had been estimated that 1,500 new cases of HPV infection could be expected in the United States each year; the lifetime risk for all children was estimated to be approximately 1/2,000. The actual number of HPV infections that have been detected in the children of HPV-infected women, however, does not support these estimates. Because the method of transmission is not known and the risk is ill defined, there is currently no consensus regarding the possibility that cesarean delivery will protect the neonate from HPV infection. Neonates born to mothers with HPV infection do not need to be managed with special precautions in the nursery.

Rubella

Prevention and Management of Infection During Pregnancy

Surveillance for susceptibility to rubella infection is essential for good prenatal care. Each patient should be screened serologically at the first prenatal visit unless she is proved to be immune by previous serologic test or documented vaccination. In a properly controlled test, any detectable antibody indicates immunity.

Seropositive women do not need further testing, regardless of their subsequent history of exposure. If seronegative pregnant women have been exposed to rubella or develop symptoms that suggest infection, however, their antibody titers should be calculated again to determine if infection occurred. Specimens should be obtained as soon as possible after exposure, 2 weeks later, and, if necessary, 4 weeks after exposure. Acute and convalescent sera specimens should be tested on the same day in the same laboratory; a fourfold or greater rise in titer or seroconversion indicates acute infection. Rubella-specific IgM testing or isolation of the virus from throat swabs rapidly establishes a diagnosis of acute rubella if the tests are available.

If rubella is diagnosed in a pregnant woman, the patient should be advised of the risks of fetal infection, and the alternative of therapeutic abortion should be discussed. Limited data indicate that the administration of immune globulin, 0.55 ml/kg, as soon as possible after exposure may prevent or modify infection in exposed susceptible persons. The absence of clinical signs in a woman who has received immune globulin does not guarantee that infection has been prevented, however; neonates with congenital rubella syndrome have been born to mothers given immune globulin shortly after exposure. If termination of pregnancy is not an option, administration of immune globulin as soon as possible after exposure should be considered.

For rubella-susceptible women of reproductive age, the RA 27/3 vaccine is highly effective and has few side effects. The puerperium is an excellent time to vaccinate susceptible women. Prevaccination serologic testing for susceptibility is not mandatory and should not impede vaccination, but sera should be tested 6-8 weeks postvaccination to confirm seroconversion.

Vaccinated women, including those vaccinated during the puerperium, should be warned to avoid conception for 3 months because of the theoretical risk that vaccine virus could be teratogenic, even though experience to date suggests that the risk of placental or fetal infection with the current RA 27/3 strain of vaccine is low. Approximately 1-2% of infants born to susceptible women immunized during pregnancy have serologic evidence of subclinical infection, but no clinical stigmata. Of 170 susceptible women vaccinated within 3 months of the estimated date of conception, none gave birth to infants who had defects compatible with congenital rubella syndrome. A woman who conceives within 3 months of rubella vaccination or who is inadvertently vaccinated in early pregnancy should be counseled that the risks to the fetus are theoretical and that data do not support an assumption that the pregnancy should be terminated. In order to assist in the development of firm recommendations for the management of this problem, physicians caring for a susceptible pregnant woman inadvertently immunized with rubella vaccine within 3 months before or after conception should report the case as soon as possible to the Division of Immunization, Centers for Disease Control.

Management of Exposed or Infected Neonates

Neonates who show signs of congenital rubella infection or who were born to women known to have had rubella during pregnancy should be managed with contact isolation, preferably in a private room. Care should be provided only by personnel known to be immune to rubella.

Every effort should be made to isolate the virus from the neonate and to document the infection. Neonates with congenital rubella should be considered contagious up to 1 year of age unless viral cultures are negative. Cases of congenital rubella syndrome or birth defects believed to be caused by rubella infection should be reported to the state health department.

Varicella-Zoster (Chickenpox)

Women with varicella during pregnancy are usually no more severely ill than other adults; they should be followed closely, however, as complications such as varicella pneumonia can be fatal. Varicella during early pregnancy is occasionally associated with congenital malformations or fetal mortality. If onset of clinical maternal infection occurs within 4-5 days of delivery (ie, prior to the maternal antibody response), subsequent infection in the newborn may be fulminant, with systemic and neurologic involvement and death. Therefore, varicella-zoster immune globulin (VZIG) should be administered directly to the neonate as soon as possible after delivery. Likewise, when maternal varicella infection is diagnosed within 4-5 days following delivery, VZIG is indicated for the neonate.

Varicella-zoster immune globulin administered to the mother within 4-5 days prior to delivery is unlikely to reach the fetus in sufficient quantities. The efficacy of VZIG administered to a pregnant woman for purposes of protecting against malformations is unknown and routine passive immunization is not recommended. VZIG is available from the American Red Cross Blood Services.

Normal full-term infants exposed postnatally are thought to be at no increased risk from complications of chickenpox than are older children, and VZIG is not indicated. Very premature infants (less than 28 weeks) who are exposed should receive VZIG (125 units) because of poor transfer of antibody across the placenta early in pregnancy.

Women with varicella must be kept in strict isolation if admitted to a hospital. Neonates exposed in utero or postnatally to varicella should be segregated and managed expectantly during the incubation period. Those neonates with varicella infection should be isolated in a private room and managed with strict isolation for the duration of illness. Neonates with congenital varicella acquired earlier in gestation do not need to be managed with special precautions.

Chlamydial Infections

Chlamydia trachomatis has been detected in the cervix of approximately 2-13% of pregnant women, but the prevalence may be as high as 25%. The prevalence tends to be highest in young women from groups that have a low socioeconomic status and a high rate of sexually transmitted diseases. Most infected women are asymptomatic, but *Chlamydia* may cause urethritis and purulent (nongonococcal) cervicitis. Chlamydial infection is also associated with postpartum endometritis and infertility. Infection may be transmitted from the genital tract of infected mothers to their neonates during birth; 60-70% of neonates born to infected mothers acquire *C. trachomatis*. Purulent conjunctivitis occurs in approximately 30-50% of neonates born vaginally to women infected with *Chlamydia,* and neonatal pneumonia occurs in 10-20%.

Important risk factors for chlamydial infection include single marital status, age less than 20 years, residence in a socially disadvantaged community (eg, inner city), presence of other sexually transmitted diseases, and late appearance for prenatal care. Although asymptomatic women are not routinely screened for *C. trachomatis,* diagnostic testing of pregnant women at high risk for this infection may be useful at the first prenatal visit and during the third trimester of pregnancy. The antenatal identification and treatment of women who have *C. trachomatis* infection in their genital tract may prevent disease in the neonate.

Treatment should be administered to women with mucopurulent cervicitis and to women whose sexual partners have nongonococcal urethritis or nongonococcal epididymitis even if diagnostic tests are not performed. Erythromycin is the drug of choice, although the optimal dosage and duration of antibiotic therapy for pregnant women have not been established. Simultaneous treatment of the male partner or partners with tetracycline or doxycycline is an important component of the therapeutic regimen.

Chlamydial infections in the neonate are generally mild and responsive to antimicrobial therapy; prophylactic cesarean delivery is not warranted. Prophylactic instillation of topical erythromycin or tetracycline into the conjuctival sac of the neonate shortly after birth helps to prevent inclusion conjunctivitis, but not chlamydial pneumonia. Neonates with inclusion conjunctivitis should be managed with drainage/secretion precautions. Those with chlamydial pneumonia should be managed similarly, but they should also be separated from neonates who are uninfected and neonates who are infected with other respiratory agents. Transmission of chlamydial infections within nurseries has been suspected, but not proved.

Gonorrhea

Maternal Gonococcal Infection

Gonorrhea is generally, but not always, asymptomatic during pregnancy. Salpingitis is rare in pregnancy; disseminated gonococcal disease (eg, with rash, fever, and arthritis) may occur more frequently. Even when asymptomatic, gonococcal infections in pregnant women may be associated with an increased incidence of perinatal morbidity and mortality, including fetal wastage, early and prolonged rupture of the membranes, premature labor, and low birth weight. The incidence of complications appears to be particularly high in women who have gonococcal infection during labor and delivery. The presence of infection at this time may result in fetal sepsis or scalp abscess if intrauterine fetal monitoring is used.

In high-risk populations, endocervical cultures for gonococci should be taken during the first prenatal visit, and a second culture should be taken late in the third trimester. Failure to treat an infected woman before or at delivery may result in the postnatal transmission of gonococcal infection to her newborn. Infected women should be treated and their newborns provided with appropriate prophylaxis or treatment. Drug regimens of choice are those for uncomplicated gonorrhea, with the exception of tetracycline type drugs, which should not be used because of their potential toxic effects on mother and fetus. Women allergic to penicillin or probenecid should be treated with spectinomycin. Women with gonococcal infection at delivery should be managed with drainage/secretion precautions until effective systemic therapy has been administered for 24 hours.

Gonococcal Infections in Newborns

The prevalence of largely asymptomatic genital gonococcal infection in pregnant women and the occurrence of gonococcal ophthalmia in approximately 28% of untreated neonates born to infected women indicate the need for prophylaxis for all neonates. Recommendations for preventing neonatal ophthalmia are discussed in Appendix D.

Neonates born to mothers with recognized gonococcal infection should receive a single injection of aqueous crystalline penicillin G, 50,000 units for full-term neonates or 20,000 units for low-birth-weight neonates; for these neonates, topical prophylaxis alone is inadequate. Neonates with clinical ophthalmia or complicated (disseminated) gonococcal infection should be hospitalized and treated with an appropriate antibiotic regimen.

Gonococcal ophthalmia is highly contagious, and infected neonates should be managed with contact isolation for 24 hours after treatment is initiated. It is especially important that gloves be used for contact with the infected area. Extraocular gonococcal infections, such as arthritis, septicemia, or meningitis, require intensive treatment. Ophthalmologic consultation is suggested for neonates with ocular infection.

Some strains of *Neisseria gonorrhoeae* are resistant to penicillin. Attempts should be made to isolate the organism from both mother and child, and the antimicrobial susceptibility of all isolates should be determined. Information on susceptibilities is then available as a therapeutic guide, should other forms of antimicrobial therapy become necessary because of a poor clinical response to penicillin.

Group B *Streptococcus* Colonization and Disease

The proportion of pregnant women and neonates colonized with group B streptococci ranges from approximately 5-35%. Colonization of women during pregnancy may be intermittent, however. Occasionally, streptococci cause significant postpartum infection (eg, endometritis, amnionitis, and urinary tract infections), but rectal or genital colonization is usually asymptomatic.

Infection is frequently transmitted from the mother to the newborn, either in utero or intrapartum; nosocomial neonatal infection (probably neonate to neonate via the hands of personnel) also occurs. Group B streptococci (types Ia, Ib, Ic, II, III) are important causes of disease in the neonate and infant. Neonatal group B streptococcal disease has an incidence of 1-5 cases per 1,000 live births, although the incidence varies widely among hospitals. Early onset disease (ie, clinical disease that appears during the first 4 days after birth) occurs in approximately 1 infant per 100-200 colonized women. The risk of early onset disease is increased by low birth weight, prolonged labor, prolonged interval between rupture of amniotic membranes and delivery, and perinatal maternal infection. Low (or absent) levels of type-specific serum antibody also may predispose neonates to disease.

No specific recommendations for the prevention of neonatal group B streptococcal disease can be made. Routine prenatal cultures to detect colonization are not recommended, because colonization may be intermittent and the sensitivity of a single rectal or vaginal culture is approximately 70%. The administration of ampicillin throughout labor to high-risk colonized women (eg, those with premature onset of labor, rupture of the membranes, or fever) has decreased rates of infection in their infants. In addition, preliminary data suggest that the intrapartum administration of ampicillin to women who have previously delivered affected neonates may be beneficial.

Studies in which a penicillin was administered to neonates shortly after birth indicate a range of effectiveness in the prevention of group B streptococcal disease. At present, programs for antimicrobial chemoprophylaxis should be considered on an individual hospital basis. Routinely obtaining specimens for cultures in order to determine whether neonates have been colonized with group B streptococci is not recommended either to identify those who could be treated or to control infection.

Neonates with group B streptococcal disease may be treated in the intensive care area if contact isolation precautions are taken to prevent the transmission of bacterial infection. In view of the high percentage of colonized neonates within many nurseries and the lack of any effective means to eradicate colonization, routine identification and isolation of asymptomatic carriers are impractical. Other methods of control (eg, treatment of asymptomatic carriers with penicillin or treatment of the umbilical cord with triple dye or hexachlorophene) are impractical or unreliable for control of group B streptococci.

Detection of a nosocomial problem caused by group B streptococci is difficult, because most neonates have late onset disease, which may not appear until days or weeks after discharge from the nursery. If a cluster of cases occurs in neonates born at a single hospital, however, an investigation is warranted. Establishing cohorts of ill and colonized neonates in the nursery may be useful. Meticulous handwashing by all personnel, sufficient personnel on all shifts, and adequate spacing between neonates may be important in limiting neonate-to-neonate transmission within the nursery.

Listeria Infection

The epidemiology of infection with *L. monocytogenes* has remained obscure. Most cases are sporadic, although there have been epidemics. Infection occurs most frequently in infants, older persons, or others who have an immunologic abnormality, including pregnant women. In adults, infection probably comes from diverse sources, including environmental sources such as plants and vegetables, and perhaps animals; the role of sexual transmission is unknown. Infection in pregnant women may be asymptomatic, or it may occur as an acute febrile illness with other constitutional signs and symptoms; amnionitis is not uncommon. Listeriosis usually occurs in the second half of pregnancy and may be associated with spontaneous abortion or premature labor.

The pathogenesis of fetal infection with *Listeria* is uncertain. It is believed that the fetus or newborn acquires the infection most often transplacentally, through ascending maternal genital tract infection, or during birth; nosocomial transmission to newborns probably occurs as well. Signs of *Listeria* infection in the newborn are highly variable and often nonspecific. The clinical picture may be similar to that of group B streptococcal infection with early and late onset syndromes. Early onset listeriosis often resembles respiratory distress or heart failure; late onset disease more often causes meningitis.

Listeria can be cultured readily, although special techniques may be necessary to isolate the organism from stool and other sites with mixed flora. Gram stain of a fecal smear from an infected newborn may show the organism in profusion.

Prompt diagnosis and antibiotic treatment of maternal infection during pregnancy may prevent fetal or perinatal infection. Because some women have had repeated fetal infection with *Listeria*, some authorities suggest that the cervix and stools of the mother of an infected infant be cultured and the mother treated if either culture is positive. Reculturing during a subsequent pregnancy has also been suggested, but the usefulness of this measure has not been evaluated.

Neonates with *Listeria* infection should be managed in the nursery with drainage/secretion precautions.

Syphilis

Pregnant women should undergo serologic screening for syphilis at the first prenatal visit and after exposure to an infected partner. As false-negative screening tests may occur in early primary infection, a repeat test for syphilis or other sexually transmitted diseases should be performed if the patient belongs to a high-risk population. Serologic and other appropriate diagnostic tests should be performed if suspicious lesions develop. The specificity of serologic testing is high if both a nontreponemal screening test and a subsequent treponemal serologic test are reactive. Dark-field and histologic examinations are the most reliable. Congenital syphilis is most often acquired through hematogenous transplacental infection of the fetus, although direct contact of the neonate with infectious lesions during or after birth can also result in infection. Transplacental infection can occur throughout pregnancy and at any stage of maternal infection.

Pregnant women with syphilis should be treated with standard regimens for acquired primary, secondary, or early latent syphilis if they are not allergic to penicillin. Patients who are allergic to penicillin should be treated with erythromycin in a dose schedule appropriate for recently acquired syphilis in nonpregnant patients. This regimen is safe for both mother and fetus, but its efficacy in preventing congenital syphilis has not been adequately documented. Neonates born after treatment of the mother with erythromycin should be examined for congenital syphilis; assessment of the cerebrospinal fluid should be included. Tetracycline and the estolate ester of erythromycin should not be used in pregnant women because of their potential toxic effects.

The results of the maternal serologic tests and treatment, if given, should be recorded in the neonate's medical record or be made available to the neonate's physician. A serologic test for syphilis should be performed on cord or venous blood of neonates for whom the results of maternal tests or treatment are unavailable or questionable.

A diagnosis of congenital syphilis is frequently difficult to establish, because clinical evidence of infection may not be apparent at birth and the result of serologic tests may be difficult to interpret. Neonates with a positive result on a serologic test for syphilis or a history of partial or questionably adequate maternal treatment for infection must be followed carefully. A reactive serologic test for syphilis (eg, VDRL or FTA-ABS) on cord or neonatal blood does not necessarily indicate that the neonate is infected. If the reaction is caused only by passively transferred antibody, the VDRL titer is usually lower than the mother's and reverts to negative in 4-6 months. A positive result on the FTA-ABS test caused by passively transferred antibody may take as long as 1 year to become negative. A persistently reactive serologic test for syphilis suggests infection, and a rising titer is almost diagnostic. The IgM FTA-ABS test is not totally specific; because false-negative results may be obtained, a negative test result does not exclude active infection in the neonate.

Clinical symptoms of early congenital syphilis may be nonspecific. Long bone roentgenograms may be useful in establishing a diagnosis. The cerebrospinal fluid of infants with suspected or proven congenital syphilis should be examined for evidence of neurosyphilis.

Moist, open syphilitic lesions are infectious. Drainage/secretion precautions and blood/body fluid precautions should be used when it is suspected that a neonate has congenital syphilis. Health care personnel (and parents) should wear gloves when handling the neonate until appropriate antibiotic therapy has been administered for 24 hours. Individuals who had close contact with the neonate before isolation precautions and treatment were instituted should be examined clinically and tested serologically for infection.

Tuberculosis

Maternal Infection

Although tuberculosis occurs infrequently in most obstetric populations, prenatal visits have traditionally been a time to perform skin testing for infection with *Mycobacterium*. This screening test is especially important for populations at high risk of infection and in areas with high endemic rates of tuberculosis. In patients with a positive skin test for tuberculosis, a chest roentgenogram should be obtained to rule out active disease. The course of the disease is not altered by pregnancy, although the clinical condition may be exacerbated during the puerperium.

Because of the social environment in which tuberculosis occurs and the risk of significant morbidity and mortality to the newborn from the disease, the local health department should be notified about a suspected or documented case in a pregnant woman, a new mother, or her family. A thorough family study should be conducted to determine if others in contact with the mother or neonate are infected. Treatment should be initiated for anyone found to be infected and continuing care arranged.

A pregnant patient with active tuberculosis or a stable (healed) lesion should be managed as other patients with tuberculosis are managed; expert consultation is recommended. Sputum specimens for mycobacterial culture should be obtained, and antimicrobial susceptibilities to the primary drugs should be determined. Prompt initiation of chemotherapy for active disease is important to protect both the mother and fetus. Pregnant patients who are receiving isoniazid should also be given vitamin B_6 (50 mg daily) to avoid pyridoxine deficiency.

Prophylactic therapy with isoniazid may be indicated for selected patients. If abnormalities are not identified on the chest roentgenogram and active tuberculosis is not suspected in any other organ system the use of preventive therapy is problematic. Although isoniazid appears to have no harmful effects on the fetus, therapy during pregnancy should be given only for those with active tuberculous disease. If possible, preventive therapy with isoniazid should be delayed until after delivery. An exception is the pregnant woman who has been recently infected; for this woman, preventive therapy with isoniazid should begin when the infection is documented, but after the first trimester.

Physicians who care for nursing mothers should be aware that isoniazid is secreted in human milk, although no adverse effects on nursing infants have been demonstrated. Isoniazid, ethambutol, and rifampin appear to be relatively safe for the fetus. The benefit of ethambutol and rifampin for the therapy of active disease in the mother outweighs the risk to the infant. Streptomycin and pyrazinamide should not be used unless they are essential to control the disease.

Management of Exposed Newborns

The care of neonates born to mothers with tuberculosis should be individualized. Tuberculosis in neonates appears to result most commonly from airborne infection during the postnatal period; mothers with active, but undiagnosed and untreated, infections are often the source. Congenital tuberculosis (transplacental infection) is rare; when it does occur, however, it results in severe disease with high mortality. Establishing a definitive diagnosis of tuberculosis in a newborn is frequently difficult. Therapy should be initiated promptly, often on the basis of clinical judgment and a high index of suspicion.

A healthy neonate born to a woman with tuberculosis that is active or of unknown infectiousness can be managed routinely without special precautions in the nursery. If possible, separation of the mother and infant should be minimized. Several widely differing circumstances must be considered.

- *Mother with a positive tuberculin skin test reaction and no evidence of current disease.* In this situation, careful investigation of each person in the household or extended family to whom the infant may later be exposed is indicated. If no current disease is found in the mother or extended family, the infant should be tested with a Mantoux test (5 TU PPD) at 4-6 weeks of age, at 3-4 months of age, and at 12 months of age. In certain difficult social situations in which the family cannot be promptly tested, isoniazid (10 mg/kg/day) should be administered to the infant until skin testing of the family has ruled out the possibility that the infant will be in close contact with a case of active tuberculosis.
- *Mother with untreated (newly diagnosed) minimal disease or disease that has been treated for 2 or more weeks and is judged to be noncontagious*

at delivery. Careful investigation of the members of the household and extended family is mandatory. The infant should have a chest roentgenogram and a 5 TU PPD skin test at 4-6 weeks of age; if findings are normal, the infant should be tested again at 3-4 and 6 months of age. Separation of the mother and infant is not necessary if the mother's compliance with treatment is assured, and the mother may breast-feed. The infant should receive isoniazid even if the tuberculin skin test and chest roentgenogram do not suggest tuberculous disease. Cell-mediated immunity of a degree sufficient to mount a significant reaction to tuberculin skin testing may develop as late as 6 months of age, even if the infant was infected at birth. Isoniazid can be discontinued if the reaction to the PPD skin test is normal at 6 months of age and there is no active disease in family members. The infant should be examined carefully at monthly intervals. If compliance is doubtful and supervision impossible, Bacille Calmette-Guérin (BCG) vaccine may be indicated for the infant; if so, the infant should be separated from the mother until a BCG-induced tuberculin response has been demonstrated.

- *Mother has current disease suspected of being contagious at the time of delivery.* The mother and infant should be separated until the mother's disease is judged to be noncontagious. Otherwise, treatment is the same as that provided when the disease is judged to be noncontagious at delivery.

- *Mother has hematogenous spread tuberculosis (ie, meningitis, miliary disease, bone involvement, and so forth).* Congenital tuberculosis in the neonate is possible. If it is suspected that the neonate has congenital tuberculosis, 5 TU PPD skin testing and chest roentgenograms should be obtained promptly, and treatment of the neonate should begin at once. If no clinical or roentgenographic findings support the diagnosis of congenital tuberculosis, the infant should be separated from the mother until her disease is judged to be noninfectious. The infant should also be given isoniazid until 6 months of age, at which time the skin test should be repeated. If the infant has a positive reaction to the skin test at this time, isoniazid should be continued for a total of 12 months.

The administration of BCG vaccine should be considered for a neonate who has a negative reaction to the tuberculin skin test, but lives in a household with untreated or ineffectively treated individuals who have sputum-positive pulmonary tuberculosis. The vaccine may be given to infants from birth to 2 months of age without tuberculin testing if the infant is known not to have been exposed to the disease; thereafter, it should be given only to infants who have a negative skin test reaction. The skin test should be repeated 2-3 months after BCG vaccination, and the vaccination repeated if the infant still has a negative reaction. Neonates given BCG vaccine should not receive isoniazid and should be separated from their mothers or other infected individuals until they have a positive reaction to the tuberculin skin test.

Toxoplasmosis

Caused by the protozoan parasite *Toxoplasma gondii,* toxoplasmosis is usually an asymptomatic or mild, nonspecific illness that resembles infectious mononucleosis when it is acquired by older children or adults. Congenital toxoplasmosis, however, ranges from asymptomatic infection to severe infection that leads to death. Clinical manifestations of fetal infection include prematurity, intrauterine growth retardation, encephalitis, microcephaly or hydrocephalus, and chorioretinitis. Survivors may have severe sequelae.

Humans acquire toxoplasmosis by consuming poorly cooked meat or by ingesting sporulated oocysts excreted in cat feces. Congenital toxoplasmosis results from acute infection of the pregnant woman. Maternal infection during the first trimester is apparently associated with a lower rate of congenital infection, but the majority of the infected neonates are severely affected. Conversely, maternal infection during the third trimester results in a high rate of congenital infection, but the majority of infected neonates have no clinical manifestations of the infection.

Serologic tests for the diagnosis of toxoplasmosis are available, but they lack sufficient specificity to be of value for screening. Because the only risk to the fetus is from acute infection during pregnancy, routine serologic testing of pregnant women is not recommended. Similarly, serologic testing of domestic cats is not useful.

Seroconversion or a fourfold or greater increase in the IgG antibody titer on serial specimens tested simultaneously suggests recent infection. Congenitally infected infants usually have high levels of IgG antibodies to *Toxoplasma* organisms; they may also have IgM antibodies, but the absence of IgM-specific antibodies does not exclude a diagnosis of congenital toxoplasmosis. IgM-specific antibodies are best detected by a capture enzyme-linked immunosorbent assay. Infant and maternal sera should be tested in parallel, as the transplacental passage of IgG results in serum antibodies in both infected and uninfected infants. In uninfected infants, the antibody concentrations decline with time.

Congenital toxoplasmosis can be averted by preventing acute infection in pregnant women. Only thoroughly cooked meats should be eaten. Cat litter should be disposed of daily, as oocysts are not infective during the first 24 hours after passage. Domestic cats should be fed only commercially prepared cat food and should not be allowed to hunt wild rodents or to eat raw or partially cooked meat and kitchen scraps. Pregnant women who are seronegative or have unknown *Toxoplasma* titers should avoid gardening or yard work in areas to which cats have access.

The regimen of choice for treating acute toxoplasmosis is the synergistic combination of pyrimethamine plus either sulfadiazine or trisulfapyrimidine. Both pyrimethamine and the sulfonamides are potentially toxic, and the former is also potentially teratogenic. Limited studies, however, indicate that the frequency of congenital toxoplasmosis can be reduced in neonates born to pregnant women acutely infected and treated after the first trimester with a combination of drugs. Treatment of infants with congenital toxoplasmosis or congenital *Toxoplasma* infection with the combination of drugs is also recommended, although the optimal dosage and duration of therapy is uncertain; consultation with experts should be sought. Early diagnosis and treatment appears to be important; treatment of infants with asymptomatic infection may prevent late sequelae. Folinic acid (calcium leucovorin) should be administered also to prevent hematologic toxic reactions. Spiramycin, an antibiotic, has frequently been used in Europe for treatment of pregnant women and infants.

Neither patients with acquired toxoplasmosis nor neonates with congenital toxoplasmosis require isolation.

OTHER INFECTIOUS PROBLEMS DURING PREGNANCY

Antepartum Infections

Pyelonephritis

Most women who develop pyelonephritis during pregnancy enter pregnancy with asymptomatic bacteriuria. Urine should be screened for bacteria in selected patients (eg, in patients with a history of urinary tract infection or renal disease). Significant bacteriuria, once detected, should be treated appropriately, and follow-up cultures should be done periodically to ensure eradication of infection and to rule out recurrence. Pregnant patients with overt pyelonephritis may go into premature labor or septic shock. Accordingly, when pyelonephritis is diagnosed in pregnancy, it should be treated vigorously in the hospital with appropriate antibiotics.

Immunization During Pregnancy

Immunizing agents are not usually indicated during pregnancy, although there is no evidence that commonly used, inactivated bacterial or viral vaccines or toxoids have an adverse effect on the mother or fetus. Live virus vaccines should not be given except in the rare case in which the patient will be exposed to yellow fever or polio and the disease poses a greater threat than does vaccination. Pregnancy is a contraindication to vaccination against rubella, measles, and mumps, because these vaccines contain live, attenuated virus. Recommendations for vaccinations during pregnancy are shown in Table 6-2.

Intrapartum Infection (Clinical Chorioamnionitis)

Chorioamnionitis is diagnosed in approximately 1% of all pregnancies; it is diagnosed in a larger percentage of pregnancies with prolonged membrane rupture. Although signs and symptoms are often nonspecific, the infection should be suspected when maternal fever, maternal or fetal tachycardia, foul odor, or uterine tenderness develops. Evaluation of infection in the mother should include a complete blood count, blood culture, and a genital culture. Therapy consists of supportive care, delivery, and administration of antibiotics. The obstetrician should inform the nursery staff of the suspected diagnosis so that the neonate's condition can be evaluated appropriately.

Postpartum Infection

Nursery staff should be informed of any suspected or confirmed maternal disease, including any sustained maternal fever.

Genital Infection (Endometritis)

Endometritis occurs after 1-3% of vaginal deliveries and complicates 10-15% of cesarean deliveries. Furthermore, genital infections are

Table 6-2. Recommendations for Active and Passive Immunization During Pregnancy*

Immunizable Disease	Vaccine/Biologic: Indications for Immunization
	Live, Attenuated Virus Vaccines
Poliomyelitis	Avoid vaccine use if possible. Live oral polio vaccine (OPV) recommended if immediate risk of exposure to wild virus is substantial.
Measles	Vaccine contraindicated. Passive immunization with immune globulin, 0.25 ml/kg (maximum dose, 15 ml) as soon after exposure as possible may attenuate infection.
Mumps	Vaccine contraindicated during pregnancy.
Rubella	Vaccine contraindicated during pregnancy.
Yellow fever	Vaccine contraindicated except for unavoidable exposure to disease before end of pregnancy.
Smallpox	No current indication.
	Inactivated Virus Vaccines
Hepatitis B	Vaccine not contraindicated during pregnancy in a susceptible woman at high risk of hepatitis B infection. Risk of vaccine to the fetus should be negligible, although data on safety are not available.
Influenza	Standard vaccine recommendations (ie, high-risk underlying conditions, such as pulmonary, cardiac, or renal disease). If possible, avoid administration during first trimester.
Rabies	Pregnancy does not alter indications for postexposure prophylaxis with rabies immune globulin and vaccine. Preexposure prophylaxis may be indicated if risk of exposure to rabies is substantial.
	Live, Attenuated Bacterial Vaccine
Tuberculosis	BCG vaccine contraindicated during pregnancy unless immediate risk of unavoidable exposure to infective tuberculosis is excessive.
	Inactivated Bacterial Vaccines
Typhoid	No information available on safety during pregnancy. Use should reflect actual risk of disease and probable benefits of vaccine.
Cholera	No information available on safety during pregnancy. Vaccinate only to meet international travel requirements.
Meningococcal infection	Vaccine safety during pregnancy not established; avoid unless risk of exposure is substantial.
Pneumococcal infection	Vaccine safety during pregnancy not established; standard vaccine recommendations should be followed (ie, high-risk underlying conditions, such as chronic pulmonary, cardiac, or immunosuppressive disease).
Plague	No information available on safety of vaccine during pregnancy. Highly selective vaccination of individuals at substantial risk of disease.
	Toxoids
Tetanus, diptheria	Booster dose of adult TD toxoid (tetanus, full dose; diphtheria, reduced dose) if primary series incomplete or no booster within 10 years. Primary series for unimmunized women.

*For all products, consult the manufacturer's package insert for instruction for storage, handling, and administration. Biologics prepared by different manufacturers may vary.

frequently more severe after cesarean delivery than after vaginal delivery. Risk factors for infection include prolonged labor or membrane rupture, lower socioeconomic status, anemia, and trauma. The results of most studies indicate that internal fetal monitoring does not directly increase infection rates in the mother. Endometritis, which usually appears within the first few days after delivery, is characterized by fever, malaise, tachycardia, abdominal pain, or foul lochia. There may be no localizing signs early in the course of infection.

The condition of febrile postpartum patients should be evaluated by means of a pertinent history; complete physical examination; blood count; and blood, genital, and urine cultures. Bacteria most likely to cause infection are the gram-negative enteric aerobes (especially *E. coli*), selected aerobic streptococci (α-hemolytic streptococci, group B β-hemolytic streptococci, and the enterococci), gram-negative anaerobic rods (especially *Bacteroides fragilis*), and anaerobic cocci (*Peptococcus* and *Peptostreptococcus*). Infections may be mixed, and anaerobic genital culture may reveal infection with some organisms that necessitate special precautions or special therapy. Isolation procedures appropriate to the suspected type of infection should be instituted promptly.

Patients usually respond promptly to antibiotic therapy, but persistent fever, retained infected placenta, septic pelvic thrombophlebitis, or pelvic abscess are occasional complications.

Mastitis

Infection of the breast usually develops during or after the second week postpartum, most often after the patient has been discharged from the hospital. Local breast inflammation, often with fever, is the predominant sign. The breast secretions should be cultured and antimicrobial susceptibilities determined. Because *S. aureus* is commonly the cause, the antibiotic given should be active against this organism, as well as others; oral agents, such as dicloxacillin or a cephalosporin, are reasonable initial choices. Local warm compresses and analgesics are helpful adjunctive measures. Frank abscesses, which occur infrequently, require drainage. Opinions vary about the advisability of continuing breast-feeding. If there is no abscess that requires drainage, feeding from the uninfected breast can usually be continued; the involved breast should be expressed manually or with a breast pump.

Epidemic Puerperal Sepsis

Although epidemic nosocomial infections on obstetric services may be caused by a number of viral and bacterial pathogens, most epidemics have involved infections with group A streptococci. Epidemics of such lethal infections were reported as late as 1927, and the threat of group A streptococcal infection has remained long after the introduction of penicillin. Because this organism is an unusual inhabitant of the vagina, the source of infection in such an epidemic is often a hospital staff member rather than a patient. After the organism has been introduced into a unit, however, infected patients serve as reservoirs, and infection is transmitted from one patient to another on the hands of personnel.

Epidemics are better prevented than controlled. Although routine cultures of specimens from personnel are not useful, cultures of specimens obtained from obstetric care personnel who have possible group A streptococcal infection (eg, pharyngitis, impetigo, or other skin infections) are necessary. Personnel found to have streptococcal infection should be treated with appropriate dosages of penicillin or erythromycin for 10 days and prohibited from providing direct patient care until cultures are negative. Patients with group A streptococcal infection should be managed with contact isolation until treatment has been initiated with appropriate dosages of penicillin or other antibiotics effective against the organism involved. Hospital personnel must observe hand-washing and isolation precautions meticulously.

If two or more cases of group A streptococcal infection develop within a short period of time, hospital infection control personnel should be notified. In addition to isolating and treating infected patients, screening patients and personnel by cultures, and possibly treating carriers, may be necessary for control. Anal and vaginal carrier-disseminators of group A streptococci have been documented. As part of the epidemiologic evaluation, isolates should be saved and submitted to the state health department laboratory for M and T typing. During severe epidemics, patients should receive prophylactic penicillin or sulfonamide, and it may be necessary to cancel elective surgery.

MANAGEMENT OF NURSERY OUTBREAKS OF DISEASE

Because many infections become apparent only after neonates leave the hospital, each hospital should establish a procedure to be used during a suspected or confirmed epidemic for disease surveillance of recently discharged neonates. Procedures for control of nursery epidemics depend on the microorganism responsible for the outbreak, the reservoir of infection, and the mode of transmission. An epidemiologic investigation should be undertaken to identify these factors. The hospital infection control committee and the proper health authorities should be notified promptly about all suspected or confirmed epidemics.

During epidemics, a comprehensive program of infection control is required. If a problem is suspected, the first step is to evaluate it promptly and carefully. The result of this initial assessment determines the need for further epidemiologic studies to define the source and means of transmission of the infections, as well as the type of specific control measures that are required. Even if an intensive investigation is not indicated, the results of the control measures should be evaluated to ensure that they have been effective and the problem has been resolved.

Infection with *Staphylococcus aureus*

Colonization of newborns by *S. aureus* is relatively common, but disease is usually sporadic; the frequency of disease is dependent on multiple factors, including the virulence of the colonizing strain. Although the prevalence of *S. aureus* colonization of neonates fluctuates and may at times be more than 50%, nurseries with good infection control practices are often able to restrict neonate colonization rates to 20% or less. Disease may occur with any prevalence of colonization in the nursery, however. The incubation period for staphylococcal lesions is highly variable. Most frequently, disease caused by infection with *S. aureus* occurs in neonates during the second week of postnatal life, after the neonates have been discharged from the nursery. Infections detected in neonates before discharge from the nursery, therefore, may represent only a small fraction of the total.

Generally, *S. aureus* is transmitted to neonates on the inadequately washed hands of personnel; colonized and infected neonates serve as the reservoir. Rarely, a personnel disseminator, with or without staphylococcal lesions, is responsbile for a cluster of infection. Most colonized personnel do not disseminate their organisms, however, and the colonization is insignificant epidemiologically. The carriers require no special treatment, and routine culturing of specimens from hospital personnel is not recommended. Fomites are not usually implicated in the transmission of *S. aureus* infections.

A presumptive epidemic in a nursery may be defined as the occurrence of cutaneous infection in two or more neonates simultaneously (or within a short period of time), the development of a breast abscess in a mother, or a deep infection in a neonate. Another

rough guideline is that no more than 3-4 full-term neonates per 1,000
live births should develop *S. aureus* infection while in the nursery. If
an epidemic or unacceptably high frequency of infection is suspected,
the following approaches should be considered:

- Infants with definite or suspected staphylococcal disease should
  be placed in strict isolation.
- Meticulous patient care techniques should be reemphasized and
  cohorts instituted for infected, colonized, and newly admitted
  neonates. All neonates in a room should be discharged and the
  room carefully cleaned before other neonates are admitted to that
  room. A strictly enforced cohort system for both neonates and
  personnel virtually eliminates contact between infected and uninfected neonates, interrupting disease transmission.
- The extent of disease in neonates recently discharged from the
  hospital should be determined, either by a survey of the physicians or health care providers who take care of most neonates
  born in the hospital or by a survey of the parents of these
  neonates. Health departments or nursing associations may provide assistance with the survey.
- Specimens obtained from the umbilical stump of infants and the
  anterior nares of personnel should be cultured to determine the
  prevalence of colonization and to identify the staphylococcal
  strains involved in the outbreak for antibiotic sensitivity testing
  and phage typing. Occasionally, it is necessary to identify personnel colonized with a strain that has been implicated in
  epidemic disease in a closed population and to remove these
  carriers from areas of patient contact. These personnel should be
  treated with topical intranasal antibiotics; sometimes, orally administered antibiotics are also necessary. The goal of therapy is to
  eliminate carriage of an epidemiologically virulent strain, which
  may be extremely difficult.
- Careful hand-washing by personnel is of paramount importance.
- During periods of epidemic disease, full-term infants may be
  bathed, in the diaper area only, with hexachlorophene (3%) as
  soon after birth as possible and daily until they are discharged.
  The hexachlorophene should be thoroughly washed off after
  bathing is completed, and should not be used for routine bathing.
  Hexachlorophene should be used only for full-term infants.
- Application of triple dye or bacitracin ointment to the umbilical
  stump of all infants twice daily throughout the nursery stay can
  be helpful.

- In unusual circumstances, it may be necessary to give oral antistaphylococcal agents to all infants and personnel who are carriers.

- Persons involved in hospital outbreaks of staphylococcal disease should be observed and warned of the possibility of delayed disease and the spread to family members.

- Surveillance in the nursery should be continued for several weeks after the epidemic has apparently terminated. Observation for disease in neonates (both in the nursery and at home for several weeks after discharge) is the most reliable index. Weekly cultures of specimens from the umbilical cord and nares of neonates in the nursery and of specimens from the nares of personnel may be valuable for a short time, but long periods of serial surveillance of neonates and personnel are not practical. Monitoring of neonates for *S. aureus* is probably the best method for determining the need for prevalence surveys in neonates or personnel.

Infectious Diarrhea: *Escherichia coli*

Measures for the management of a nursery epidemic of diarrheal disease caused by *E. coli* are also appropriate for the management of diarrheal disease caused by other bacterial (eg, *Salmonella*) or viral pathogens. The reservoir of infection is usually the intestinal tract of ill or colonized neonates, and infection is usually transmitted from neonate to neonate on the inadequately washed hands of personnel. Occasionally, other sources, such as extrinsically contaminated formula, may be found.

Epidemic enteric disease may be caused by 1) strains of enterotoxin-producing *E. coli* that may or may not be agglutinated by commercial antisera or 2) specific enteropathogenic *E. coli* that do not usually produce known enterotoxins. Strains of *E. coli* can be identified by their colony characteristics and antimicrobial susceptibility patterns; when a single strain is predominant or pure in cultures from ill neonates, when the strain is isolated from ill neonates much more often than from those who remain well, and when there is no other obvious pathogen such as *Shigella* or *Salmonella*, that strain is likely to be the epidemic strain. It should be serotyped and tested for enterotoxin production if this can be done quickly and reliably by available laboratories.

Because asymptomatic carriage of an identifiable pathogen may perpetuate an outbreak, a rectal specimen for culture should be obtained from neonates in proximity to the index case or to other symptomatic neonates.

Diseased and colonized neonates should be placed into strict cohorts and segregated from the other neonates; personnel providing care for the culture-positive neonates should not provide care for neonates who have not been infected or colonized. If possible, it is helpful to reduce the number of neonates in the nursery. If multiple cases occur, the nursery room should be closed to admissions and not reopened until all neonates in the room have been discharged and the room has been cleaned. Newborns should be discharged home, not transferred to other nurseries. In some outbreaks, it may be necessary to close the entire nursery to all new admissions and to make other arrangements for newborns.

Appropriate antibiotics should be administered to all neonates excreting the epidemic strain. If serotype information is not available to identify the epidemic strain, all symptomatic neonates, as well as those in the same room or cohort, should be treated. Antibiotic selection should be based on susceptibility tests. Colistin (10-15 mg/kg/day) or neomycin (100 mg/kg/day), administered orally in three or four doses for 5 days, may be useful. Although treatment of this duration may be adequate, neonates who must remain in the nursery should be retreated if they continue to carry the pathogenic strain (as determined by fluorescent antibody study or culture of three consecutive specimens obtained after completion of antibiotic therapy). During an outbreak, prophylactic administration of colistin or neomycin to all neonates may be appropriate, although efficacy may be variable.

Personnel who are carriers of the epidemic organism have been implicated only rarely as the source of an epidemic, but they should be identified by culture of stool specimens. Carrier-disseminators should be removed from the nursery until they have been treated and are culture-negative.

Antiseptic and aseptic techniques should be reviewed and strictly observed. Particular emphasis should be placed on hand-washing by personnel after each contact with each neonate. Requiring personnel to wear gowns when caring for infected or colonized neonates and to wash their hands, even if they wore disposable gloves, after handling infected neonates and contaminated materials may reduce the degree of contamination of hands and clothing by the infecting pathogen.

Although *E. coli* is seldom transmitted from neonate to neonate by means of contaminated fomites, nursery practices should be evaluated; equipment that may be contaminated, especially solutions or articles that would have contact with the gastrointestinal tract of neonates, may need to be cultured. After all infected or colonized neonates have been discharged, the nursery, including the equipment, should be thoroughly cleaned and disinfected. Neonates recently discharged should be surveyed. All symptomatic neonates should be examined, specimens obtained for culture, and treatment provided. Surveillance by periodic examination of cultures from neonates, personnel, and other sources of contamination should be continued for a short period after the outbreak has been controlled. If the pathogen is not recovered from cultures, surveillance can be ended.

Klebsiella and Other Gram-Negative Bacteria

Gram-negative bacteria, especially *Klebsiella pneumoniae*, frequently cause infections in nurseries, particularly in intensive care nurseries. Strains of these bacteria that are resistant to various antibiotics, including gentamicin, kanamycin, and chloramphenicol, are becoming increasingly common. Thus, these organisms may be virulent, invasive, and unusually difficult to eradicate.

The physician in charge of the nursery should be aware of all illness in the neonates and the nature of infections in personnel so that clusters of infections are recognized and appropriately investigated. Because nursery-acquired infections may become evident only several weeks to months after discharge, this physician should be notified by other physicians in the community of serious infections in infants who have recently been discharged from the nursery.

Several cases of infection occurring in infants in physical proximity or caused by an unusual pathogen may indicate an epidemic, in which case epidemiologic or bacteriologic surveys may be necessary to identify the source. When these surveys confirm an epidemic, infection control procedures should be instituted promptly. Although clinical infection with *Klebsiella* and other gram-negative bacteria may occur at various sites, the intestinal tract is the most frequent site of colonization; therefore, stool cultures (and perhaps cultures of specimens from other sites) should be obtained from all neonates in the nursery to identify rapidly those who are colonized. Selective media containing antibiotics may be used to simplify isolation of the specific pathogen.

The infected neonates should be segregated and managed with appropriate isolation precautions (eg, contact isolation or enteric precautions). Neonate isolation techniques should include the use of disposable diapers and gloves. A strict cohort system should be established immediately. Personnel providing care for infected or colonized neonates should not provide care for uninfected neonates, as transmission appears to occur despite careful hand washing. The pattern of antibiotic use in the nursery may have to be altered periodically to avoid bacterial resistance.

Necrotizing Enterocolitis

Occasionally, neonates in the nursery develop necrotizing enterocolitis. This illness may be defined by pathologic examination, by compatible findings on an abdominal roentgenogram, and by a symptom complex that includes abdominal distention, gastrointestinal bleeding, gastric retention, and palpable loops of bowel. Necrotizing enterocolitis occurs predominantly in preterm neonates; although neonates at high risk of disease can be identified, the etiology and pathophysiology are poorly understood. Cases often occur in clusters, and several investigators have noted that neonates whose bowel has been colonized by specific strains of bacteria are more likely to develop necrotizing enterocolitis than are neonates colonized by different strains.

These data suggest that it may be prudent to manage neonates with suspected or confirmed necrotizing enterocolitis with enteric precautions, including the use of gown and gloves when working directly with the neonate or articles likely to be contaminated with feces. A cluster of cases may require the establishment of a strict cohort of neonates colonized with a common bacterial strain. A cohort of personnel should also be established to care for the affected neonates.

Administration of prophylactic oral or systemic antibiotics in an effort to prevent necrotizing enterocolitis in neonates has not been successful and is likely to result in the emergence of resistant bacteria.

Group A *Streptococcus*

Epidemics of infection with strains of group A streptococci are uncommon at present. If this problem should arise, the following steps are recommended:

- Determine the extent of the epidemic by culturing any lesions and the umbilical stumps of all neonates in the nursery.
- Institute a cohort system. The nursery need not be closed to new admissions.
- Employ the various approaches that have been used to control epidemics, including isolation and treatment of all culture-positive neonates (cohort isolation is satisfactory), fomite control, and careful hand-washing. A complete epidemiologic investigation with isolation or treatment of carriers is essential to control.

Use isolation techniques (eg, drainage/secretion precautions, physical segregation in cohorts) for all neonates who have had contact with infected persons in order to reduce the number of colonized neonates in the nursery who may serve as a reservoir for infection.

- Provide prophylaxis for all neonates with benzathine penicillin G (50,000 units/kg); treat neonates with disease caused by group A streptococci with penicillin G (50,000-100,000 units/kg/day in two or three divided doses) for 10 days.

- Conduct a telephone survey of the parents or pediatricians of recently discharged, exposed neonates to determine whether any neonate is ill, although most neonates carrying group A streptococci will be free of disease or will have only a mild omphalitis. Examine symptomatic neonates and obtain specimens for culture; institute antibiotic treatment, if appropriate.

- Obtain culture specimens from the nose, throat, and any cutaneous lesion of all nursery personnel. Anal carriage of group A streptococci has been implicated as the cause of epidemics of surgical wound infections; to avoid the need for anal cultures from all nursery personnel, epidemiologic techniques should be used in an effort to identify those few personnel most likely to be disseminating infection. Personnel with positive cultures should be removed from the nursery and treated until cultures are negative.

- Continue surveillance in the nursery for several weeks after the epidemic has ended. Obtain specimens for culture from neonates just before they are discharged. If the problem persists, weekly nose and throat cultures of nursery personnel may be indicated.

THE ENVIRONMENT: CLEANING, DISINFECTION, AND STERILIZATION

The physician in charge and the nursing supervisor of the obstetric and nursery areas should work with the infection control officer and other groups as appropriate (eg, representatives of the respiratory therapy service, central supply, and housekeeping) to establish an environmental control program for the labor, delivery, and nursery areas. This program should include specific procedures in a written policy manual for cleaning and disinfection or sterilization of patient care areas, equipment, and supplies. Consultation for specific details and problems is essential. Nursing supervisors should ensure that these procedures are carried out correctly.

Methods of Sterilizing and Disinfecting Patient Care Equipment

All medical and hospital personnel should understand the difference between sterilization and disinfection. Sterilization is the destruction of all microorganisms, including spores; disinfection is simply a reduction in the number of contaminating microorganisms. High-level disinfection is the elimination or destruction of all microorganisms, except spores. Cleaning is the physical removal of organic material or soil, including microorganisms, from objects.

Equipment that enters normally sterile tissue or the vascular system should be sterile. For neonates, equipment that comes into contact with mucous membranes or that has prolonged or intimate contact with skin should also be sterile. Much of the equipment required in perinatal care areas can be used safely if it is satisfactorily cleaned and disinfected, however; clean, dry surfaces do not support the growth of microorganisms.

It is sometimes necessary to decontaminate equipment before it is cleaned and sterilized or disinfected in order to allow processing without the risk of exposure of personnel to hazardous microbes. The equipment must be cleaned thoroughly to remove all blood, tissue, secretions, food, and other residue. Without thorough cleaning, no method of sterilization or disinfection can be effective. Furthermore, some chemical disinfectants are inactivated by organic materials.

Sterilization

Methods of sterilization include steam autoclaving, dry heat, and gaseous (ethylene oxide) or liquid chemical (eg, 2% glutaraldehyde) techniques. The preferred method of sterilization is steam autoclaving, because this is the least expensive method and provides the greatest margin of safety. Some equipment may be damaged by steam, however, and must be sterilized by another method.

Equipment made of material that absorbs ethylene oxide usually requires 8-12 hours of aeration after sterilization with ethylene oxide before it can be used again. Ethylene oxide sterilization of supplies or equipment should be preceded by a comprehensive review of authoritative data on the aeration time required for each material to be processed and the extent to which toxicity standards have been established. An ethylene oxide sterilization plan requires the presence of sufficient backup equipment to allow time for aeration.

Equipment that cannot be sterilized with steam or ethylene oxide may be satisfactorily sterilized after cleaning by immersion for 10 hours in 2% glutaraldehyde or other acceptable liquid sporicide; this should be followed by three rinses with sterile water (or tap water with at least 10 mg of hypochlorite per ml), thorough drying, and packaging in sterile wrappers.

High-Level Disinfection

Equipment that does not need to be sterilized may be subjected to high-level disinfection. Both hot water pasteurization and chemical disinfection are satisfactory. Pasteurization of equipment requires immersing it in water at 80°C-85°C (176°F-185°F) for 15 minutes or 75°C (167°F) for 30 minutes. After air drying (preferably in a cabinet with heated, filtered air), disinfected items should be aseptically wrapped and stored until needed. Although spores are not eradicated by this method, bacterial and viral decontamination is adequate. The original reports of the equipment manufacturer should be consulted for a list of any parts or materials that may be warped or damaged at these temperatures.

The choice of liquid chemicals for high-level disinfection depends on the type of equipment to be disinfected. In many instances, immersion of the equipment for 30 minutes in 2% glutaraldehyde or an environmental iodophor solution (500 ppm available iodine),followed by three rinses with sterile water (or tap water with at least 10 mg of hypochlorite per liter) and thorough drying, is satisfactory.

Cleaning and Disinfecting Noncritical Surfaces

Selection of Disinfectants

Although numerous disinfectants are available, no single agent or preparation is ideal for all purposes. Consideration should be given to the agent and its special use as well as to the types of organisms likely to be contaminating the object that is to be disinfected. Special attention should be given to the recommended concentration of each disinfectant and its time of exposure. Unnecessary exposure of neonates to disinfectants should be avoided, and strict adherence to manufacturers' recommendations is essential.

Hexachlorophene preparations are not disinfectants and should not be used on equipment or environmental surfaces. Iodophors, chlorine compounds, phenolic compounds, and glutaraldehyde are satisfactory disinfectants. Only iodophor or quaternary disinfectant-detergent products registered by the U.S. Environmental Protection Agency and recommended by the manufacturer for nursery surfaces with which neonates have contact should be used. Phenolic compounds, especially if used in inappropriate concentrations or on surfaces with which neonates have direct contact, have been associated with hyperbilirubinemia. Information about specific label claims of commerical germicides can be obtained by writing to the Disinfectants Branch, Office of Pesticides, Environmental Protection Agency, 401 M Street, SW, Washington, DC 20460.

General Housekeeping

The following order of cleaning is recommended:

1. Patient areas
2. Accessory areas
3. Adjacent halls

It is not known if floor bacteria are a source of nosocomial infection, but regular cleaning prevents the accumulation of pathogenic bacteria. Disinfectant-detergents have been shown to be more effective than soap and water alone in cleaning floors, although hospital floors are rapidly recontaminated after disinfection. Available disinfectant-detergents may differ in effectiveness.

In the cleaning procedure, dust should not be dispersed into the air. Removal of dust by a dry vacuum machine, followed by wet vacuuming, is effective in cleaning and disinfecting hospital floors. Once dust has been removed, scrubbing with a mop and disinfectant-detergent solution should be sufficient. Mop heads should be machine-laundered and thoroughly dried daily.

Standard types of portable vacuum cleaners should not be used in nurseries or delivery areas because particulate matter and microbial contamination in the room may be disturbed and distributed by the exhaust jet. Vacuum cleaners that discharge outside the patient care area (ie, central vacuum cleaning systems or portable vacuums) should be used so that only the cleaning wand, floor tool, and vacuum hose are brought into the patient care area. Central vacuum cleaning systems are most efficiently installed during extensive remodeling or construction of new units.

Cabinet counters, work surfaces, and similar horizontal areas may be subject to heavy contamination during routine use. These areas should be cleaned at least once a day with a disinfectant-detergent and clean cloths; friction cleaning is important to ensure physical removal of dirt and contaminating microorganisms. Surfaces that are contaminated by patient specimens or accidental spills should be carefully cleaned and disinfected; iodophors formulated for environmental cleaning, phenolic compounds, or hypochlorite are useful disinfectants for this type of surface decontamination.

Walls, windows, and storage shelves may be reservoirs of pathogenic microorganisms if grossly soiled or if dust and dirt are allowed to accumulate. These areas—particularly windowsills and other horizontal surfaces—and similar noncritical surfaces should be scrubbed periodically with a disinfectant-detergent solution as part of the general housekeeping program. Aerosols of phenolic or other disinfectants are not reliable for disinfecting hard surfaces; this method is not recommended.

Faucet aerators may be useful to reduce water splashing in sinks, but they are notoriously susceptible to contamination with a variety of water-loving bacteria. Removing aerators periodically for cleaning and disinfection or sterilization should reduce contamination, at least temporarily. Sinks and drain traps are usually heavily contaminated, frequently with the same bacteria that cause infections in patients; epidemiologically, however, these bacterial reservoirs have only rarely been implicated as the source of bacterial infection in neonates. Sinks should be scrubbed clean daily with a disinfectant-detergent; drain traps should not need routine cleaning or disinfection.

Written policies should be established for the removal and disposal of solid wastes. Sturdy plastic liners should be used in trash receptacles; these liners should be sealed before they are removed from the trash receptacles. In patient care areas, trash receptacles should be cleaned and disinfected regularly. Infectious material requires special handling and disposal.

Special housekeeping personnel should be assigned to clean the nursery. If the nursery is small, they may also be assigned to work in the obstetric areas or other "clean" areas of the hospital (eg, offices, psychiatric services, or elective surgical areas). Housekeeping personnel assigned permanently to the obstetric or nursery areas should wear scrub uniforms, as should other full-time personnel; those not assigned to these areas exclusively should wear clean gowns when entering the areas. Daily cleaning of the nursery should take place when most neonates are not present.

Cleaning and Disinfecting Patient Care Equipment

Incubators, Open Care Units, and Bassinets

After a neonate has been discharged, the care unit used by that neonate should be cleaned and disinfected thoroughly. An iodophor or quaternary ammonium disinfectant-detergent registered by the U.S. Environmental Protection Agency is recommended for this purpose. Manufacturers' directions should be followed carefully. A bassinet or incubator should never be cleaned when occupied. Infants who remain in the nursery for an extended period should be transferred to a cleaned and disinfected unit periodically.

When a care unit is being cleaned and disinfected, all detachable parts should be removed and scrubbed meticulously. If the incubator has a fan, it should be cleaned and disinfected; manufacturer's instructions should be followed to avoid equipment damage. The air filter need not be discarded each time the incubator is cleaned, but it should be removed and autoclaved weekly or each time the unit is cleaned. Mattresses should be replaced when the surface covering is broken, because such a break precludes effective disinfection or sterilization. Mattresses may be sterilized by heat or gas. Portholes and porthole cuffs and sleeves are easily contaminated, often heavily; cuffs should be replaced on a regular schedule or cleaned and disinfected frequently with freshly prepared mild soap or quaternary ammonium disinfectant-detergent solutions. Incubators not in use should be thoroughly dried by running the incubator "hot" without water in the reservoir for 24 hours after disinfection.

Evaporative humidifiers in incubators usually do not produce contaminated aerosols, but contaminated water reservoirs may be responsible for direct rather than airborne transmission of infection. Reservoirs should be filled only with sterile water; they should be drained and refilled with sterile water every 24 hours. In many areas of the United States or in hospitals with a central ventilation system, environmental humidity may be sufficiently high to eliminate the need for additional humidification in most cases and water reservoirs may be left dry. If humidification is necessary, a source of humidity external to the incubator may be preferable to incubator humidifiers, because an external humidifier can be changed daily and the equipment sent for cleaning and sterilization or disinfection.

Nebulizers, Water Traps, and Respiratory Support Equipment

Because nebulizers are easily contaminated, nebulizers and attached tubing should be replaced by clean, sterile equipment (or equipment that has been subjected to high-level disinfection) every 12-24 hours. Failure to replace tubing may result in contamination of freshly cleaned equipment. Water traps should also be replaced daily by autoclaved or disinfected equipment. Only sterile water should be used for nebulizers or water traps; residual water should be discarded when these containers are refilled. Water condensed in tubing loops should be removed and discarded and should not be allowed to reflux into the container.

Other Equipment

Cleaning and disinfection or sterilization of equipment should be performed between use on successive patients. Equipment that is used for only one patient should be replaced, cleaned, and disinfected or sterilized according to an established schedule. For many types of equipment, this may be at least once a day. Disposable equipment should be replaced with approximately the same frequency as reusable equipment is recycled. Disposable equipment should never be reused.

Resuscitators, face masks, and other items used in direct contact with neonates should be dismantled, thoroughly cleaned, and sterilized, if possible. Alternately, the equipment may be subjected to high-level disinfection with liquid chemicals or by pasteurization. Equipment such as tubing for respiratory or oxygen therapy should be either sterilized or discarded after use.

Stethoscopes and similar types of diagnostic instruments should be wiped with iodophor or alcohol before use. Tubing, connectors, and jars of suction machines should be replaced daily with cleaned and sterilized equipment.

Procedures should be established to ensure that the neonate warmers used for resuscitation in the delivery areas are cleaned regularly, as well as after each use; they should always be stocked with clean, sterile equipment and supplies, available and ready for use when needed.

Cultures of Environmental Surfaces and Equipment

Routine cultures of equipment after cleaning and disinfection are expensive and time consuming; they should not be a substitute for specific, clearly written, and carefully followed procedures for cleaning and disinfection. Cultures of environmental surfaces and equipment may be useful as part of epidemiologic investigations, however, and an occasional, selective bacteriologic survey of particular patient care areas or equipment may help determine the effectiveness of existing procedures. These studies should be coordinated with the infection control committee and the microbiology laboratory.

Neonatal Linen

Procedures for laundering, making up packs, and delivering linen to the nursery should be established by the medical, nursing, laundry, and administrative staffs of the hospital.

Each delivery of clean linen should contain sufficient linen for at least one 8-hour shift. Linen should be brought to the nursery from the laundry in a closed cabinet that can also serve as the storage unit. If this system is not used, the linen should be stored in specifically designated cabinets in a clean area of the laundry. Traditionally, linen used in the intensive care, intermediate care, continuing care, and admission/observation areas is autoclaved, but the need for this to prevent infections in newborns has not been established by any studies. Autoclaved linen is probably not necessary in normal newborn care areas.

No new garments or linen should be used for neonates without prior laundering. In order to prevent methemoglobinemia, garments should not be marked with aniline dyes.

Disposable Diapers

It is acceptable to use disposable diapers rather than cloth diapers in a nursery. The significance of nonsterile diapers in the epidemiology of neonatal disease has not been established. Disposable diapers not labeled as sterile may be acceptable for most neonates. Presterilized diapers are probably preferable for small neonates, for those with a diaper rash, and for those with other skin lesions that are prone to secondary infection. Clinical data are not available, however, to support this assumption.

Care of Soiled Linen

An established procedure for the disposal of soiled linen should be strictly followed. Chutes for the transfer of soiled linen from patient care areas to the laundry are not acceptable unless they are under negative air pressure. Soiled linen should be discarded into impervious plastic bags placed in hampers that are easy to clean and disinfect. Soiled diapers should be placed into special diaper receptacles immediately after removal from the neonate; they should never be rinsed in the nursery. All personnel should be aware that handling dirty diapers with bare hands can result in heavy contamination and transient colonization of the hands with microorganisms that cannot be eliminated easily with hand-washing and can be readily transmitted to the next neonate for whom they provide care.

Plastic bags of soiled diapers (reusable or disposable) and other linen should be sealed and removed from the nursery at least every 8 hours. Individuals who collect the bags of soiled diapers or linen need not enter the nursery if all bags are placed outside the nursery. Sealed bags of reusable, soiled nursery linens should be taken to the laundry at least twice each day; sealed bags of disposable diapers should also be taken away at least twice a day.

Laundering

Diapers and soiled linen from the nurseries should not be removed from their sealed bags until they reach the laundry. They should be washed separately from other hospital linen. It is important that nursery linen remain soft. Acidification neutralizes the alkalis used in the washing process and is responsible for the greatest bacterial destruction.

Fatal poisoning has been observed when an antimildew agent that contained a high concentration of the sodium salt of pentachlorophenol was used in the final rinse in a laundry. Similarly, the chemical trichlorcarbanilide should not be used in hospial laundering because it may be harmful.

In order to avoid such potential hazards associated with chemicals or enzymes used in the hospital laundry, the physician in charge should know of all agents in use and should be informed before any changes are made in laundry chemicals or procedures. Currently, there are no legal requirements for testing laundry or cleaning agents for special hazards to neonates. Therefore, caution should be exercised when new laundry or cleaning agents are introduced into the nursery or when procedures are changed.

RESOURCES AND RECOMMENDED READING

American Academy of Pediatrics, Committee on Infectious Disease: Report of the Committee on Infectious Disease, 21 ed. Elk Grove Village IL, AAP, 1988

American College of Obstetricians and Gynecologists: Genital Human Papillomavirus Infections (ACOG Technical Bulletin 105). Washington DC, ACOG, 1987

American College of Obstetricians and Gynecologists: Herpes Simplex Virus Infections (ACOG Technical Bulletin 102). Washington DC, ACOG, 1987

American College of Obstetricians and Gynecologists: Immunization During Pregnancy (ACOG Technical Bulletin 64). Washington DC, ACOG, 1982

American College of Obstetricians and Gynecologists: Perinatal viral and parasitic infections (ACOG Technical Bulletin 114). Washington DC, ACOG, 1988

American College of Obstetricians and Gynecologists: Human Immunodeficiency Virus Infections (ACOG Technical Bulletin). Washington DC, ACOG, 1988

Bernbaum J, Anolik R, Polin RA, et al: Development of the premature infant's host defense system and its relationship to routine immunization. Clin Perinatol 11(1):73-84, 1984

Public Health Service, Department of Health and Human Services: Guideline for infection control in hospital personnel. HHS Publication No (CDC)83-8314. Atlanta, Centers for Disease Control, 1983

Public Health Service, Department of Health and Human Services: Guideline for isolation precautions in hospitals. HHS Publication No (CDC)83-8314. Atlanta, Centers for Disease Control, 1983

Smolen P, Bland R, Heiligenstein E, et al: Antibody response to oral polio vaccine in premature infants. J Pediatr 103(6):917-919, 1983

Vohr BR, Oh W: Age of diphtheria, tetanus and pertussis immunization of special care nursery graduates. Pediatrics 77(4):569-571, 1986

7

MATERNAL AND NEWBORN NUTRITION

Over the past 15 years, concern about the nutritional status of pregnant women has increased because of the possible association of nutritional deficiencies with the delivery of low-birth-weight and preterm infants. Thus, maternal nutrition and, by extension, fetal nutrition are important factors that can be influenced in efforts to reduce perinatal mortality.

NUTRITIONAL RISK FACTORS

During the initial or later prenatal visits, a pregnant woman should be asked about her food intake. Any major or potential nutritional risk factors should be identified. If necessary, the patient may be referred to a registered dietitian or nutritionist for dietary counseling. In addition, educational materials on nutrition that are available from the American College of Obstetricians and Gynecologists, the US Public Health Service, and the March of Dimes may be given to the patient. If economically unable to meet her nutritional needs, the patient should be referred to public agencies or to the Women, Infants, and Children (WIC) program for assistance.

DIETARY RECOMMENDATIONS

The recommended dietary allowances and recommended energy intakes for adolescent and young adult women when nonpregnant, pregnant, and lactating are listed in Table 7-1. These recommendations should be considered a general guide to nutrition in formulating a balanced diet.

193

Table 7-1. Recommended Daily Dietary Allowances for Adolescent and Adult Nonpregnant, Pregnant, and Lactating Women

Nutrient (unit)	Non pregnant			Pregnant	Lactating
	15-18 yr	19-22 yr	23-50 yr		
Energy (kcal)	2,100	2,100	2,000	+300	+500
Protein (g)	46	44	44	+30	+20
Calcium (mg)	1,200	800	800	+400	+400
Phosphorus (mg)	1,200	800	800	+400	+400
Magnesium (mg)	300	300	300	+150	+150
Iron (mg)	18	18	18	+30-60	+30-60
Zinc (mg)	15	15	15	+5	+10
Vitamin A (μg retinol equivalents)	800	800	800	+200	+400
Vitamin D (μg)	10	7.5	5	+5	+5
Vitamin E (mg)	8	8	8	+2	+3
Vitamin C (mg)	60	60	60	+20	+40
Thiamin (mg)	1.1	1.1	1.0	+0.4	+0.5
Riboflavin (mg)	1.3	1.3	1.2	+0.3	+0.5
Niacin (mg)	14	14	13	+2	+5
Vitamin B_6 (mg)	2	2	2	+0.6	+0.5
Folacin (mg)	400	400	400	+400	+100
Vitamin B_{12} (μg)	3	3	3	+1	+1

Adapted from National Research Council, Food and Nutrition Board: *Recommended Dietary Allowances,* 9 ed. Washington, DC, National Academy of Sciences, 1980

Caloric Intake

The average recommended caloric intake for a pregnant woman is 2,300 kcal/day, in a patient over 23 years of age. This may be excessive for a sedentary woman, but inadequate for a very active and growing adolescent. Thus, energy intake should be regulated on the basis of weight gain. The usual pattern is to gain 1-2 kg in the first trimester, 0.4 kg/week in the second and early third trimesters, with a decrease to 0.35 kg/week toward the end of pregnancy.

Women who are underweight before pregnancy and who gain less than 9 kg by the end of gestation have a relatively high incidence of low-birth-weight infants. Obese women with weight gains of 7-8 kg by the end of gestation, however, may have normal-sized infants. The lowest frequencies of low-birth-weight infants have been associated with weight gains during pregnancy of 13.5 kg for underweight women, 9 kg for women of average weight, and 7 kg for women overweight at the start of pregnancy.

Obese women should not be advised to lose weight during pregnancy. Many of these women are malnourished before pregnancy; caloric restriction compromises protein utilization, and the ketonemia that results from rapid fat mobilization may be detrimental to the fetus. Weight loss after pregnancy should be encouraged, however.

Iron

Even in the presence of normal hemoglobin and hematocrit levels, the iron stores of many women are depleted because of blood loss during their menstrual periods. A woman requires more iron during pregnancy because of the iron needs of fetal tissue and the increase of the maternal circulating hemoglobin mass. As it is difficult to meet these needs by dietary means alone, pregnant women should take a supplement of 30-60 mg/day of elemental iron in the form of simple ferrous salts.

Folic Acid

Additional folic acid is required in pregnancy because of increased maternal erythropoiesis, rapid synthesis of DNA in fetal and maternal tissues, and increased maternal urinary excretion. Folic acid deficiency can cause megaloblastic anemia. As it is difficult to meet the increased requirements by diet alone, a folic acid supplement of at least 400 ug/day is needed.

Protein

The recommended intake of protein for pregnant women approximates 1.5 g/kg/day. One study in which the diet of nutritionally deprived pregnant women was supplemented with large amounts of protein showed no beneficial effect on pregnancy outcome and possible adverse effects on fetal growth and the incidence of premature delivery. Other studies, however, have shown that supplementation of calories and moderate amounts of protein can increase birth weight and length of gestation in undernourished pregnant women.

Calcium and Phosphorus

In order to ensure that the calcium and phosphorus needed for fetal bone mineralization are available, pregnant adult women need 1,200 mg/day of each. For pregnant adolescents, the recommended amount of each is 1,600 mg/day; in these patients, the calcium and phosphorus are needed not only for fetal bone mineralization, but also for maternal growth. Adults can meet their calcium intake requirement by consuming 1 quart milk per day. Adolescents need calcium and phosphorus supplementation or additional milk.

Other Vitamins and Minerals

The increased amounts of other vitamins and minerals recommended during pregnancy (see Table 7-1) can usually be obtained through dietary intake, and the routine use of a multivitamin supplement is not necessary. If there are doubts about the adequacy of a patient's diet, however, a vitamin and mineral supplement that provides the recommended dietary allowances can be given safely. It is important to avoid excessive vitamin and mineral intakes (ie, more than twice the recommended dietary allowances) during pregnancy because both fat-soluble and water-soluble vitamins may have toxic effects. Large amounts (ie, 10-90 times the recommended dietary allowance) of vitamin A, for example, may cause fetal bone deformities; similarly, large amounts of vitamin D may cause renal damage in the fetus.

LACTATION AND THE NURSING MOTHER

Breast milk is the ideal food for all healthy, full-term neonates, and mothers should be encouraged to breast-feed. In addition to promoting maternal-neonatal interaction, breast-feeding alone can satisfy the infant's nutritional needs for the first 4-6 months of life.

At birth, the resistance of the neonatal intestinal tract to bacterial and viral agents is incompletely developed. Colostrum and human milk contain a number of antiinfectious factors, including macrophages, secretory IgA, lactoferrin, and lysozyme, that help to protect the infant from infection until the infant's own antiinfectious agents are operational. In families with a strong history of allergy, breast-feeding is likely to be especially beneficial, and the ingestion of solid foods should be delayed until the infant is 6 months of age.

If a mother decides to feed her newborn with formula, the reasons for that decision should be explored in the event that the decision is based on a misconception. Encouragement will sometimes convince a hesitant mother, who may then be able to nurse successfully. If the mother chooses not to breast-feed, however, she should be supported in her decision.

Nutritional Requirements

An additional energy intake of 500 kcal/day and increases in the intake of protein, calcium, and phosphorus are recommended for lactation (see Table 7-1). The mother should also drink at least 2 liters water daily. The precise dietary management of a lactating patient should be determined by her daily milk volume, her level of daily activity, and her intrapartum history. In general, consumption of 1 quart milk and 1 egg each day, together with a balanced healthy diet, meets the dietary needs of a lactating mother. The maternal diet strongly influences the water-soluble vitamin content of the milk. In addition, the maternal intake of large amounts of vitamin D may be reflected in the milk. The mother at nutritional risk should be given a multivitamin supplement, but such a supplement is not needed routinely. Because the iron intake of the mother has little effect on the iron content of the milk, iron should be administered to the mother only if she herself needs it.

Initiating Lactation

The successful management of lactation begins during pregnancy. In providing prenatal care, the obstetrician should discuss feeding plans and breast care with the patient. The breasts should be examined to determine whether the nipples are inverted or flat; if so, the patient should wear a shield in her brassiere to facilitate eversion. The areolar glands provide adequate lubrication during pregnancy and lactation, and the use of special soaps and ointments is not required. During prenatal visits to the pediatrician, the decision to breast-feed should be reinforced and questions answered about the integration of breast-feeding into the total care of the infant in the first months of life.

The mother should be offered the opportunity to nurse her newborn as soon after delivery as possible. She should be allowed to nurse her newborn in any position that she and the baby find comfortable, and she should be guided so that she can help the newborn grasp the breast properly. Enough of the areola should be in the infant's mouth to permit the tongue to stroke the areola over the collecting ductals against the hard palate in the act of sucking. After a brief sucking period of 3-4 minutes, the mother should break the suction by slipping her clean finger into the corner of the infant's mouth. A brief sucking period is then initiated on the second breast.

After the mother and newborn have been transferred to the postpartum unit, they should be together as much as possible. When awake, the newborn should be encouraged to feed frequently to stimulate milk production. Usually, it is wise to alternate the side used to initiate the feeding and to equalize the time spent at each breast over the day. By the third day, a feeding may take 10 minutes or more on each side.

Breast and Nipple Care

The nipples should be kept dry, and ointments or lotions should not be used. Irritation of the nipple can be treated by dry heat provided by a low-wattage goose neck lamp placed 1.5-2 feet away for 20 minutes after each feeding, or by a hair dryer set on low heat and held approximately 6 inches from the breast.

Bottle Feedings and Supplements

Under normal conditions, bottle feedings should not be offered to a breast-fed neonate for the first 2 weeks of life. The neonate may be confused by a rubber nipple. Furthermore, if the infant's appetite is partially satisfied by water or formula supplements, the infant will take less from the breast, and milk production will be diminished. Water supplements for either the breast-fed or bottle-fed newborn have not been shown to limit hyperbilirubinemia in the neonatal period.

Monitoring the Breast-Fed Infant

An adequately nourished infant is usually considered to be one who takes at least 6 feedings per day and sleeps well between feedings. It is also important to be sure that the infant urinates at least 6 times each day and gains weight over a period of time. The healthy infant may actually feed 12-14 times each day and have a small moist stool with many of the feedings, however. A physician or nurse should examine the neonate at 10-14 days of age, especially if the mother is a primipara. Weight loss after 10 days of age or failure to regain birth weight by 3 weeks of age indicates a failure to thrive and requires a careful evaluation of the feeding techniques being used and the adequacy of lactation.

CONTRAINDICATIONS TO BREAST-FEEDING

Maternal Illnesses

Only after they are receiving adequate therapy and considered to be noninfectious should mothers with active tuberculosis breast-feed their infants (see Tuberculosis, Chapter 6). The infant should be examined for infection and provided with appropriate treatment, if necessary.

Cytomegalovirus (CMV) is excreted in human milk. Mothers with identified primary CMV infection should probably not breast-feed their infants during the acute phase of illness. Mothers who are chronic carriers of hepatitis B virus, as demonstrated by the presence of hepatitis B surface antigen (HBsAg), excrete the virus in their milk and may infect their infant through this route. Prevention of this infection through the administration of hepatitis B immune globulin and vaccine to the newborn (see Hepatitis Infections, Chapter 6) should markedly diminish any risk of infection through this route.

Human immunodeficiency virus (HIV) has been found in the milk of a small number of women whose milk was cultured. The relative risk of infection of newborns from this source is unknown (see HIV Infection, Chapter 6). In the United States and in other developed countries where formula is safe and readily available, women infected with HIV should be counseled not to breast-feed their infants.

Mothers with active herpes simplex virus infections may breast-feed their infants if they have no vesicular lesions in the breast area and all active cutaneous lesions are covered.

Maternal Medications

Studies of the effects on the infant of most medications taken by a nursing mother have been inadequate. A few drugs are known to be contraindicated in the breast-feeding mother, however (Table 7-2). It is important that the mother discuss the use of medications with her obstetrician and pediatrician if she wishes to continue breast-feeding. In such a case, the infant should be carefully monitored to detect any adverse effect.

BREAST MILK COLLECTION AND STORAGE

Many mothers wish to provide their milk for their sick or preterm infants, and they should be encouraged to do so. Some hospitals have human milk banks that collect and provide milk for infants from unrelated heterologous donors. Because of concern about the safety of providing milk from multiple donors to one infant, however, it is no longer acceptable to pool milk from multiple donors. Careful screening of potential donors and the establishment of additional controls (ie, controls that are not required when a mother provides milk for her own infant) are important aspects of these programs.

Table 7-2. Drugs Contraindicated During Breast-Feeding

Drug	Reported Sign or Symptom in Infant or Effect on Lactation
Amethopterin*	Possible immune suppression; unknown effect on growth or association with carcinogenesis
Bromocriptine	Suppression of lactation
Cimetidine†	Possible suppression of gastric acidity in infant, inhibition of drug metabolism, and CNS stimulation
Clemastine	Drowsiness, irritability, refusal to feed, high-pitched cry, neck stiffness
Cyclophosphamide*	Possible immune supression; unknown effect on growth or association with carcinogenesis
Ergotamine	Vomiting, diarrhea, convulsions (doses used in migraine medications)
Gold salts	Rash, inflammation of kidney and liver
Methimazole	Potential interference with thyroid function
Phenindione	Hemorrhage
Thiouracil	Decreased thyroid function (not applicable to propylthiouracil)

*Data not available for other cytotoxic agents.

†Drug is concentrated in breast milk.

American Academy of Pediatrics, Committee on Drugs: The transfer of drugs and other chemicals into human breast milk. Pediatrics 72(3):375-383, 1983

Mothers with positive results on a test for HIV antibody or HBsAg, should not provide milk for their infants. Although mothers who are HBsAg-positive may breast-feed their infants after the infants have received hepatitis B immune globulin and vaccine, it is preferable not to use milk potentially contaminated with hepatitis B virus in the nursery.

Women who donate milk for other infants should be interviewed carefully regarding their history of past and current infectious diseases, their use of drugs and medicines, and other factors that may impair the quality or safety of the milk that they provide. In addition, before they are accepted as milk donors, they should be tested for HIV and CMV antibody, HBsAg, and tuberculosis. Women whose test results are positive should not be accepted as donors. These tests should be repeated annually for donors who continue to provide milk or who seek reinstatement as a donor. The potential risks should be explained to mothers whose infants are receiving donated milk.

All women who provide milk for infants should be instructed in the proper techniques of milk collection in order to prevent bacterial contamination of the milk. Careful hand-washing is critical, and the nipples should be wiped with cotton and plain water before the milk is expressed. The first 5-10 ml milk contain a larger number of bacteria; discarding this portion greatly decreases the contamination of the expressed samples. Although manual expression, when performed correctly, yields relatively clean milk, many women prefer to use a breast pump. All parts of the pump that are in contact with milk should be washed carefully with hot soapy water after each use and sterilized by boiling for 10-15 minutes each day.

Expressed milk can be refrigerated in sterile glass or plastic containers for 24 hours without an increase in bacterial contamination. If it must be stored for longer periods, it can be frozen in the freezing compartments of refrigerators for 2-3 weeks, or in a deep freeze at -18°C to -23°C for several months.

Frozen milk should be thawed quickly under running water, with precautions taken to avoid contamination from the water, or gradually in the refrigerator at 4°C. It should not be left at room temperatures for long periods, nor should it be subjected to extremely hot water or to microwave ovens. The very high temperatures that may be reached with the latter methods can destroy valuable components of the milk. Once milk has been thawed, it may be refrigerated for 24 hours, but it should not be refrozen.

There is no consensus on microbiologic quality standards for expressed milk. In general, each milliliter of expressed breast milk contains 10^3-10^4 colony-forming units (CFU) of normal skin bacteria, such as *Staphylococcus epidermidis* and diphtheroids; this milk can be fed to infants with no ill effects. The presence of gram-negative rods in the milk indicates a problem in the collection technique. When there are more than 10^2 CFU/ml gram-negative bacteria, feeding intolerance has been reported, and higher levels have been associated with suspected sepsis. Bacteria levels in the milk can be controlled by heat treatment. Even mild Holder pasteurization, which involves heating the milk to 62°C to 65°C for 30 minutes, leads to a 25-30% loss of host resistance factors and a decrease in milk lipase activity, however.

Expressed milk samples are seldom routinely screened for bacterial count. Such screening should be carried out, however, when there are concerns about the expression techniques, when intestinal intolerance of the milk is suspected, and when the milk is to be given by continuous infusion at room temperature over many hours, thus creating a risk of bacterial proliferation in the container and tubing.

FORMULA PREPARATION

Physicians and nursing staff should support the decision of a mother who wishes to bottle-feed her newborn. The mother certainly should not be made to feel inadequate because she chooses not to breast-feed. Like mothers who breast-feed their newborns, those who bottle-feed their newborns should wash their hands carefully and should feed their infants in a comfortable position.

Formula selection and control should be a physician-directed activity. New formulas should be reviewed by the appropriate hospital committees and the director of the nursery before use. The physician should write orders for the formula to be used and the amount to be given at each feeding.

The composition of formulas currently used in many nurseries are listed in Table 7-3. Data on the types and amounts of protein, fat, and carbohydrate, as well as the concentrations of sodium, potassium, phosphorus, and calcium, have been provided by the manufacturers. Values may vary slightly from one lot to the next, and various features of the formulas may be changed by the manufacturers as new nutritional information becomes available.

If infant formulas are prepared from concentrated liquids or powders either terminal heating or aseptic technique should be used. Terminal heating involves heating the prepared formula in a clean feeding container by autoclaving at 230°F for 10 minutes, or placing the container in boiling water and maintaining the water temperature at 212°F for 25-30 minutes. The formula should be cooled and refrigerated within 1 hour after heating. Aseptic technique involves mixing concentrated liquid or powder with clean water (boiled for 5 minutes) in clean containers using clean utensils. Containers and utensils are considered clean after they have been boiled for 5 minutes and then allowed to cool for 1 hour. Information regarding the risk of using unboiled municipal tap water is not available. Aseptic technique can be most safely carried out in a laminar flow hood, although such a hood is not specifically recommended by formula manufacturers. Aseptic technique is not likely to damage any nutrients in the formulas, whereas heat treatment, especially autoclaving, may caramelize the sugars, reduce the levels of heat-labile vitamins, and decrease the availability of lysine.

Most hospitals now use prepared formula units with separate nipples that are readily attached to the bottles just before use. These units need not be refrigerated; they may be stored in a convenient, clean, cool area. The sterile cap should be kept on the nipple until the neonate is ready to be fed. If there is a special area where nipples are uncapped and placed on the bottle, it should be kept very clean and should be used only for formula preparation. Alternatively, nipples may be uncapped and attached to bottles at the mother's bedside just prior to feeding. The formula should be used as soon as possible, certainly within 4 hours after the bottle is uncapped.

VITAMIN AND MINERAL SUPPLEMENTATION

Infants who are breast-fed may show evidence of vitamin D deficiency if their mothers have a low vitamin D intake or little exposure to sunlight, either antepartum or postpartum. If it is suspected that the mother's vitamin D status is not optimal, the infant should receive 400 IU/day supplemental vitamin D. This is particularly important if the infant is dark skinned or if there is little possibility of significant exposure to sunlight.

Because of the poor passage of fluoride into the milk, breast-fed infants should receive supplemental fluoride even in areas with fluoridated water supplies. The Committee on Nutrition of the American Academy of Pediatrics recommends that the supplementation begin shortly after birth. Formula-fed infants should be given supplemental fluoride if they do not live in an area with a fluoridated water supply.

The iron content of human milk is low, but the bioavailability is high; 50% of the iron is absorbed by infants who are exclusively breast-fed. It is recommended that these infants be given 2-3 mg/kg/day supplemental elemental iron when they reach 4-6 months of age. Iron-containing formulas have 12 mg/dl elemental iron, and further supplementation is not necessary if such formulas are used. Preterm infants require 2-3 mg/kg/day elemental iron supplementation after their weight reaches approximately 2 kg or after they are discharged from the hospital.

Preterm infants should be given supplemental vitamins unless they are fed one of the formulas that are specifically designed for preterm infants (eg, Similac Special Care or Enfamil Premature Formula); high levels of vitamins have already been added to these special formulas. Human milk and most formulas contain insufficient vitamins to meet the preterm infant's needs. The combination of formula and vitamin supplements should provide the preterm infant with a daily intake of 20-50 mg vitamin C, 400 units vitamin D, and 5-10 IU vitamin E. Preterm infants do not absorb folate well, and 50-100 μg/day supplemental folic acid is recommended.

Table 7-3. Source and Composition of Infant Formulas

Formula/milk	Calories/oz	Protein Source	g/dl	Fat Source	g/dl	Carbohydrate Source	g/dl	Na (mEq/liter)	K (mEq/liter)	Phosphorus (mg/dl)	Calcium (mg/dl)	Osmolality (osm/kg Water)
						Feeding at Infancy						
Human milk	20	Human milk	1.0–1.2	Human milk	4.5	Lactose	7.0	7	13	16	34	300
Enfamil	20	Skim milk, whey	1.5	Soy oil, coconut oil	3.8	Lactose	6.9	8	18	32	46	300
Enfamile Premature	24	Whey, casein	2.4	MCT, corn oil	4.1	Lactose, corn syrup solids	9.0	14	23	48	95	300
Isomil	20	Soy protein isolate with L-methionine	1.8	Soy oil, coconut oil	3.7	Corn syrup, sucrose	6.8	14	24	51	71	250
Nursoy	20	Soy isolate with L-methionine	2.1	Oleo, coconut oil, olein, soy oil	3.6	Sucrose	6.9	9	18	42	60	296
Nutramigen	20	Casein hydrolysate	1.9	Corn oil	2.6	Sucrose, tapioca starch	9.1	14	18	43	63	480
Portagen	20	Casein	2.3	MCT, corn oil	3.2	Corn syrup solids, sucrose, lactose	7.8	14	22	48	63	236
Pregestimil	20	Casein hydrolysate	1.9	MCT, corn oil	2.7	Tapioca starch, corn syrup solids	9.1	14	19	42	63	350
Prosobee	20	Soy protein isolate with L-methionine	2.0	Soy oil, coconut oil	3.6	Corn syrup solids	6.8	13	20	50	63	200

Similac	20	Skim milk	1.5	Coconut oil, soy oil	3.6	Lactose	7.2	11	21	39	51	290
Similac PM 60/40	20	Whey, casein	1.5	Coconut oil, corn oil	3.8	Lactose	6.9	7	15	19	38	260
Similac-LBW	24	Skim milk	2.2	MCT, coconut oil, soy oil	4.5	Lactose, corn syrup solids	8.5	16	31	57	73	290
Similac Special Care	24	Whey, casein	2.2	MCT, corn oil, coconut oil	4.4	Lactose, corn syrup solids	8.6	18	29	73	146	300
SMA	20	Whey, skim milk	1.5	Oleo, coconut oil, safflower oil, soy oil	3.8	Lactose	7.2	7	14	28	42	300
SMA Preemie	24	Whey, casein	2.0	Oleo, coconut oil, olein, soy oil, MCT	4.4	Lactose malto-dextrins	8.6	14	19	40	75	280
Soyalac	20	Soybean, solids with L-methionine	2.1	Soy oil	3.7	Sucrose, corn syrup solids	6.8	13	20	37	63	240
I-Soyalac	20	Soy protein isolate with L-methionine	2.1	Soy oil	3.7	Sucrose, tapioca starch	6.8	12	20	48	69	270
Advanced Feeding Beyond Infancy												
Cow's milk	20	Cow's milk	3.4	Cow's milk	3.8	Lactose	4.8	22	40	96	123	290

FEEDINGS FOR LOW-BIRTH-WEIGHT INFANTS

Infants who weigh more than 1,500 g at birth grow adequately if they are fed a regular 67 kcal/dl (20 cal/oz) infant formula designed for full-term infants or their mother's milk, although they retain calcium and phosphorus at rates slower than the fetal accretion rates. Very low birth weight infants are better nourished if they are fed a 67-80 kcal/dl formula especially designed for preterm infants or their own mother's milk fortified by a commercial mixture. Special formulas for small preterm infants contain easily digested and absorbed lipids (15-50% medium chain triglycerides), additional protein, easily absorbed carbohydrates (glucose polymers and lactose), and enough added calcium and phosphorus to achieve a rate of bone mineralization faster than the rate that can be achieved by means of regular infant formulas or unfortified mother's milk. Sufficient sodium is added to prevent hyponatremia, while additional trace metals and vitamins are included to meet, at least in part, the special needs of the preterm infant.

Human milk has a number of special features that make its use desirable in feeding preterm infants. It contains antiinfectious factors, and the triglyceride structure results in excellent fat absorption. The lipase in human milk facilitates fat digestion and supplements the deficient quantity of pancreatic lipase of the preterm infant. The milk does not provide amounts of protein, calcium, and phosphorus adequate to meet the needs of rapidly growing small preterm infants, however. These shortcomings can be corrected by the addition of nutritionally well-balanced and commerically available dry or liquid human milk fortifiers.

NUTRITIONAL COUNSELING

Ideally, each perinatal care center should have a nutritional counseling program. Dietitians and nutritionists can educate patients at nutritional risk about ways to correct problems that are dangerous to the health of their fetuses and themselves. Specialized programs for a wide range of nutritional disorders should be available to those who need them.

RESOURCES AND RECOMMENDED READING

American Academy of Pediatrics, Committee on Drugs: The transfer of drugs and other chemicals into human breast milk. Pediatrics 72(3):375-383, 1983

American Academy of Pediatrics, Committee on Fetus and Newborn: Standards and Recommendations for Hospital Care of Newborn Infants, 6 ed. Evanston IL, AAP, 1977, pp 75-81

American Academy of Pediatrics, Committee on Nutrition: Pediatric Nutrition Handbook, 2 ed. Elk Grove Village IL, AAP, 1985

American College of Obstetricians and Gynecologists: Assessment of Maternal Nutrition. Washington DC, ACOG, 1978

American Hospital Association: Procedures and Layout for the Infant Formula Room. Chicago, AHA, 1965

Committee on Dietary Allowances, Food and Nutrition Board, Division of Biological Sciences, Assembly of Life Sciences, National Research Council: Recommended Dietary Allowances, 9 ed. Washington DC, National Academy of Sciences, 1980

Committee on Nutrition of the Mother and Preschool Child: Nutrition Services in Perinatal Care. Washington DC, National Academy Press, 1981

Dwyer J: Maternal nutrition in pregnancy with emphasis on adolescence. In: Grand RJ, Sutphen JL, Dietz WH Jr (eds): Pediatric Nutrition—Theory and Practice. Boston, Butterworth, 1987, pp 205-220

Greer FR, Tsang RC: Calcium, phosphorus, magnesium, and vitamin D requirements for preterm infants. In: Tsang RC (ed): Vitamin and Mineral Requirements in Preterm Infants. New York, Marcel Dekker, 1985, pp 99-136

Jacobson HN: Nutrition and pregnancy. In: Walker WA, Watkins JB (eds): Nutrition in Pediatrics—Basic Science and Clinical Application. Boston, Little Brown & Co, 1985, pp 373-388

Lawrence RA: Breast-Feeding: A Guide for the Medical Profession. St Louis, CV Mosby, 1980

Neville NC, Niefert MR: Lactation, Physiology, Nutrition and Breast-Feeding. New York, Plenum Press, 1983, pp 309-311

Sauve R, Buchan K, Clyne A, et al: Mothers' milk banking: Microbiologic aspects. Can J Publ Health 75(2):133-136, 1984

8

INTERHOSPITAL CARE OF THE PERINATAL PATIENT

The transport of pregnant women, new mothers, and neonates between hospitals is recognized as an essential component of modern perinatal care. As noted in Chapter 1, transport is one part of the systems approach to improved obstetric and newborn care. There are three types of patient transport:

1. *Maternal-fetal transport:* Pregnant women are transferred from one facility to another for special care or delivery.
2. *Neonatal transport:* A team is deployed from one facility to evaluate and stabilize the condition of a neonate at another facility with the intent of transferring the neonate to the team's facility for more intensive care.
3. *Return transport:* Patients are returned to the facility to which they were originally admitted or to their local hospital for further care when the problems that required transport have been resolved. A return transport is an important benefit to both the individual patient and the system.

Level II neonatal care units should have ongoing liaison with a level III neonatal intensive care unit. The concept of a network of neonatal care units can logically be extended to apply to all perinatal care services. Regional perinatal care networks should have specific guidelines for the referral of high-risk mothers, as well as sick newborns, to regional centers for care.

The goal of interhospital transport is to care for high-risk perinatal patients in a facility appropriate to their needs. A successful regional referral program is based on:

1. Risk identification and assessment of problems that will benefit from consultation and transport
2. Knowledge of the available resources and the ways to gain access to them
3. Availability of an organized, appropriate, transport service that has adequate economic and political support
4. Recognition that care is continuous
5. Evaluation and analysis of performance

From the recognition of a perinatal problem to the resolution and follow-up of the problem, there should be a continuum of care that includes the community of origin. Because disease processes do not become static while a patient is being transferred, management during transport is necessary.

INDICATIONS FOR TRANSPORT

The decision to transfer a perinatal patient should be made by the primary physician in conjunction with a consultant. Both should be well-informed about the resources at each perinatal care center, as not all centers have facilities for every type of referral. In general, transport should be considered when the resources immediately available to the maternal, fetal, or neonatal patient are not adequate to deal with the patient's actual or anticipated condition. Maternal transport that would benefit the fetus, but could seriously jeopardize the mother's well-being, should be avoided.

The following conditions require specialized care and may require patient transfer:

I. Maternal Conditions
   A. Obstetric complications (especially at less than 34 weeks of gestation or less than 2,000 g expected birth weight)
      1. Premature rupture of membranes
      2. Premature labor
      3. Severe preeclampsia or other hypertensive complication
      4. Multiple gestation
      5. Third trimester bleeding

B. Medical complications
   1. Infections
   2. Severe heart disease
   3. Poorly controlled diabetes mellitus
   4. Thyrotoxicosis
   5. Renal disease with deteriorating function or increased hypertension
   6. Drug overdose
C. Surgical complications
   1. Trauma requiring intensive care or surgical correction or requiring a procedure that may result in the onset of premature labor
   2. Acute abdominal emergencies at less than 34 weeks of gestation or with a fetus weighing less than 2,000 g

II. Fetal Conditions
   A. Anomalies that may be amenable to intervention.
   B. Rh disease with or without hydrops
   C. Anomalies that will require postnatal surgery
   D. Intrauterine growth retardation (IUGR)

III. Neonatal Conditions
   A. Gestation less than 34 weeks or weight less than 2,000 g
   B. Sepsis or meningitis
   C. Persistent respiratory distress
   D. Blood loss
   E. Hypoglycemia
   F. Hemolytic disease of the newborn
   G. Neonatal drug withdrawal
   H. Neonates of diabetic mothers
   I. Seizures
   J. Congenital malformations requiring surgical care or observation
   K. Shock or asphyxia persisting beyond 2 hours
   L. Cardiac disorders
   M. Physiologic instability

These examples are to be considered guidelines only; they vary with individual patient needs or institutional capabilities.

THE ORGANIZED APPROACH TO TRANSPORT

Medical, surgical, and technical advances in perinatal care continue to alter the management of many anomalies and illnesses previously considered lethal. Community physicians should consider seeking help from their referral center when faced with complex, difficult clinical decisions, especially those decisions involving the use of neonatal life support. Depending on the details of the particular case, consultation may involve either telephone communication or inter-hospital transfer for further evaluation.

In certain circumstances, the referring physician may manage the transfer personally. Maternal-fetal transports are frequently conducted in this fashion. Transports that originate at the referring hospital, frequently termed one-way transports, function effectively in some locations; however, two-way transport systems, which operate from a base at the center, are more common. Any transport procedure is acceptable if it follows the guidelines given here and attains its goals and objectives.

The provision of adequate life support during the transport of critically ill perinatal patients requires considerable knowledge, skill, experience, and specialized equipment not readily available in all hospitals. Many perinatal care centers that provide level III services have developed two-way transport systems for their service regions because only such a regional system gives personnel experience with a large enough number of patients to maintain the skills required for care during transport. Assistance should be solicited as soon as the need for transport becomes apparent. This practice ameliorates the immediate problems and reduces the time that the transport team must be in the referring hospital.

Because the demand for tertiary care beds sometimes exceeds the number available, regional centers should have contingency plans. An agreement between centers in neighboring regions that each will accept referrals from the other is probably the most efficient way to resolve this problem. Interunit coordination should be the responsibility of the neonatal/perinatal care staff at each referral center. During periods of high demand, regular communication between the neonatal intensive care units, for example, can provide an up-to-date status report on available beds, preventing a time-consuming last minute search and allowing the transport team to focus on a prompt and efficient interhospital transfer.

Informal, poorly organized interhospital care is hazardous. In order to avoid compromising the patient's condition, to ensure a predictable response to transport requests, and to provide the highest quality of care, the approach to transport should be logical and organized. An interhospital care system has five identifiable components: 1) organization, 2) communications, 3) personnel, 4) equipment, and 5) transport vehicles.

Organization

Interhospital care should be available 24 hours/day through a program in which the response time and minimum capabilities of personnel have been defined. The director of the transport service should be a subspecialist in maternal-fetal medicine or neonatal medicine, or a board-certified obstetrician or pediatrician with a special interest in these subspecialty areas. The director's responsibilities are

1. Quality control of patient care through regular case review
2. Personnel training and supervision
3. Development and use of patient care protocols
4. Development and use of record-keeping systems and subsequent collation of data for evaluation and analysis
5. Review of operational aspects of the program (eg, response times, effectiveness of communications, and equipment maintenance)

Communications

The transfer of a patient from one hospital to another and from one care team to another requires a reliable communications system. It is essential that the referring physician provide the receiving physician with specific clinical information on the patient being referred.

Maternal-fetal transfers are generally made in anticipation of complications in the mother or her infant. Because the decision is usually based on information derived from some combination of maternal medical records, ultrasound or amniotic fluid studies, and electronic fetal monitoring, these records (or copies of them) should be transferred with the patient. A tube of the mother's blood should accompany the records. A delay in the transfer of the records or failure to transfer them at all may lead to an unnecessary repetition of studies with concomitant delays in care and risks to both mother and infant. Complete neonatal and appropriate maternal records should accompany the newborn patient who is being transferred. For a neonatal patient, this information should include the following items:

Gestational age
Birth weight
Perinatal history
Temperature
Color
Hematocrit
Oxygen requirement and blood gas levels
Respiratory activity (particularly the presence of apnea or the need for assisted ventilation)
Blood glucose level or Dextrostix result
Pertinent radiologic findings
Reasons for transfer
Therapy administered, including drugs

Possession of the appropriate information will enable the receiving facility to prepare for the patient's stabilization, transfer, and admission. Appendixes E and F contain sample record formats for information that can be provided conveniently by telephone. Referral centers in large service areas may establish toll-free lines for referring physicians and families. In metropolitan areas or in small service areas, direct hotlines may link referring obstetric units and nurseries to the perinatal care center. These lines should be open 24 hours/day and should be well publicized throughout the service region. Communications between the referring and the receiving facilities should include telephone or radio contact during stabilization and transfer.

Dispatching services should provide rapid coordination of vehicles and personnel, as well as communication links between the referring and receiving hospitals and the transfer team. Referring physicians should be given the estimated arrival time of the transport team so that they can arrange for laboratory studies on which to base therapy in transport. The receiving hospital should also be given an estimated arrival time so that the staff can prepare for the patient's admission. When flights must connect with ground ambulances, it is desirable for a single dispatching center to coordinate the movement of all vehicles. The complexity and sophistication of the dispatching operation vary considerably with the nature of the transport service.

Personnel

The interhospital care team should have the collective expertise necessary to provide supportive care for a wide variety of emergency conditions in high-risk mothers and neonates. Team members should be drawn from appropriately trained physicians, registered nurses, respiratory therapists, and emergency medical technicians. Usually, one team member is a physician or a registered nurse. Transport teams are often staffed by neonatal nurse-clinicians. In addition to being highly knowledgeable in the care and procedures required by perinatal patients, transport personnel should be thoroughly familiar with the transport equipment, as any malfunction en route must be handled without the assistance of hospital maintenance staff.

Equipment

The safety and efficiency of a patient transfer are highly dependent on the equipment available to the transport team. The type of transport (maternal or neonatal), the distance of the transfer, the type of transport vehicle(s) used, and the resources available at the referring medical facility determine the kinds and amounts of equipment, drugs, and supplies needed by the transport team.

In the past, many authorities have felt that all transport equipment should be battery-operated throughout the transport. In many transport situations, this is still true. Many ambulances and aircraft are now equipped with converters/inverters that provide 100/110 volt 400 Hz AC or 24/28 volt DC power during transport, however, and the equipment on these vehicles requires only enough battery power for the portions of the transport that take place outside the vehicles. This arrangement makes it possible to use much less cumbersome, light-weight equipment. The integration of multiple modules into the transport vehicle with a single transformer and battery supply greatly reduces space requirements, but may lock the transport team into a system that is not easily upgraded.

The equipment needed for transport of a neonate includes an incubator especially designed for transport. It is essential that the transport team be able to monitor the neonate's heart rate, temperature, and blood pressure. An intravenous pump capable of continuous microinfusion is necessary. If ventilator-dependent patients are to be transferred, it should be possible to monitor ventilator pressures and inspired oxygen levels during transport. Devices used to assess blood oxygen levels may be helpful, especially during a long transport.

In addition to equipment for monitoring, resuscitation, and support of both mother and neonate, a transport kit that contains essential drugs and special supplies should be continuously available during stabilization and transfer of the patient. A list of the equipment and drugs that should be contained in the transport kit is found in Appendix G.

Transport Vehicles

Several factors should be considered in the selection of vehicles for an interhospital transport system. Ground ambulances are adaptable to most short-range transport situations; fixed-wing aircraft facilitate coverage of a large referral area, but are more expensive, require skilled operators and specially trained crews, and may actually prolong the time required for response and transport over relatively short distances because of the time needed to prepare for flight; helicopters can shorten response and transport time over intermediate distances or in highly congested areas, but are very expensive to maintain and operate.

The decision to use aircraft in a patient transport system requires special commitments from the director and members of the transport team. During air transport, the pilot should be considered an integral part of the transport team. Therefore, the pilot should be included in appropriate decision making and should have the authority to change, modify, or cancel the mission for safety reasons. All equipment should be tested to ensure its accuracy and safety in flight. The US Air Force School of Aerospace Medicine maintains records of all medical equipment tested and approved for military aircraft. The American Society for Hospital Based Emergency Air Medical Services, the Aerospace Association, the Federal Aviation Administration, and the Emergency Care Research Institute can also offer assistance regarding medical equipment suitable for use in aircraft.

TRANSPORT PROCEDURE

Evaluation

The referring physician should carefully evaluate the patient's condition, both in regard to the primary diagnosis and in regard to the development of complicating conditions. Steps should be taken in consultation with staff at the receiving facility to correct these conditions to the extent possible before the transfer.

Stabilization

Maternal patients sometimes require hemodynamic stabilization before transport; it may be necessary to administer tocolytic agents, anticonvulsants, or antihypertensive agents. A patient with active bleeding, rapidly progressive preeclampsia, or rapidly progressive labor should not be transported until her safety can be ensured.

In some situations, maternal transport may not be advisable; neonatal transport may be preferable. If so, the referring physician may arrange for the transport team to arrive at the referring hospital in time to attend the birth. By prior agreement between the referring physician and the dispatch center, the transport team may participate in the initial stabilization of the neonate. Temperature, blood gas levels, blood pressure, and blood glucose level are normal in the fully stabilized neonate. Complete stabilization of a newborn is not always possible, but transport of an extremely unstable newborn is contraindicated.

Although there have been no controlled trials, experience indicates that stabilization of the patient before departure from the referring hospital is probably the most critical aspect of interhospital care, because it minimizes subsequent deterioration in transit.

Medicolegal Concerns

Many legal details of perinatal transport are not well defined, but all involved parties (eg, the referring hospital and personnel, the receiving hospital and personnel, and commercial ambulance and aircraft charter corporations) assume responsibilities. As spokesperson for the transport team, the physician should thoroughly explain the patient's condition and reasons for transfer to the patient or to the parents of the newborn. Informed consent for transfer, admission to the receiving hospital, and care should be obtained. The newborn should be clearly identified.

Perinatal transport teams are involved in very special transport situations, and prior attention to potential legal problems is advisable. In most situations, the institution that employs the team is responsible for its actions, and a physician at that institution directs the team's professional activities. Individual hospitals and regions should investigate the use of transfer agreements, which may include the granting of emergency privileges to members of transport teams.

The departure of the transport team from the premises of the referring hospital may be considered the official point of transfer of responsibility from the referring physician to the transport team.

Many hospitals consider patients who are en route and under the care of the transport team to have been admitted to their institution. Physician-directors and hospital administrators should identify and address the potential administrative or legal problems that may arise in certain situations, for example, when transport teams cross one or more state lines during a transport. Each institution should establish its own policy.

INTERACTION AT THE REFERRING HOSPITAL

If possible, the referring physician should be at the hospital when the transport team arrives and should remain at the hospital while the team is there in order to ensure complete communication.

The referral center should receive a report on the patient's condition prior to departure. If the patient being transferred is a newborn, the mother and father should be offered the opportunity to see and touch their neonate before the transfer, even if the neonate is in a transport incubator or on a respirator. An instant picture of the neonate taken prior to transport has proved particularly helpful when parents are to be separated from their newborn for a long period or when the mother is recovering from a cesarean delivery and may not remember the time that she spent with the neonate. The parents should also be given written information about the receiving hospital, including the names of staff members, visiting hours, telephone numbers, and places to stay in the hospital's vicinity. Brochures about the hospital can be useful. If the mother wishes to breast-feed her newborn, she should be taught how to express her milk until nipple feeding becomes possible. Early attention to family needs and concerns at this critical time can reduce anxiety and ease the transition to a new medical center.

Records are essential for the continuing care of the patient and for the evaluation of the referral transport process. Records should include the following information:

Patient's name
Referring hospital
Receiving hospital
Referring physician
Attendants' names and professional status
Mode of transport
Time data, including the time of the transport team's arrival at
    the referring hospital, the time of departure, ground or air

ambulance time, and the time of arrival at the receiving hospital
Patient's age, weight, gestational age, and sex
Diagnosis and condition
Procedures performed
Medication administered
Periodic vital signs
Special comments

PATIENT CARE IN TRANSIT

A patient in a stable condition requires little or no intervention during
transport, but should be under continuous observation. The key
factors to be monitored in the maternal patient include uterine
contractions, cardiopulmonary status, fetal heart rate, deep tendon
reflexes, infusion rate of intravenous fluids, and the administration of
tocolytic agents or anticonvulsants. In the newborn patient, the
transport team should frequently and noninvasively monitor temperature, respiration, heart rate, blood pressure, color, activity, and
oxygen concentration. A neutral thermal environment should be
maintained. It may be necessary to monitor other parameters as well,
such as the blood glucose level. Furthermore, the availability of
portable transcutaneous monitoring devices has made it feasible to
monitor blood gases during transport.

The patient, attending personnel, and all equipment should be
safely secured inside the transport vehicle. Although it may be
necessary to respond rapidly to an emergency, there is generally little
need for excessive speed if the patient is stabilized.

INTERACTION AT THE RECEIVING HOSPITAL

The staff of the receiving hospital should be prepared to deal with any
unresolved problems or emergencies that involve the transferred
patient. Transport personnel should inform the receiving staff of the
patient's history and clinical status, as well as all the current plans for
management. The receiving physician should not change therapies
provided during transport without consulting the transport team.

Family members are extremely anxious when a patient is transferred. If they have not been able to accompany or follow the patient,
they should be called as soon as possible after the patient has arrived
at the receiving hospital and informed of the patient's condition. The
referring physician and the nursing staff at the referring hospital not

only should be informed of the patient's arrival, but also should be kept up-to-date on the patient's progress throughout the patient's stay at the receiving hospital.

The transfer is not complete until the equipment on the transport vehicle has been restocked and prepared for the next call. Reusable equipment that has come into contact with the transported patient should be appropriately sterilized or decontaminated.

RETURN TRANSPORT

Referred infants who have received the maximal benefits of tertiary care, but are not yet ready for discharge, are transported back to the hospital to which they were originally admitted. This allows the infants to complete their convalescence as close as possible to the family members who will be responsible for care after discharge. Furthermore, beds at tertiary centers are most efficiently used for the most critically ill infants. Return transports are an integral part of a regional transport program.

OUTREACH EDUCATION AND THE REGIONAL TRANSPORT SYSTEM

Because interhospital care of the high-risk perinatal patient requires the cooperation and coordination of many skilled persons, outreach education efforts should reinforce that cooperation and coordination. One of the most often overlooked segments of outreach education associated with the regional transport system is the follow-up report to the referring physician. A prompt and complete report to the referring physician, describing the patient's condition, the events of transport, and planned therapy, is an invaluable source of information and experience. The referring physician should also receive periodic updates on the patient's condition. At discharge, a detailed summary of the patient's condition with recommendations for ongoing care is essential. A complete set of medical records is as important in the return transport as it was in the initial transport.

Outreach education related to transport should focus on the following objectives:

1. Informing perinatal care providers in the region of the specialized resources available to them through the perinatal care network

2. Assisting primary physicians in developing their abilities to anticipate complications, to identify high-risk perinatal patients, and to stabilize these patients before transport
3. Facilitating effective quality assurance through the continuing education of perinatal care providers
4. Establishing 24-hour consultation and referral sources
5. Promoting a regionalized care system designed to ensure high-quality care to all patients in a cost-effective fashion

PROGRAM EVALUATION

The creation of regional advisory councils with representatives from the various perinatal care programs facilitates evaluation of a region's transport system, as such a group can identify and verify the particular region's needs for interhospital perinatal care. The characteristics of the successful transport system, as described earlier, can be used as a guide for program evaluation. Other criteria should also be considered in evaluating the transport system:

1. Availability: Does the system provide all services that may be needed by the perinatal patient?
2. Accessibility: Is it possible to "connect" the patient quickly and appropriately with the services needed? Do those who will need the services know where to get them?
3. Responsiveness: Is there a mutual commitment from referring care providers and specialized care providers to honor and accommodate each other's special needs as they arise?
4. Effectiveness: Are perinatal patients being given the appropriate care in the appropriate setting? Do physicians and patients regard the perinatal transport service as useful and effective?

As basic as these questions may appear, their answers are often assumed rather than tested. The purpose of an evaluation of the transport system is to collect the evidence to confirm that the system provides high-quality care to high-risk mothers and neonates.

RESOURCES AND RECOMMENDED READING

Merenstein GB, Pettett G, Woodall J, et al: An analysis of air transport results in the sick newborn: II. Antenatal and neonatal referrals. Am J Obstet Gynecol 128(5):520-525, 1977

Modanlou HD, Dorchester WL, Freeman RK, et al: Perinatal transport to a regional perinatal center in a metropolitan area: Maternal versus neonatal transport. Am J Obstet Gynecol 138(8):1157-1164, 1980

Paneth N, Kiely JL, Susser M: Age at death used to assess the effect of interhospital transfer of newborns. Pediatr 73(6):854-861, 1984

Paneth N, Kiely JL, Wallenstein S, et al: The choice of place of delivery. Effect of hospital level on mortality in all singleton births in New York City. Am J Dis Child 141(1):60-64, 1987

Pettett G, Merenstein GB, Battaglia FC, et al: An analysis of air transport results in the sick newborn infant: I. The transport team. Pediatrics 55(6):774—782, 1975

Segal S (ed): Manual for the Transport of High-Risk Newborn Infants: Principles, Policies, Equipment, Techniques. Ottawa Ont, Canadian Paediatric Society, 1972

Sinclair JC, Torrance GW, Boyle MH, et al: Evaluation of neonatal-intensive-care programs. N Engl J Med 305(9):489-494, 1981

9

EVALUATION OF PERINATAL CARE

Whether in a hospital, a region, a state, or a nation, the evaluation of perinatal care depends on precise definitions and the availability of accurate data. A complete evaluation of perinatal events is best done on a state and national level; however, such evaluation should begin at the local level and should focus on the following goals:

1. Reduce maternal, fetal, and neonatal morbidity and mortality
2. Identify problem areas that require improvement and provide a focus for continuing education of the perinatal care team
3. Improve local care through a systems approach, with special emphasis on the process of risk assessment and management and its effect on the regional approach to perinatal care
4. Provide standard data for hospital-to-hospital comparisons of outcome, evaluations of programs, and studies of comparative epidemiology
5. Document the long-term outcome of perinatal care and practices

Evaluation techniques that are based on information recorded on official certificates (eg, matching birth and death certificates) are not always adequate for judging the quality of care and detecting problem areas at the local level. Not only are the data on these certificates sometimes insufficient, but also it is difficult for most state data centers to provide local hospitals with timely feedback. In addition, a hospital that specializes in the care of a high-risk population is not directly comparable to a hospital that serves primarily a low-risk population. Williams and associates have devised a method that allows each hospital to compare its perinatal mortality statistics with those of other institutions in its region by partially correcting for certain characteristics of the population it serves. Finally, as mortality rates fall, morbidity evaluation becomes increasingly important, and statistics concerning morbidity are even more difficult to obtain than are statistics concerning natality and mortality.

DEFINITIONS

Appendix H, Standard Terminology for Reporting of Reproductive Health Statistics in the United States, represents the joint efforts of organizations concerned with the statistical uniformity and accuracy of perinatal care data.

In addition to collecting those measures listed in Appendix H, it may be useful in a perinatal care evaluation to collect data on certain characteristics of the mother, the father, the prenatal care provided, the delivery, and the newborn. Following is a partial list of characteristics that may be included in a hospital perinatal data base:

1. **Maternal:** age, gravidity, parity, education, marital status, economic status, race, drug exposure, ingestion of alcohol and smoking, occupational environment, and the presence of concurrent medical-surgical disease.

2. **Paternal:** age, education, marital status, economic status, race, and the presence of concurrent medical-surgical disease.

3. **Prenatal care:** date of the initial visit to the physician, the number and timing of subsequent visits, the type of facility where the visits occurred, the fetal evaluation methods used, and the medications administered.

4. **Delivery:** nature of the labor initiation, divided into spontaneous and nonspontaneous (induced) groups; the use of monitoring in labor; timing of the rupture of the membranes; duration of labor; medications administered; and the type of anesthesia administered for delivery. The route of delivery should be designated. Vaginal delivery should be classified as spontaneous or instrumental, and a vaginal birth after a previous cesarean birth should be noted. Abdominal delivery should be further classified as a primary or repeat procedure. The fetal presentation, any obstetric complications, and indication for operative deliveries should also be recorded.

5. **Newborn:** birth weight; gestational age, including method of calculation; sex; Apgar scores; head circumference; length; and any anomalies.

STATISTICAL EVALUATION

Uniformity in recording and reporting data is extremely important to intergroup comparisons. Several standard rates and ratios are widely used for evaluation of local and regional perinatal care (see Appendix H). In addition to these, accuracy and completeness of data make it possible to calculate specific perinatal mortality rates for any clinical entity, age, weight, or time period. The denominator must clearly define a population to which the deaths in the numerator belong, and the study period in the numerator and denominator must coincide. Mortality rates of population subsets can thus be determined, as illustrated in the following examples:

Example 1: Clinical entity, maternal diabetes

$$\text{Perinatal Mortality Rate} = \frac{\text{Fetal Deaths } (\geq 500 \text{ g, Diabetic Mothers}) + \text{Neonatal Deaths (Diabetic Mothers)} \times 1{,}000}{\text{Total Live Births (Diabetic Mothers)} + \text{Fetal Deaths } (\geq 500 \text{ g, Diabetic Mothers})}$$

Example 2: Weight-specific neonatal mortality rate

$$\text{Mortality Rate of Neonates } 1{,}000 \text{ to} < 1{,}500 \text{ g} = \frac{\text{Neonatal Deaths } (1{,}000 \text{ to} < 1{,}500 \text{ g}) \times 1{,}000}{\text{Total Live Births } (1{,}000 \text{ to} < 1{,}500 \text{ g})}$$

Example 3: Age-specific fetal mortality rate

$$\text{Fetal Mortality Rate } (32\text{-}36 \text{ weeks}) = \frac{\text{Fetal Deaths } (32\text{-}36 \text{ weeks}) \times 1{,}000}{\text{Total Live Births } (32\text{-}36 \text{ weeks}) + \text{Fetal Deaths } (\geq 500 \text{ g}, 32\text{-}36 \text{ weeks})}$$

The fetal mortality rate plus the neonatal mortality rate does not equal the perinatal mortality rate, because the denominators are different. The differences, however, are small. These differences may be avoided by expressing each of these with the same denominator (ie, live births).

LOCAL HOSPITAL EVALUATION

The major concern of the practicing physician and the local hospital is to provide the best possible quality care for patients. Regional and national statistics rarely pinpoint local problems; the most meaningful evaluation originates at the local hospital. The process of evaluation at the local level should be simple in design, should involve minimal paperwork and maximal visibility, and should provide for input from all members of the health care team. There is no single solution to the problem of local evaluation, but the following suggestions may be helpful.

All clinical information should be recorded on a single, multicopy obstetric and neonatal discharge summary that provides complete information for patient charts, for the obstetrician, for the pediatrician, and for a hospital body charged with concurrent review of care. In addition, a simple monthly tabulation of delivery and nursery statistics should be available to all staff members of the obstetric and newborn units. Deaths should be recorded on a separate form that shows the date, hospital unit number, name, birth weight, and presumptive cause of death. This allows for regular local peer review.

Periodically, the health care team should meet to review summaries and address key questions regarding each death. Ultimately, each death should be classified as preventable or nonpreventable. If the death is classified as preventable in retrospective review, the means of prevention should be identified. The results of such deliberations should be communicated to the chief(s) of service and to those directly involved with the care. The team may also discuss specific procedures or diagnoses. Yearly review can provide further critical evaluation as well as important learning experiences for all members of the health care team. Trends in care can easily be documented by simple tabulation, graphic illustration, and display of several years of data. Many hospitals are now using computers for the storage, retrieval, and analysis of data.

QUALITY ASSURANCE

The quality of health care services provided under the auspices of the institution should be monitored, evaluated, and continually improved through quality assurance activities. One essential element of quality assurance is the ongoing identification of existing or potential problems by a systematic review of health care services in terms of valid criteria. The second essential element of quality assurance is a direct link between problems identified through this review process and definitive actions designed to resolve the identified problems, including the development of appropriate continuing professional education programs. Each problem area should be continuously monitored to help ensure that the desired objective is achieved. All patient care review activities should be coordinated and directed through the quality assurance program. The American Hospital Association has issued guidelines to underscore the responsibility for quality assurance, to outline the elements of a program, and to identify ways in which the results should be integrated and utilized to enhance the quality of care.

Providers of perinatal care have by the nature of their field of endeavor focused on outcome. The birthing event culminates in a clearly demonstrated endpoint, and the product is visible and definable in terms of life or death. Such specificity permits the measurement of mortality outcome with relative ease. Morbidity is less easily defined and thus more difficult to measure; however, it is very important in the evaluation of perinatal care.

Accreditation procedures of the Joint Commission on Accreditation of Healthcare Organizations (JCAHO) in the past have focused on structure and process. Evaluation of structure encompasses the availability of equipment such as fetal monitors, the credentialing of physicians in perinatal care, and the scheduling of periodic meetings such as mortality/morbidity reviews. Evaluation of process focuses on the appropriate performance of examinations and tests, as well as the accuracy with which results are recorded. These activities emphasize capability, on the assumption that quality results from capability.

Outcome assessment is currently receiving a new emphasis through the JCAHO. Clinical indicators are used to direct attention to specific situations in which there is a possibility of unsatisfactory outcome or deficient quality. Structure and process criteria are then applied to those situations for further evaluation. With this approach, both clinical performance and capability are assured.

The additional emphasis on outcome assessment in quality assurance and accreditation processes is compatible with traditional individual care of perinatal patients and regional programs. Concepts such as risk assessment and tools such as regional data systems are integral parts of perinatal care and newer directions in quality assurance.

RESOURCES AND RECOMMENDED READING

American Hospital Association: Quality Assurance in Health Care Institutions (Policy and Statement). Chicago, AHA, 1981

Schroeder SA: Outcome assessment 70 years later: Are we ready? N Engl J Med 316(3):160-162, 1987

Williams RL, Cunningham GC, Norris FD, et al: Monitoring perinatal mortality rates: California, 1970 to 1976. Am J Obstet Gynecol 136(5):559-568, 1980

10

SPECIAL
CONSIDERATIONS

ADOPTION

Neonatal adoptions in the United States number close to 25,000/year. The number of neonates who are available for adoption is far lower than that of couples who seek to adopt infants, however. Private independent adoptions (now constituting approximately one-third of infant adoptions), foreign adoptions, and adoptions of handicapped children are becoming common alternatives to agency adoptions. "Open" adoption, rather than the secret and totally anonymous adoption of the past, is a growing trend.

The physician's participation in all these circumstances is increasing. The physician's role is to see that all parties are given as much truthful information, counseling, and support as possible so that they can make informed and thoughtful choices. The data base developed for the infant should be very complete, as the information transferred in the neonatal period may be the only personal and family history available to the child for a lifetime. Therefore, physicians should work closely with other professionals who work in this specialized area.

ADOPTION PROCEDURES

Couples often turn first to the obstetrician-gynecologist for advice concerning adoption. If the couple is seeking an adoption because of primary or secondary infertility, both the husband and the wife should have had a complete workup, and the alternatives should have been discussed with them. The physician should understand that the couple may need help in dealing with the grief, anger, and loss of self-esteem that the inability to conceive a child frequently causes. Consultation with a mental health professional skilled in this field may be helpful.

Once a couple has decided to seek a child via adoption, they are usually anxious and impatient to begin the procedure, although the waiting time may be 3-10 years. They often ask the physician to explain the procedures required and to refer them to the best resources available. Moreover, adoption agencies look to the physician for a conscientious and thorough appraisal of the applicants' physical and emotional capacity for parenthood. Thus, it is essential that physicians, nurses, and medical social workers involved in adoption have a thorough knowledge of local procedures, resources, and the laws and regulations regarding adoption in their state.

There is little uniformity in the adoption laws from state to state. Every state requires an assessment of adoptive parents, and most states have specific residency requirements. Legal counsel may be helpful. Experienced attorneys and adoption agencies protect the rights of both the birth and adoptive parents and ensure that the adoption is properly executed, thus avoiding subsequent legal, emotional, and financial difficulties.

Independent (ie, private) adoptions are legal in some states, and their number is increasing dramatically, particularly among well-educated, older couples with greater financial resources. In such cases, prospective adoptive parents may pay for the pregnant woman's food, housing, and medical care; any additional payment is strictly prohibited by law. In some states, intervention by a third party is also illegal, and a physician or attorney who acts as an intermediary may be liable for prosecution. Familiarity with local law in this specialized area is mandatory.

The majority of adoptions are still arranged by agencies. In addition to preparing a couple for adoptive parenthood, agencies should provide counseling and support services to the birth mother in order to make certain that her decision to surrender her child for adoption was made with careful thought and without pressure or haste. (In private adoptions, this responsibility is assumed by the physician.) The birth mother may be allowed to review the files on prospective parents, choose her child's placement, and even to meet the prospective family prior to the infant's birth. Through careful home study, agencies reduce the risk of inappropriate placement of a child. The physician should support the agency by keeping complete, thorough records, as such records may reduce the likelihood of later anxiety and searches for birth parents. Physicians may also work with agencies to help prospective adoptive couples evaluate medical data on a child. Postadoptive counseling should be available to both the birth parents and the adoptive parents. Issues such as the postbirth care of the neonate, visitation, and access to information should be resolved in a way that conforms both to legal requirements and to hospital procedures *prior to* the infant's birth. If that is not possible, these issues should be clarified as soon as possible after the birth.

In both independent and agency adoptions, the wishes, background, and health of the birth father should be clearly addressed. Many states require a custody release from the father, if the mother has identified him, before the child can be adopted. The birth mother should be told that the father's health and family medical history is important to the child's record and that this information can be recorded while preserving his anonymity.

EXAMINATION OF THE ADOPTIVE NEONATE

Some state laws do not allow the adoptive newborn to be placed with the adoptive parents until 48 hours after birth, and agencies may not place newborns less than 3 days old. Although adoptive newborns should be united as soon as possible with their new parents, at least 48 hours of in-hospital observation is desirable to ensure that the neonate is stabilized fully. This does not preclude adoptive parents' visitation and participation in care if legally permissible and acceptable to all parties.

Nursing and medical observations of the adoptive newborn should be identical to those of any newborn. Laboratory studies, diagnostic procedures, and screening procedures performed on the neonate should be determined by basic medical needs, not by the adoption process. It is the physician's responsibility to assess the newborn's physical status and report this information to the agency or adoptive family for their careful consideration. When medical problems have been identified and the adoption is to proceed, disclosure should be complete, including possible treatments, prognosis, and extent of care required. Questions concerning the condition and care of the neonate should be answered fully. A schedule of periodic neurodevelopmental assessments should be planned for children with high-risk or handicapping conditions. Complete medical documents should be provided to the placement resource. Test results that are not available at the time of discharge should be reported to the adoption agency and to the physician who will have continuing medical responsibility for the newborn; this is particularly important in the presence of infectious disease, because test results in this instance may affect the immediate care and follow-up of the neonate.

After a thorough review of the obstetric chart and the family history, a verification of the birth mother's wishes, and a conference with the social worker, the physician should give the birth mother a summary of the newborn's status. At this time, the baby's physician should confirm the prenatal history, which should include family history, status of previous children born to the mother, chemical exposure, genetic diseases, and other related factors, with the birth mother. A sensitive inquiry into the possibility of consanguinity is essential. When the infant is the product of father-daughter or brother-sister incest, genetic consultation is mandatory. A history of past and present drug or alcohol abuse, or of high-risk conditions (eg, infection with hepatitis B virus, human immunodeficiency virus, or sexually transmitted disease) should be addressed. The birth mother's responses may be more truthful if these questions are asked by the infant's physician, who is addressing the health concerns of the child.

Physicians and nurses should be sensitive to the birth mother's needs and desires. Although she should not be overly pressured to do so, she should be encouraged to see her newborn at least once. The birth mother should be informed of any problems related to the baby. Studies suggest that long-term adjustment of the birth mother is improved if she sees and holds her newborn and discusses the infant with the baby's physician.

The use of an adoption communication sheet (see example in Appendix I) facilitates consistent, sensitive care during the perinatal period. Care should be taken not to disclose the birth mother's identity to the adoptive parents if that is the agreed upon plan. An obstetric social worker who has no other connection to the care should provide counsel to the birth mother concerning the adoption plans in order to ensure that the mother's needs and wishes are being met.

Whatever the birth mother's original intent, she normally feels some ambivalence after the birth. She should be allowed and encouraged to see and hold her baby until she has formally waived parental rights.

Nursing and medical care provided to the birth mother should be identical to that provided to other new mothers. Room assignment off the obstetric floor should be considered if possible, appropriate, and desired by the mother. The emotional turmoil, grief, anger, and sense of isolation may require special support.

RESPONSIBILITY TO THE ADOPTIVE PARENTS

Without appropriate legal clearance, adoptive parents have no right to any contact with the baby. When clearance has been obtained, hospital personnel should facilitate contact between adoptive parents and their baby. In some states, unfortunately, legal clearance is not given until at least 30 days after birth; the child is placed in a foster home in the interim. Foster parents should be provided with complete information on the baby's medical condition so that they can anticipate the baby's needs and can convey them to the future adoptive parents.

In states that allow direct placement, it may be permissible for the adoptive parents to visit their baby in the hospital. The wishes of the birth parents should not be overshadowed by the wishes of the adoptive parents, however. Parents adopting through independent placement may know the identity of the birth parents and may have had contact prior to birth ("open" adoptions). In states where this is prohibited, care should be taken to preserve the birth parents' anonymity.

The need of the adoptive parents to learn parenting skills should be recognized and honored. Like any new parents, prospective adoptive parents may feel uncomfortable and anxious. They should be encouraged to attend child care classes and should be provided with the opportunity for a prenatal interview with the child's prospective physician.

Given information on a child after birth, adoptive parents often turn to a physician to help them evaluate the information in a very short time (see Appendix J). Such a consultation can be a vital service to the parents. Physicians should not be judgmental when evaluating conditions in the child's background that may have both genetic and environmental components (eg, schizophrenia, alcoholism). Information—not decisions—are the proper domain of professional consultation.

RESOURCES AND RECOMMENDED READING

American Academy of Pediatrics, Committee on Adoption and Dependent Care: The role of the pediatrician in adoption with reference to "The right to know": An update. Pediatrics 67(2):305-306, 1981

American Academy of Pediatrics, Committee on Adoption and Dependent Care: Intercountry adoption. Pediatrics 68(4):596-597, 1981

American Academy of Pediatrics, Committee on Adoption and Dependent Care: Adoption of the hard-to-place child. Pediatrics 68(4):598-599, 1981

American Academy of Pediatrics, Committee on Early Childhood, Adoption, and Dependent Care: How and when to tell the adoptee (AAP Policy Statement). News and Comment 34(8):8, 1983

Auerbach KG, Avery JL: Induced lactation: A study of adoptive nursing by 240 women. Am J Dis Child 135:340-343, 1981

Baran A, Pannor R, Sorosky A: The lingering pain of surrendering a child. Psychology Today 11(1):58, 1977

Concerned United Birthparents: Understanding the Birthparent. Milford, MA, CUB, 1977

Frank DA, Graham JM, Smith DW: Adoptive children in a dysmorphology clinic: Implications for evaluation of children before adoption, letter. Pediatrics 68(5):744-745, 1981

Lawrence R: Induced lactation and relactation. In: Breastfeeding: A guide for the medical profession, 2 ed. St Louis, CV Mosby, 1985, pp 409-428

Melina CM, Melina L: The family physician and adoption. Am Fam Physician 31(2):109-118, 1985

National Committee for Adoption (private): Adoption Fact Book: United States data, issues, regulations, and resources. Washington DC, NCA, 1985

Scarr S, Weinberg RA: The Minnesota adoptive studies: Genetic differences and malleability. Child Dev 54(2):260-267, 1983

Sokoloff B: Adoption and foster care: The pediatrician's role. Pediatrics in Review 1(2):57-61, 1979

ANTENATAL DETECTION OF GENETIC DISORDERS

Human genetics is now recognized as an integral component of medical practice. It is, however, a field in which scientific understanding and technologic advances are occurring so rapidly that not all practitioners can remain completely up-to-date. The goal of practitioners should be to maintain a knowledge of current developments that may benefit their patients and to identify those families and pregnancies for which the new or specific genetic knowledge is critical. Well-informed and trained practitioners may handle many of the counseling situations that arise in their practice, but they should recognize those situations in which genetic referral is appropriate.

Historically, obstetricians and pediatricians have done much of the clinical and investigative work in genetic services. Other professionals have also made important contributions to clinical human genetics, and these activities will continue. Regional genetic programs are now functioning in some areas. Close coordination, perhaps integration, of programmatic and individual clinical activity involving genetic and perinatal concerns is necessary.

IDENTIFICATION AND COUNSELING OF COUPLES AT INCREASED RISK FOR GENETIC DISORDERS

Couples at increased risk for producing genetically abnormal offspring are usually identified on the basis of advanced parental age or the presence of a birth defect in the prospective father or mother, their previous offspring, or a near relative. Repetitive abortions or stillbirths also constitute grounds for genetic investigation. Certain autosomal recessive diseases are sufficiently common to warrant screening for heterozygosity. For example, Jews should be screened to identify carriers of Tay-Sachs disease; blacks, to identify carriers of sickle cell anemia; and individuals of Italian, Greek, or Oriental descent, to identify carriers of thalassemia. In addition, a family history of autosomal dominant (eg, Huntington's disease) or X-linked disease (eg, hemophilia) is an indication for genetic investigation.

In order to facilitate identification of such couples, brief questionnaires are available (see Appendixes K and L). Couples at increased risk may or may not need formal genetic consultation. Sometimes, the problem is relatively uncomplicated; for example, the primary physician can readily explain the well-known relationship between advanced maternal age and chromosomal abnormalities (Table 10-1). In other cases, complexities may justify referral. Whatever the situation, counseling is obligatory before antenatal diagnostic studies are performed.

Genetic counseling, whether done by the primary care physician or by the medical geneticist, is defined as a communication process that

Table 10-1. Risk of Having a Liveborn Child with Down's Syndrome by 1-Year Maternal Age Intervals from 20-49 Years

Maternal Age	Risk of Down's Syndrome
20	1/1923
21	1/1695
22	1/1538
23	1/1408
24	1/1299
25	1/1205
26	1/1124
27	1/1053
28	1/990
29	1/935
30	1/885
31	1/826
32	1/725
33	1/592
34	1/465
35	1/365
36	1/287
37	1/225
38	1/177
39	1/139
40	1/109
41	1/85
42	1/67
43	1/53
44	1/41
45	1/32
46	1/25
47	1/20
48	1/16
49	1/12

Data from Hook EB, Chamber GM: Estimated rates of Down's syndrome in live births by 1-year maternal age intervals for mothers aged 20-49 in a New York state study—implications of the risk figures for genetic counseling and cost-benefit analysis of prenatal diagnosis programs. Birth Defects 13:124, 1977 deals with the occurrence, or the risk of occurrence, of a genetic disorder in a family. In this process, one or more appropriately trained persons attempts to help the individual or family 1) comprehend the medical facts, including the diagnosis, the probable course of the disorder and the available management; 2) appreciate the way in which heredity contributes to the disorder and the risk of occurrence in specified relatives; 3) understand the options for dealing with the risk of recurrence; 4) choose the course of action that seems appropriate in view of the risk and the family goals, and act in accordance with that decision; and 5) make the best possible adjustment to the disorder in an affected family member and to the risk of recurrence in another family member. The key elements in this definition are diagnosis, communication, and options. When a genetic disorder has been diagnosed in a family member, the counselor should communicate to the family a range of available options; the counselor's function is not to dictate a particular course of action, but to provide information that will allow couples to make an informed decision.

ANTENATAL DIAGNOSTIC TECHNIQUES

The efficacy of visualization of the fetus by ultrasonography is well established, and nuclear magnetic resonance imaging is under active investigation. Antenatal diagnosis of certain birth defects with these methods is feasible. Ultrasonography plays a role in dating pregnancies and excluding multiple gestations whenever antenatal studies are planned. High-resolution ultrasonography has been used to diagnose hydrocephalus, neural tube defects, renal abnormalities, skeletal abnormalities, and cardiac anomalies. Expert ultrasonographers have often been able to predict fetal outcomes correctly on the basis of midtrimester studies, although neither the sensitivity nor the specificity of such studies is well defined. Fetal blood sampling is used for the diagnosis of hemoglobinopathies, hemophilia, and other disorders. Moreover, fetoscopic or ultrasonographic directed skin biopsies have been used to diagnose certain serious congenital skin disorders that have an unknown metabolic basis.

The scope of the antenatal detection of genetic disorders has been expanded further by recent rapid advances in molecular biology. Because the deoxyribonucleic acid (DNA) complement is identical in every cell of an organism, any hereditary defect detectable at the DNA level should be found in any nucleated cell from that organism.

It is possible to identify mutant genes directly with the use of specific restriction endonucleases (enzymes that cleave DNA within specific base-sequence recognition sites), as an enzyme no longer recognizes its cut site if a single nucleotide has changed. Thus, application of restriction enzymes and DNA probes permits detection of α-thalassemia, sickle cell anemia, and often β-thalassemia in chorionic villi or amniotic fluid cells solely on the basis of DNA sequence.

Amniocentesis

Antenatal diagnosis of genetic disorders usually requires fetal cells. Until recently, the only method to obtain fetal cells was amniocentesis. Transabdominal amniocentesis for genetic purposes usually is performed by the 16th week, but it recently has been performed earlier in pregnancy. An ultrasound examination should be performed prior to amniocentesis to confirm fetal viability, determine fetal age, localize the placenta, and identify multiple gestations. A 20- to 22-gauge spinal needle is placed transabdominally to aspirate 20-35 ml amniotic fluid. With simultaneous ultrasound guidance, an experienced obstetrician can obtain the required volume of fluid in essentially all cases. Cultures usually require 2-4 weeks, and cytogenetic and biochemical analyses are almost always accurate (99%).

Amniocentesis is not without some risk for mother and fetus. Although significant maternal injury rarely occurs, abortion sometimes follows the procedure. Unexplained differences in the abortion rates have been observed in several collaborative studies, all involving centers in which amniocentes were performed in large numbers by a relatively few, skilled individuals; however, the procedurally related risk of spontaneous abortion is in the range of 0.5%. Injury to the surviving fetus is extremely rare.

Chorionic Villus Sampling

A technique for obtaining fetal cells, chorionic villus sampling (CVS) is an alternative to amniocentesis. Samples of tissue obtained between 9 and 12 weeks of gestation provide sufficient tissue for chromosome analysis, enzyme determination, and DNA analysis.

Prior to CVS, a sonogram is done to verify the fetus' gestational age, to assess fetal cardiac activity, to determine the placental implantation site, and to identify multiple gestations. The sampling instrument, a long plastic catheter with a solid flexible obturator, is then guided sonographically to the site of placental development; a small sample is aspirated, and the villi are dissected free from decidual tissue with the aid of a dissection microscope. The villus material is then placed in culture or assayed directly. An alternative technique is transabdominal CVS, whereby a spinal needle is directed into the placenta under continuous ultrasonographic monitoring and a sample removed by aspiration.

The major advantage of CVS is that it permits an earlier diagnosis of a genetic disorder. Disadvantages of the procedure are related to potential complications. The incidence of spontaneous abortion due to the procedure is unknown, but preliminary data suggest that it may be 1% (ie, two times the risk of spontaneous abortion associated with amniocentesis). This risk appears to be related to operator experience. The long-term effects of CVS are likewise unknown. Theoretically, it could lead to intrauterine growth retardation, prematurity, Rh isoimmunization, or placental abruption. The effect of the procedure on the subsequent growth, development, and intellectual function of infants will need to be assessed, just as it was for amniocentesis. In over ten thousand pregnancies that have now gone to term following CVS, however, these potential problems have not occurred.

Chorionic villus sampling has the potential to become a major tool in the prenatal diagnosis of genetic disorders. Transabdominal CVS is another alternative method for obtaining fetal cells. Chorionic villus sampling does not allow alpha-fetoprotein (AFP) determination to detect fetuses at increased risk for a neural tube defect. Accordingly, women undergoing CVS should be offered maternal serum alpha-fetoprotein screening between 15 and 20 weeks of gestation, and optimally between 16 and 18 weeks.

Percutaneous Fetal Blood Sampling

The technique of percutaneous umbilical cord or hepatic vein fetal blood sampling is accomplished by the placement of a 20- to 25-gauge spinal needle under direct ultrasound guidance. The safety and accuracy of this technique, however, have not been systematically evaluated. The use of fetoscopy for visualization of the fetus or for fetal blood sampling has largely been replaced by percutaneous umbilical cord blood sampling.

Laboratory Studies

Physicians should be aware that many laboratories perform cytogenetic (chromosome) analyses, but relatively few perform certain metabolic tests. Before obtaining specimens, physicians should make arrangements with reliable laboratories to ensure that proper preparations have been made to perform the necessary diagnostic studies.

Maternal Serum AFP Screening

Neural tube defects are disorders of polygenic-multifactorial inheritance that occur in 1-2 of every 1,000 live births in the United States. History of such a defect in either parent's family increases the risk of occurrence in the offspring.

Alpha-fetoprotein crosses the placenta and appears in maternal serum. The relative concentrations and general trends in the levels of AFP in fetal serum, amniotic fluid, and maternal serum at 15-24 weeks of gestation are important. The concentration in fetal serum (milligram levels) is highest at 15 weeks of gestation and slowly declines during the remainder of pregnancy. During a normal pregnancy, AFP concentrations in amniotic fluid (microgram levels) follow a similar pattern, but at lower levels. The AFP concentration in maternal serum (nanogram levels) is low early in pregnancy, but rises to a peak value at approximately 30 weeks of gestation (Fig. 10-1). In the second trimester, the level of amniotic fluid AFP is approximately 100 times that of maternal serum AFP.

Levels of AFP in maternal serum and amniotic fluid are usually elevated in the presence of an open neural tube defect; however, closed defects, including those associated with hydrocephalus, are not associated with abnormal AFP findings. Elevated AFP levels also occur with multiple pregnancy and certain fetal abnormalities (eg, omphalocele, congenital nephrosis, Turner's syndrome with cystic hygroma, fetal bowel obstruction, and teratoma). Moreover, small-for-date fetuses and fetal death may be associated with high levels of AFP in amniotic fluid or maternal serum. Incorrect assessment of gestational age may create falsely high (or low) AFP levels, particularly of maternal serum AFP, because the rapidly changing range of normal AFP values depends so critically on gestational age. Normal values should be established by individual laboratories, and correction for various factors (eg, maternal weight, diabetes mellitus, and race) may be appropriate. The values should be interpreted by reference to that laboratory's standards. Regardless of the cutoff value used, however, false-negative and false-positive results occur.

A comprehensive maternal serum screening program that detects elevated AFP levels at 16-18 weeks of gestation can identify fetuses with a neural tube defect. The successful implementation of a screening program for maternal serum AFP should include the

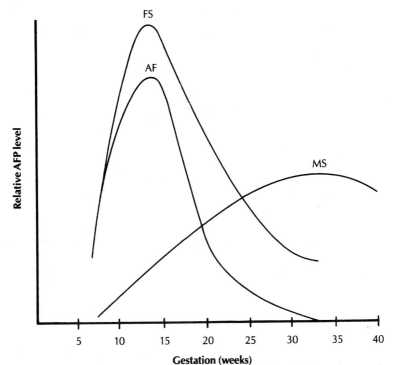

Fig. 10-1. *Relative levels of AFP in fetal serum (FS), amniotic fluid (AF), and maternal serum (MS) throughout a normal singleton pregnancy. (Modified from Milunsky A (ed): Genetic Disorders and the Fetus. New York, Plenum Press, 1979)*

provision of information to the patient, accurate and prompt laboratory testing, access to consultants for sonography and for complex prenatal diagnosis, support services, and competent counseling on the available options, including pregnancy termination. Success is further dependent on the proper coordination of these components so that the time span from screening to decision making is relatively short. Because 90-95% of neural tube defects occur in families without a history of such defects, maternal serum AFP screening is appropriate provided the aforementioned prerequisites are in place.

Recently, low maternal serum AFP levels have been found to be associated with pregnancies in which the fetus has a chromosomal disorder, particularly trisomy 21 (Down syndrome). Thus, maternal serum AFP screening programs should make it possible to detect both high and low values and to develop protocols for responses to abnormal results.

INDICATIONS FOR PRENATAL DIAGNOSTIC TESTS
FOR CONGENITAL DEFECTS

After consideration of both the potential benefits and the potential risks, the following indications for prenatal diagnostic tests for birth defects have been generally accepted:

1. Cytogenetic indications
   a. Advanced maternal age (35 years or older at the expected time of delivery)
   b. Previous offspring with a chromosomal aberration, particularly autosomal trisomy
   c. Chromosomal abnormality in either parent, particularly a translocation
   d. Need to determine fetal sex when there is a family history of a serious X-linked condition for which specific intrauterine diagnosis is not available

2. Single gene disorders (ie, conditions such as inborn errors of metabolism, hemoglobinopathies, cystic fibrosis, and Duchenne muscular dystrophy that are detectable in chorionic villi, amniotic fluid, or amniotic fluid cells) in a sibling or risk of such disorders because of parents' carrier status

3. Multifactoral disorders in a first-degree relative
   a. Neural tube defects
   b. Insulin-dependent maternal diabetes

Antenatal cytogenetic studies may be appropriate in many other circumstances, depending on the preferences of patients and the availability of scientific expertise. It is unrealistic to expect all primary physicians to be familiar with all genetic advances. Therefore, practitioners should seek consultations with specialists in antenatal diagnosis whenever they are in doubt.

RESOURCES AND RECOMMENDED READING

American College of Obstetricians and Gynecologists: Prenatal Detection of Neural Tube Defects (ACOG Technical Bulletin 99). Washington DC, ACOG, 1986

Antonarakis SE, Phillips JA, Kazazian HH: Genetic diseases: Diagnosis by restriction endonuclease analysis. J Pediatr 100(6):845-856, 1982

Davis RO, Cosper P, Huddleston JF, et al: Decreased levels of amniotic fluid alpha-fetoprotein associated with Down syndrome. Am J Obstet Gynecol 153(3):541-544, 1985

DiMaio MS, Baumgarten A, Greenstein RM, et al: Screening for fetal Down's syndrome in pregnancy by measuring serum alpha-fetoprotein levels. N Engl J Med 317(6):342-346, 1987

Golbus MS, Harrison MR, Filly RA: Prenatal diagnosis and treatment of fetal hydronephrosis. Semin Perinatol 7(2):102-108, 1983

Manning FA, Harrison MR, Rodeck C: Catheter shunts for fetal hydronephrosis and hydrocephalus: Report of the International Fetal Surgery Registry. N Engl J Med 315(5):336-340, 1986

Merkatz IR, Nitowsky HM, Macri JN, et al: An association between low maternal serum alpha fetoprotein and fetal chromosomal abnormalities. Am J Obstet Gynecol 148(7):886-894, 1984

Mibashan RS, Rodeck CH, Thumpston JK, et al: Plasma assay of fetal factors VIIIC and IX for prenatal diagnosis of haemophilia. Lancet 1(8130):1309-1311, 1979

Simoni G, Brambati B, Danesino C, et al: Efficient direct chromosome analyses and enzyme determinations from chorionic villi samples in the first trimester of pregnancy. Hum Genet 63(4):349-357, 1983

CLINICAL CONSIDERATIONS IN THE USE OF OXYGEN

The hazards associated with the administration of oxygen to the premature neonate have been recognized for many years. The prolonged use of supplemental oxygen in neonates of low birth weight, especially those weighing less than 1,500 g, has been associated with an increased incidence of retinopathy of prematurity (ROP, also called retrolental fibroplasia). Short-term hyperoxia has not been shown to increase the incidence of ROP, however. Therefore, when the association between oxygen and ROP was first suspected, many clinicians tried to restrict oxygen use. Although the incidence of ROP decreased with restricted oxygen use, the mortality rate of neonates with hyaline membrane disease increased, as did the incidence of spastic diplegia and other neurologic disorders among premature neonates who survived. Thus oxygen was seen as an effective treatment with potential risks.

Although it appears that vasospasm and ischemia of the retina, particularly of the immature retina, may initiate the vasoproliferative process that leads to ROP, many factors other than simple hyperoxia may play an important role in the pathogenesis of ROP. Apnea, sepsis, nutritional deficiencies, and blood transfusions, as well as prolonged oxygen therapy and ventilatory support (especially when accompanied by episodes of hypercapnia and hypoxia) have each been associated with ROP.

Thus far, it has been difficult to see a clear relationship between the partial pressure of oxygen (PaO_2) in the premature neonate's blood and the incidence of ROP. Retinopathy of prematurity has occurred in neonates who have never received supplemental oxygen, in neonates with cyanotic congenital heart disease whose PaO_2 could never have been greater than 50 mm Hg, and in full-term neonates. Conversely, many small premature neonates have undergone sustained periods of hyperoxia without developing ROP. Some neonates have developed severe changes in one eye with little or no disease in the other. Neonates who have been monitored continuously with skin surface electrodes have developed ROP, even when extraordinary attempts have been made to maintain the PaO_2 levels within a recommended range.

METHODS OF OXYGEN ADMINISTRATION AND MONITORING

In an emergency, oxygen in high concentration may be administered by face mask or endotracheal tube to a pale or cyanotic neonate. If the neonate requires supplemental oxygen beyond the emergency period, oxygen should be warmed, humidified, and delivered via a system capable of regulating the concentration (usually by mixing 100% oxygen with variable proportions of compressed air). These principles apply whether the oxygen is delivered by means of a head hood with continuous positive pressure or by means of a ventilator. A calibrated oxygen analyzer should be used frequently, if not continuously, to monitor the concentration of oxygen delivered.

It is necessary to determine the arterial oxygen tension (PaO_2) in order to monitor oxygen therapy. The neonate's color changes from cyanotic to pink as the PaO_2 increases from 20 mm Hg to 35 or 40 mm Hg, but it is not possible to distinguish between a PaO_2 of 40 and a PaO_2 of 140 mm Hg on the basis of color alone. With the development of transcutaneous oxygen electrodes, the skin surface PO_2 level can be measured continuously for relatively long periods. Although these electrodes have made it easier to maintain the neonate's PaO_2 within target limits, they may not always reflect the PaO_2 accurately, especially in the presence of poor perfusion, hypovolemia, or shock. Because perfusion artifacts and sensor drift can occur with transcutaneous instruments, regular correlation of transcutaneous monitors with direct measures of the PaO_2 is recommended.

Recently developed neonatal pulse oximeters provide a continuous estimation of arterial blood oxygen saturation via skin sensors. These devices can be very helpful in the detection of low oxygen saturations (which correlate with oxygen tensions), but lose sensitivity as the PaO_2 rises above 50 mm Hg. So far, there is no noninvasive method for determining the PaO_2 that can completely replace intermittent arterial sampling. The sampling procedure is simple when the neonate has an in-dwelling arterial catheter, but it becomes more difficult when no arterial catheter is in place. Intermittent arterial punctures have been used to verify the validity of the skin surface measurements; however, this technique is not always possible in very small neonates. Arterialized capillary measurements have been used in such cases. These measurements produce fairly reliable estimates of the arterial pH and carbon dioxide pressure ($PaCO_2$), but the PO_2 measurements obtained with this approach tend to produce an underestimation of the PaO_2, especially when the values exceed 50 or 60 mm Hg or when perfusion is compromised.

CONCLUSIONS AND RECOMMENDATIONS

Current knowledge about the hazards and benefits of oxygen therapy is not complete. Nevertheless, the following conclusions can be supported:

1. ROP is not currently preventable in some neonates, especially among those of very low birth weight, and the efficacy of proposed treatments of ROP is still being evaluated.
2. Many factors other than simple hyperoxia can be important in the pathogenesis of ROP in a given neonate.
3. Transient elevations of the PaO_2 alone cannot be considered sufficient to cause ROP.
4. There are as yet no standards of care for the use of oxygen that can totally prevent its complications or side-effects.

With consideration of the current, but incomplete, understanding of the effects of oxygen administration, the following recommendations are offered:

1. Supplemental oxygen should not be used without a specific indication, such as cyanosis, respiratory distress, or a low PaO_2.
2. The use of supplemental oxygen beyond the emergency period should be monitored by means of regular estimates of the PaO_2. When this is not possible, oxygen should be delivered in concentrations just sufficient to abolish cyanosis. If neonates delivered after less than 36 weeks of gestation require oxygen therapy, they should be transferred immediately to a facility with the means to monitor the PaO_2. For more mature neonates, it may be reasonable to administer oxygen for a few hours without such monitoring before making a decision on their transfer. Measurements of the blood pressure, blood pH, and PCO_2 should accompany those for the PaO_2 in neonates who require oxygen therapy. In addition, a record should be maintained of blood gas and ambient oxygen concentrations.
3. When supplemental oxygen is administered to a premature neonate, attempts should be made to maintain the PaO_2 be-

tween 50 and 80 mm Hg. Oxygen tensions in this range should be adequate for tissue needs, given normal hemoglobin concentrations and blood flow. Even with careful monitoring, however, the PaO_2 may fluctuate outside this range, especially in neonates with cardiopulmonary disease. If hyperoxia occurs, it is sometimes prudent to maintain the PaO_2 above 100 mm Hg, especially if attempts to decrease the inspired oxygen concentration dramatically reduce the PaO_2 to very low levels. This is a common occurrence in the care of newborns with pulmonary hypertension. The concomitant increased risk of ROP may be unavoidable during such periods. The medical record should reflect the physician's observations, concerns, and decisions relating to oxygen administration, as well as the discussion with the parents about these decisions and the associated risks and benefits.

4. Hourly measurement and recording of the concentration of oxygen delivered to the neonate is recommended. The oxygen analyzer should be recalibrated every 8 hours with the use of room air and 100% oxygen.

5. Except in emergencies, air-oxygen mixtures should be warmed and humidified before they are administered to neonates.

6. An individual experienced in neonatal ophthalmology and indirect ophthalmoscopy should examine the retinas of all premature neonates (ie, those who were delivered after less than 35 weeks of gestation or who weigh less than 1,800 g) who require supplemental oxygen. Infants that are less mature at birth (ie, those less than 30 weeks of gestation or who weigh less than 1,300 g) should be examined regardless of oxygen exposure. The examination is best done prior to discharge or at 5-7 weeks of age if the infant is still hospitalized and should be repeated according to the schedule appropriate to the original findings. Annual follow-up is recommended for those who have had significant active disease.

RESOURCES AND RECOMMENDED READING

American Academy of Pediatrics, Committee on Fetus and Newborn: Vitamin E and the prevention of retinopathy of prematurity. Pediatrics 76(2):315-316, 1985

Farrell PM, Taussig LM (eds): Bronchopulmonary Dysplasia and Related Chronic Respiratory Disorders. Report of the 90th Ross Conference on Pediatric Research. Columbus OH, Ross Laboratories, 1986

Flynn JT: Acute proliferative retrolental fibroplasia: Multivariate risk analysis. Trans Am Ophthalmol Soc 81:549-591, 1983

Long JG, Philip AG, Lucey JF: Excessive handling as a cause of hypoxemia. Pediatrics 65(2):203-207, 1980

Lucey JF, Dangman B: A reexamination of the role of oxygen in retrolental fibroplasia. Pediatrics 73(1):82-96, 1984

Martin RJ, Klaus MH, Fanaroff AA: Respiratory problems. In: Klaus MH, Fanaroff AA (eds): Care of the High Risk Neonate, 3 ed. Philadelphia, WB Saunders, 1986, pp 171-178

Martin RJ, Robertson SS, Hopple MM: Relationship between transcutaneous and arterial oxygen tension in sick neonates during mild hyperoxemia. Crit Care Med 10(10):670-672, 1982

Yu VY, Hookham DM, Nave JR: Retrolental fibroplasia: Controlled study of 4 years' experience in a neonatal intensive care unit. Arch Dis Child 57(4):247-252, 1982

//

DIAGNOSTIC RADIATION

It has not been established that any particular level of radiation can be considered completely safe, although no ill effects have been proved to occur when the annual level of exposure is below 5 rad. The National Council on Radiation Protection and Measurements recommends maximum permissible limits for occupational and nonoccupational exposure, but these limits are not applicable to medical radiation, which is expected to yield a net health benefit to the individual. In attempts to compare the risk associated with medical radiation to other risks in life, it has been estimated that a bone marrow dose of 10 mrad in an adult carries a risk of death of 2 in 10 million, the same risk that driving 3.6 miles in a car carries. The average loss of life expectancy from medical roentgenograms is estimated to be 6 days, from natural background radiation, 8 days; from motor vehicle accidents, 207 days; and from cigarette smoking by men, 2,250 days.

For perinatal patients, ultrasonography has eliminated the need for many diagnostic radiologic studies, including studies with iodinated media and air. Many pathologic states can now be evaluated noninvasively by ultrasound examination. Thus far, no untoward effects of ultrasound examinations have been demonstrated unequivocally in humans, despite substantial experimental and clinical efforts to detect such effects.

MATERNAL-FETAL EXPOSURE TO RADIATION

Exposure of the embryo or fetus to radiation most commonly results from diagnostic radiologic studies. Most diagnostic studies expose the fetus to very low levels of radiation, however. Fetal exposure with a maternal chest roentgenogram is 8 mrad; upper gastrointestinal series, 550 mrad; intravenous pyelogram, 400 mrad; abdominal computed tomography, 250 mrad per slice. Generally, any study that exposes the fetus to less than 5 rad of ionizing radiation is not thought to be teratogenic. In contrast, exposure of the developing embryo to more than 15 rad ionizing radiation during the first trimester may cause abortion, malformations of the central nervous system, and growth and mental retardation.

It is advisable to avoid fetal exposure to diagnostic ionizing radiation whenever feasible. When X-ray pelvimetry of the mother or X-ray examination of the fetus is necessary, a radiologist should be consulted so that the needed information can be obtained with a minimum of ionizing radiation. Magnetic resonance imaging involves no ionizing radiation and holds great promise for the future evaluation of maternal and fetal abnormalities, but data are still insufficient to establish its safety and efficacy in the fetus.

Although diagnostic radioisotope studies, like diagnostic x-rays, are not hazardous to the fetus, they should be used only when clearly indicated. The fetal thyroid has a greater affinity for radioiodine than does the maternal gland. Because iodine 123 and technetium 99m are generally used today, however, this factor is of importance only when iodine 131 is administered at therapeutic levels (ie, for hyperthyroidism or thyroid cancer).

Women who are scheduled for radiologic studies should be questioned about the possibility of pregnancy. If they are or may be pregnant, alternative methods of obtaining diagnostic information should be considered. When a radiologic procedure is clearly indicated, the physician should consult a radiologist about its extent. There is no contraindication to a diagnostic imaging technique that could prove beneficial to the patient.

RADIATION ASSOCIATED WITH NEONATAL INTENSIVE CARE

A sick newborn may be exposed to two major types of medical radiation: 1) ionizing, such as radiography, fluoroscopy, radionuclide scanning, and computed tomography; and 2) nonionizing, such as ultrasonography and magnetic resonance imaging.

The skin dose from a newborn chest radiograph is approximately 5 mrad; that from a newborn barium enema, 2.3 rad. Skin doses reflect the maximum dose to the body; as radiation is attenuated internally, doses to the bone marrow and specific organs are lower. There are no data indicating that pediatric patients exposed to numerous diagnostic radiologic studies (eg, premature neonates who have many chest and abdominal radiographs or neonates with congenital heart disease who undergo repeated cardiac catheterization) have a higher incidence of leukemia or other malignancy than does the general population. Nevertheless, because there is a theoretical risk of delayed effects and because young children seem more sensitive to late effects, ionizing radiation is best used only when there is no satisfactory alternative.

Most ultrasound applications in the newborn involve real-time pulse-echo scanning and Doppler studies of fluid velocity. Although ultrasonography appears to be safe, it seems appropriate to apply to its use in the neonate the principles outlined by the American Institute of Ultrasound and Medicine, the National Council on Radiation Protection and Measurements, and the Consensus Development Conference on Diagnostic Ultrasound Imaging in Pregnancy: "Until more is known, it is recommended that diagnostic ultrasound utilization be limited to that extent necessary to obtain sufficient clinical information in each patient. At this time, however, the benefits to patients of use of diagnostic ultrasound appear to outweigh whatever risks may be present."

Abdominal ultrasound examinations are used in a variety of clinical settings in the neonatal period. Such an examination is often the only imaging modality required for evaluation of the solid viscera and major blood vessels. Even when further imaging is necessary, ultrasound findings are valuable in selecting subsequent diagnostic studies.

Many neonates in the intensive care unit undergo imaging studies of the brain for diagnosis and follow-up of intracranial hemorrhage. Less frequently, infants undergo such studies for the evaluation of congenital anomalies or trauma to the brain. Three imaging modalities, each with different advantages and limitations, may be used in diagnostic studies of the brain: 1) ultrasonography, 2) computed tomography, and 3) magnetic resonance imaging. The energy delivered to the body in the form of sound waves (diagnostic ultrasonography) or radio frequency waves (magnetic resonance imaging) has not been demonstrated to cause tissue damage in humans or animals at the power levels of intensity used in diagnostic imaging.

Ultrasonography has several advantages in imaging studies of the brain. It uses portable equipment, can be performed rapidly, and does not require absolute immobilization of the patient. The examination can be performed while the patient is in the incubator which avoids excessive handling and cooling of the neonate. Intraventricular-periventricular hemorrhage, as well as ventricular size and a variety of congenital anomalies, are well demonstrated. Ultrasonography is playing an increasing role in the evaluation of cerebral ischemia and other disorders in full-term neonates and has become the screening procedure of choice.

Computed tomography is superior to ultrasonography in the demonstration of subarachnoid and subdural hemorrhage, both of which are much less common in the premature neonate than in intraventricular-periventricular hemorrhage. Computed tomography and ultrasonography are complementary in the evaluation of cerebral ischemia in the full-term infant. In the follow-up of ventricular shunt placement, ultrasonography suffices in many cases; in others, computed tomography may provide useful additional information. The well-collimated fourth-generation computed tomography unit gives a skin dose of approximately 1.4 rad in a standard study of the newborn brain.

Magnetic resonance imaging of the brain in adults and older children has been shown to provide anatomic detail superior to that provided by computed tomography. Its present application to the newborn is restricted by technical considerations, however. For example, magnetic resonance imaging takes more time than does computed tomography. Because the subject must be absolutely still for several minutes, most neonates require heavy sedation before they undergo this procedure. Metal objects, such as respirators and cardiorespiratory monitors, cannot be brought near the magnet, which limits its application for critically ill newborns. On the other hand, studies in stable newborns indicate that magnetic resonance imaging demonstrates fine anatomic detail of the brain parenchyma that cannot be achieved with any other technique.

RADIATION EXPOSURE TO PERSONNEL

At a distance of more than 1 foot from the primary vertical roentgen beam, radiation exposure to personnel is negligible. Because most neonatal radiography is done with vertical beams, it is generally unnecessary for personnel to leave the room during roentgen exposures. Horizontal beam radiography, used for decubitus and cross-table lateral films, may expose other patients and personnel, however. Care should be taken to ensure that only the patient being examined is in the primary beam.

The strong magnetic field in magnetic resonance imaging units may cause cardiac pacemakers to malfunction and various metallic implants to move. Therefore, personnel who have such devices should not accompany patients to magnetic resonance imaging examinations.

RESOURCES AND RECOMMENDED READING

American College of Obstetricians and Gynecologists: Guidelines for Diagnostic X-Ray Examination of Fertile Women (ACOG Statement of Policy). Washington DC, ACOG, 1977

American Institute of Ultrasound in Medicine, Bioeffects Committee: Safety Considerations for Diagnostic Ultrasound. Bethesda MD, AIUM, 1984

Evans JS, Wennberg JE, McNeil BJ: The influence of diagnostic radiography on the incidence of breast cancer and leukemia. N Engl J Med 315(13):810-815, 1986

National Council on Radiation Protection and Measurements: Radiofrequency Electromagnetic Fields: Properties, quantities and units, biophysical interaction, and measurements. Report No 67. Washington DC, NCRP, 1981

National Council on Radiation Protection and Measurements: Radiation Protection in Pediatric Radiology. Report No 68. Washington DC, NCRP, 1981

National Council on Radiation Protection and Measurements: Protection in Nuclear Medicine and Ultrasound Diagnostic Procedures in Children. Report No 73. Bethesda MD, NCRP, 1983

National Council on Radiation Protection and Measurements: Biological Effects of Ultrasound: Mechanisms and clinical implications. Report No 74. Bethesda MD, NCRP, 1983

National Council on Radiation Protection and Measurements: Biological Effects and Exposure Criteria for Radiofrequency Electromagnetic Fields. Report No 86. Bethesda MD, NCRP, 1986

Poznanski AK, Kanellitsas C, Roloff DW, et al: Radiation exposure to personnel in a neonatal nursery. Pediatrics 54(2):139-141, 1974

Robinson A, Dellagrammaticas HD: Radiation doses to neonates requiring intensive care. Br J Radiol 56(666):397-400, 1983

US Department of Health and Human Services, Public Health Service, National Institutes of Health: Diagnostic Ultrasound Imaging in Pregnancy. NIH Publication No 84-667. Washington DC, US Government Printing Office, 1984

Whalen JP, Balter S: Radiation Risks in Medical Imaging. Chicago, Year Book Medical Publishers, 1984

ETHICS

Bioethical dilemmas have always been present in perinatal medicine but the degree of interest and concern associated with them seems to be intensifying. The continuing emergence of new technology enables new approaches to fetal and newborn diagnosis and treatment. Developments in reproductive medicine, such as in vitro fertilization or embryo transplantation, are also of direct concern to providers of perinatal care. Bioethical dilemmas can arise at all levels of care, however, and do not necessarily involve new or extraordinary technology.

Over the past 5 years, there has been intense debate and maneuvering over the perinatal bioethical problems associated with decisions on treatment versus nontreatment of newborns with severe birth defects. The debate focused on two legal cases: the index case, referred to as "Baby Doe," from an infant born April 1982, in Bloomington, Indiana, and a later case, known as "Baby Jane Doe," that involved an infant born on Long Island with neural tube defects.

The issue came to the forefront when the federal government tried to intervene in these decisions by imposing regulations based on Section 504 of the Rehabilitation Act of 1973. After judicial rejection of that effort, the federal government attempted to establish new regulations, but they were rejected by the Supreme Court in 1986. While the court did not uphold the process based on that particular act, other developments occurred that have had what seems likely to be a more lasting impact.

The diverse and often conflicting viewpoints of individuals, government agencies, and groups representing various constituencies (eg, medical and other professional groups, prolife organizations, and disabled citizens) gradually merged into a generally accepted approach to treatment/nontreatment decisions in the care of the newborn. The existing Child Abuse Prevention and Treatment Act was amended in 1984 to require the involvement of state, not federal, protective service agencies in cases in which children are allegedly not receiving needed medical care. The involvement of state child abuse agencies represents an attempt 1) to balance the rights of neonates with the rights of parents to make decisions regarding their children and 2) to avoid inappropriate or unreasonable government intervention into the practice of medicine.

In a March 1983 report, the President's Commission for the Study of Ethical Problems in Medicine and Biomedical and Behavioral Research suggested that "seriously erroneous decisions" about the treatment of newborns were very rare, but that there were apparent "shortcomings" in the decision-making process. The Commission made a number of suggestions, including establishment of explicit hospital policies on decision-making procedures and the possible formation of an "ethics committee" or similar body for select or difficult cases. As the newborn case debate evolved, many of these suggestions, particularly the recommendation that local input into decisions be increased through the use of a committee, were put into practice.

The use of committees to assist in bioethical decision-making is not new. Sterilization and abortion have been subject to review committee action in the past. The use of institutional review boards for biomedical research was intensely debated at first, but is now widely accepted. Although the committees have been empowered to make decisions, not all ethics committees have such authority. Bioethical review committees or the more limited in scope infant care review committees appear to have increased rapidly in number, and extensive reviews of their experience, which has generally been positive, are now appearing in the literature. Many organizations, including the American Academy of Pediatrics, the American College of Obstetricians and Gynecologists, the Nurses Association of the American College of Obstetricians and Gynecologists, the National Association of Children's Hospitals and Related Institutions, the American Nurses Association, the Catholic Health Association, and the American Medical Association, have endorsed the concept.

Institutions and providers of perinatal care should review the way in which they deal with bioethical issues and dilemmas. Traditional values, such as the importance of patient confidentiality, parental rights, the physician-patient relationship, and community or local opinion, can and should remain strong. The rare possibility of a decision that is not in the best interest of a patient and the need for conflict resolution through expression of opinion should be recognized, however. A process that facilitates functions or objectives such as consultation (prospective and retrospective review), policy development, and education is recommended.

Bioethics committees can be a means of attaining the objectives mentioned. The precise details associated with the establishment of such a committee are the prerogative of local institutions and organizations. Discussion of details regarding their structure and function is available in the literature. The proliferation of such committees has provided a broad base of experience with the many details and considerations that should be confronted.

RESOURCES AND RECOMMENDED READING

American Academy of Pediatrics: Principles and treatment of disabled infants (Joint Policy Statement). Pediatrics 73(4):559-560, 1984

American College of Obstetricians and Gynecologists: Withholding or Withdrawing Life-Sustaining Medical Therapy (ACOG Committee Opinion). Washington DC, ACOG, 1985

American College of Obstetricians and Gynecologists: Endorsement of Institutional Ethics Committees (ACOG Committee Opinion). Washington DC, ACOG, 1985

Bowes WA Jr, Selgestad B: Fetal versus maternal rights: Medical and legal perspectives. Obstet Gynecol 58(2):209-214, 1981

Cranford RE, Doudera AE (eds): Institutional Ethics Committees and Health Care Decision Making. Ann Arbor MI, Health Administration Press, 1984

Kliegman RM, Mahowald MB, Younger SJ: In our best interests: Experience and workings of an ethics review committee. J Pediatr 108(2):178-188, 1986

Lantos J: Baby Doe five years later: Implications for child health. N Engl J Med 317(7):444-447, 1987

Michaels RH, Oliver TK Jr: Human rights consultation: A 12-year experience of a pediatric bioethics committee. Pediatrics 78(4):566-572, 1986

Nicholson EB, Horowitz RM, Parry J: Model Procedures for Child Protective Service Agencies Responding to Reports of Withholding Medically Indicated Treatment from Disabled Infants with Life-Threatening Conditions. Washington DC, American Bar Association National Legal Resource Center for Child Advocacy and Protection, 1986

President's Commission for the Study of Ethical Problems in Medicine and Biomedical and Behavioral Research: Deciding to forego life-sustaining treatment. Washington DC, US Government Printing Office, 1983

Stahlman MT: Ethical dilemmas in perinatal medicine. J Pediatr 94(3)516-520, 1979

FETAL THERAPY

With technologic advances in perinatal medicine, the fetus has become more accessible to
diagnostic procedures and to treatment. In or-
der to offer effective therapy to any patient, it is necessary to make an
accurate diagnosis, to understand the pathophysiology leading to the
diseased state, and to know the natural history of the disease in
question. Prior to any attempt at in utero intervention, these factors
should be considered; furthermore, they should be considered within
the context of the unique dynamics of the maternal-fetal relationship.
In some instances, a pregnant woman may be asked to assume
significant risk for the welfare of the fetus. It is important to weigh the
risks and benefits to both patients and to make every reasonable effort
to protect the fetus while preserving the pregnant woman's auton-
omy or right to choose or refuse recommended treatment. Acts of
coercion to obtain consent or to impose a course of action limit
maternal freedom of choice, threaten the physician-patient relationship, and violate the principles underlying the informed consent
process. The use of court orders to resolve conflicts is almost never
warranted.

Active fetal intervention can be divided into medical and surgical
therapy. The modern era of fetal medical therapy began with the
introduction of intrauterine transfusion for the treatment of erythroblastosis fetalis. Subsequently, medical therapy has been extended to
select fetal problems, including some inborn errors of metabolism and
cardiac arrhythmias.

In some instances, fetal therapy involves the timing of delivery.
The risk of premature delivery and its inherent problems should be
weighed against the benefit of early delivery in preventing the
progression of the disease process. The value of this approach is
well-known in pregnancies complicated by diabetes, Rh sensitization,
or intrauterine growth retardation. Early delivery may also play a role
in the management of the fetus with either significant obstructive
uropathy or progressive ventriculomegaly, however. In most conditions detected prenatally, the best course of action is expectant
management with appropriate correction after term delivery.

Fetal surgical therapy is investigational. Interventions have so far
been limited to hydrocephalus, urinary tract obstruction, diaphrag-

matic hernia, and sacrococcygeal teratoma associated with congestive heart failure (placentomegaly or hydrops). These and other structural defects are now being discovered more frequently and at earlier stages of gestation, largely because of the increased use and precision of obstetric ultrasonography. The detection of a single anatomic defect by ultrasound examination should stimulate a careful search for associated conditions (eg, chromosomal abnormalities, metabolic disorders, severe heart defects, or neurologic anomalies) prior to attempt at intervention, as any associated abnormality may significantly alter the prognosis. In addition, there should be an assessment of any irreversible damage to the target organ (eg, kidney, lung) that would make attempted correction in utero of no benefit.

Experimental approaches to treatment of fetal structural defects have generally involved the placement of a catheter to drain abnormal fluid collections. An even more experimental approach to management is the possibility of fetal surgical repair following hysterotomy. Research in this area may play a greater role in future fetal corrective surgery.

Fetal therapy is likely to involve the technique of in utero transplantation in the future. At a molecular level, gene transplantation may be feasible. Disorders such as the hemoglobinopathies or immunodeficiency diseases may be treated by stem cell transplantation, a procedure not greatly different from intrauterine transfusion.

In utero fetal therapy remains an experimental form of medicine. Extreme caution should be exercised in the choice of candidates and disease processes during these developmental stages of fetal therapy. Because it is impossible to determine absolutely when a situation is harmful to the fetus and to guarantee absolutely that the pregnant woman will not be harmed, great care should be exercised to present a balanced evaluation of maternal and fetal expectations.

RESOURCES AND RECOMMENDED READING

American College of Obstetricians and Gynecologists: Patient Choice: Maternal-Fetal Conflict (Committee Opinion 55). Washington DC, ACOG, 1987

Harrison MR, Golbus MS, Filly RA: Management of the fetus with a correctable congenital defect. JAMA 246(7):774-777, 1981

HYPERBILIRUBINEMIA

The factors that determine the toxicity of bilirubin to the brain cells of neonates are many, complex, and incompletely understood. They include those that inhibit the penetration of bilirubin into the brain, as well as cell resistance to the toxic effects of bilirubin. In addition, the interrelationships among serum bilirubin concentrations, kernicterus (a condition characterized by a yellow discoloration of the brain with specific yellow staining of the nuclear areas), and bilirubin encephalopathy (brain damage due to bilirubin) in full-term and low-birthweight neonates are not clear. Yellow discoloration of the brain has been equated with bilirubin encephalopathy in the past, but recent experiments have challenged the theory that they are always associated. The two phenomena may be independent of each other. The incidence of mild neurologic impairment due to bilirubin is not known, nor is it known at what bilirubin concentration or under what circumstances the risk of brain damage exceeds the risk of treatment. Therefore, there are no simple solutions in the management of jaundiced neonates.

BILIRUBIN TOXICITY

A direct association among severe, unconjugated hyperbilirubinemia, kernicterus, and bilirubin encephalopathy has been demonstrated in neonates with erythroblastosis fetalis. In the past, survivors often manifested serious sequelae, particularly the athetoid form of cerebral palsy, hearing loss, paralysis of upward gaze, and dental dysplasia. Observations made some 30 years ago suggested that encephalopathy was unlikely to occur in full-term neonates with erythroblastosis fetalis if serum bilirubin concentrations were kept below 20 mg/dl (342 μmol/liter). Subsequent experience in the care of such neonates has justified these conclusions. In other studies, a correlation was found between elevated serum concentrations of bilirubin during the neonatal period and developmental disabilities, but the designs of those studies do not exclude several other causes for the developmental problems.

With the increasing success of neonatal intensive care, much concern has been expressed regarding the risk of kernicterus in sick, low-birth-weight neonates. As a result of reported autopsy findings of yellow-stained cerebral tissues in premature neonates whose bilirubin concentrations never exceeded 10 mg/dl (171 μmol/liter), published guidelines for the management of jaundice in such neonates have suggested early phototherapy and exchange transfusion at bilirubin concentrations as low as 10 mg/dl (171 μmol/liter). It has been assumed that, if kernicterus can be documented (at autopsy) at very low bilirubin concentrations, bilirubin-related brain damage may be occurring in some surviving neonates whose serum bilirubin concentrations did not exceed 10 mg/dl (171 μmol/liter). Several studies of low-birth-weight neonates have failed to confirm a relationship between serum bilirubin concentrations and later neurodevelopmental handicap, however, particularly if serum bilirubin concentrations did not exceed 20 mg/dl (342 μmol/liter). The number of patients in these studies may not have been large enough to detect a small effect, if one existed.

Studies of low-birth-weight neonates have failed to identify a specific serum bilirubin concentration as a risk factor for kernicterus. In addition, risk factors such as sepsis, hypothermia, asphyxia, acidosis, hypercapnia, hypoxia, hypoglycemia, and hypoalbuminemia, when present, did not significantly increase the risk of kernicterus at a given serum concentration of bilirubin. In neither of these studies could any single factor or combination of factors (including serum bilirubin concentrations) be associated with an increased risk for kernicterus. These studies underscore the extreme complexity of attempting to correlate serum concentrations of bilirubin and subsequent neurologic status. Nevertheless, there is legitimate concern that subtle neurodevelopmental impairment may represent part of a continuum of neurologic damage associated with hyperbilirubinemia.

Theoretically, bilirubin must be "free" (ie, not bound to albumin) in order to cross the normal blood-brain barrier. An increase in free bilirubin in the presence of normal or low total serum bilirubin concentrations is the explanation most frequently advanced for the lack of correlation between total serum bilirubin concentrations and autopsy evidence of kernicterus in low-birth-weight neonates. Although there is evidence from animal studies to support this theory, it has not been tested critically in neonates. Furthermore, the correlation between measured free bilirubin concentrations and the presence of kernicterus at autopsy is not consistent. (It is questionable whether free bilirubin actually can be measured, as the methodology is fraught with difficulties. A better term for clinical use is apparent unbound bilirubin concentration.) Finally, recent animal studies have provided direct proof that, when the blood-brain barrier is disrupted, albumin-bound bilirubin can color brain tissue. Thus, one possible explanation for the lack of correlation between total (or free) bilirubin concentrations and the development of kernicterus is that other factors (eg, hypoxic-ischemic encephalopathy) alter the permeability of the blood-brain barrier to albumin-bound bilirubin. Whether yellow staining through this mechanism also indicates an impairment of brain function is not known.

CLINICAL MANAGEMENT OF THE JAUNDICED NEONATE

When carefully reviewed, the data from numerous studies of bilirubin toxicity are so complex that it is difficult to derive a single rational approach to jaundiced neonates. One principle is well accepted; if there is any evidence that a neonate's jaundice is not physiologic, the cause should be investigated prior to the initiation of treatment. Although bilirubin binding tests theoretically may make it possible to determine the risk of bilirubin encephalopathy, they have not yet been validated well enough to be recommended for general use.

Numerous guidelines for the management of jaundiced neonates have been published, but their effectiveness has not been validated by properly designed experiments. Over the past two decades, clinical observations (not experiments) in full-term neonates with hemolytic disease of the newborn have confirmed that the occurrence of clinical kernicterus is highly unlikely if serum unconjugated bilirubin concentrations are kept below 20 mg/dl (342 μmol/liter). However, there are no properly designed studies or even observational data in low-birth-weight or full-term neonates without hemolytic disease on which to base clinical guidelines for the treatment of neonates with serum bilirubin concentrations below 20 mg/dl (342 μmol/liter). Many European centers perform exchange transfusions for hyperbilirubinemia on infants without hemolytic disease only when the serum bilirubin concentration exceeds 25 mg/dl (428 μmol/liter) and report no apparent ill effects from these higher concentrations.

Many physicians currently use published guidelines that recommend aggressive treatment of jaundice in low-birth-weight neonates, initiating phototherapy early, and performing exchange transfusions in certain neonates with very low bilirubin concentrations (less than 10 mg/dl). Nevertheless, this approach will not prevent kernicterus consistently. Some pediatricians prefer to adopt a more conservative therapeutic stance and allow serum bilirubin concentrations to approach 15-20 mg/dl (257-342 μmol/liter), even in low-birth-weight neonates, before considering exchange transfusions. At present, both these approaches to treatment should be considered rational. In either case, the finding of low bilirubin kernicterus at autopsy in certain low-birth-weight neonates cannot necessarily be interpreted as a therapeutic failure or equivalent to bilirubin encephalopathy. Like retinopathy of prematurity, kernicterus is a condition that cannot be prevented in certain neonates, given the current state of knowledge.

Although there is some evidence of an association between hyperbilirubinemia and neurodevelopmental handicaps less severe than those associated with classic bilirubin encephalopathy, a cause-and-effect relationship has not been established. Furthermore, there is no information presently available to suggest that treating mild jaundice will prevent such handicaps.

Hemolytic Disease

In the presence of hemolytic disease, serial determinations of the serum concentration of bilirubin, not the cord blood concentration of hemoglobin or bilirubin, indicate the appropriate time for the first exchange transfusion (unless the neonate is hydropic or has a life-threatening anemia). The physician may elect to perform an exchange transfusion before the serum bilirubin concentration reaches 20 mg/dl (342 μmol/liter), if it appears that the concentration is likely to reach that point. Women who are likely to deliver severely affected, hydropic neonates should be managed in perinatal centers capable of the full range of obstetric and neonatal intensive care.

Breast-Feeding and Jaundice

Many pediatricians have had the impression that breast-fed neonates have higher serum bilirubin concentrations during the first week of life than do bottle-fed neonates. This association of jaundice with breast-feeding, which must be distinguished from true breast milk jaundice, rests on a body of data that is by no means secure. The composite data from several recent studies reveal that breast-fed neonates have a higher incidence of serum bilirubin concentrations greater than 12 mg/dl (205 μmol/liter) than do bottle-fed neonates, however, and the decline in bilirubin concentrations is slower.

There is some indication that frequent feeding (more than seven times per day) may reduce the incidence of hyperbilirubinemia, but supplemental feedings of water to breast-fed neonates do not reduce serum bilirubin concentrations. Furthermore, when an elevated indirect serum bilirubin concentration is due to some pathologic cause, there is no reason to discontinue breast-feeding. The finding of an association between breast-feeding and increased serum concentrations of bilirubin does not imply a causal relationship.

Breast Milk Jaundice

Approximately 1-2% of breast-fed neonates develop the syndrome of breast milk jaundice. The serum unconjugated bilirubin concentration rises progressively after approximately the fourth day of life and reaches a maximum concentration of 10-30 mg/dl (171-513 μmol/liter) by 10-15 days of life. If breast-feeding continues, elevated concentrations may persist for several days, then decline slowly, and reach normal values by 3-12 weeks of age. If breast-feeding is interrupted at any stage, however, the serum bilirubin concentration declines within 48 hours. With the resumption of nursing, the bilirubin concentration may rise slightly, but it does not reach the previous level.

Although no cases of overt bilirubin encephalopathy related to breast milk jaundice have been reported, there have been no prospective studies of a possible relationship in either full-term or preterm neonates. Furthermore, there is no reason to believe that significant elevations of serum bilirubin in the breast-fed neonate are less threatening than are similar elevations in the bottle-fed neonate. If the bilirubin concentration in a breast-fed neonate is rising and seems likely to reach 20 mg/dl (342 μmol/liter), nursing may be interrupted for 48 hours. This is usually followed by a prompt decline in bilirubin concentration, and nursing may then be resumed.

Mothers who must temporarily cease nursing should be given positive and enthusiastic support, and they should be encouraged to maintain lactation by using a breast pump or manual expression during the period of interrupted nursing. They should also be reassured that there is nothing wrong with them or their milk. Cessation of nursing under these circumstances is rarely permanent and does not affect the mother's subsequent ability to nurse her neonate (see Chapter 7).

Phototherapy

Used extensively throughout the world, phototherapy is an effective means of producing a prolonged reduction of serum bilirubin concentrations in neonates with nonhemolytic jaundice. Exchange transfusion, however, remains the only certain way to decrease the serum bilirubin concentration rapidly and is the treatment of choice when the bilirubin concentration appears to pose an imminent threat to the health of the neonate. Phototherapy is less effective in ABO and Rh hemolytic disease; it reduces, but does not eliminate, the overall need for exchange transfusions. (It is unknown whether phototherapy improves the ultimate neuropsychological function of neonates.)

Characteristics of Light Source and the Dose-Response Relationship

Various types of fluorescent light, as well as a quartz halide light, have been used for phototherapy. A minimum irradiance of 4 µW/cm^2/nm in the blue spectrum (as measured by a photometer) appears to be necessary for effective phototherapy. The response increases as the dose increases until a saturation point is reached at approximately 10-12 µW/cm^2/nm. Because various instruments provide readouts in different units, caution should be exercised in interpreting measurements from photometers. Blue and green lights are most effective; unfortunately, these lights produce undesirable color changes in the neonates, and blue light may cause discomfort and vertigo in the nursery staff. A combination of four special blue lamps placed in the center of the phototherapy unit with two daylight lamps on either side has been found to provide excellent irradiance without producing significant discomfort to personnel. Less information is available on the use of green light.

Indications for Phototherapy

A suggested guideline for the use of phototherapy is to decide on the serum bilirubin concentration at which exchange transfusion will be performed and to initiate phototherapy if the concentration increases to a level 5 mg/dl below that point. In the presence of hemolytic disease, however, it may be appropriate to start phototherapy earlier. In many nurseries, phototherapy is used at much lower bilirubin concentrations, particularly in very small neonates. At present, there is no evidence to show that this is either helpful or harmful. If the diagnosis is breast milk jaundice, it is more effective to interrupt nursing temporarily than to initiate phototherapy.

Toxicity

Phototherapy has no known toxic effects in the human neonate. Nevertheless, phototherapy has many biologic effects, and long-term follow-up studies of neonates who have undergone phototherapy are needed. Because animal experiments have produced documentation of retinal damage from phototherapy, it is recommended that neonates' eyes be covered with opaque patches during phototherapy. These patches can become displaced and obstruct the nares, however, causing apnea and even asphyxia. Constant supervision is necessary because of this potential hazard.

Lamp Life

The life of a lamp varies widely, depending on the circumstances and the type of lamp. Overheating in the light chamber causes the phosphorus to deteriorate and shortens lamp life. With adequate cooling, lamp life is usually several thousand hours. In order to ensure lamp effectiveness, however, it is useful to measure the energy output with a photometer.

RESOURCES AND RECOMMENDED READING

American Academy of Pediatrics, Committee on Fetus and Newborn: Home Phototherapy. Pediatrics 76(1):136-137, 1985

Bjure J, Liden G, Reinand T, et al: A follow-up study of hyperbilirubinemia in full-term infants without isoimmunization. Acta Paediatrica 50(5):437-443, 1961

Kim MH, Yoon JJ, Sher J, et al: Lack of predictive indices in kernicterus: A comparison of clinical and pathological factors in infants with or without kernicterus. Pediatrics 66(6):852-858, 1980

Lewis HM, Campbell RHA, Hambleton: Use or abuse of phototherapy for physiological jaundice of newborn infants. Lancet 2(8295):408-410, 1982

Poland RL, Ostrea EM Jr: Neonatal hyperbilirubinemia. In: Klaus MH, Fanaroff AA (eds): Care of the High-Risk Neonate, 3 ed. Philadelphia, WB Saunders, 1986, pp 239-261

Turkel SB, Guttenberg ME, Moynes DR, et al: Lack of identifiable risk factors for kernicterus. Pediatrics 66(4):502-506, 1980

PERINATAL DEATH

The death of a fetus after 20 weeks of gestation or of a liveborn baby is a traumatic event for parents. The way in which the medical, nursing, and social service staff of the hospital manage this situation during the mother's hospitalization, as well as after discharge, has a critical impact on the parents' ability to adjust adequately to their loss. The goals of the health care team should be to acknowledge the parents' grief and to help each family come to terms with their loss so that grieving can be successfully accomplished and pathologic adjustments avoided. A structured approach that clearly designates the responsibilities of the members of the health care team, establishes a suggested schedule for follow-up meetings, and utilizes written materials concerning such matters as autopsy and funeral arrangements can be most helpful in achieving these goals.

The neonatal mortality rate (number of deaths of liveborn neonates at the age of 28 days or less per 1,000 live births) was approximately 7/1,000 in 1984 in the United States. As there were nearly 3.7 million live births that year, approximately 26,000 liveborn infants died. The stillbirth rate (number of deaths of fetuses who were delivered after more than 20 weeks of gestation or who weighed more than 350 g per 1,000 pregnancies) was even higher at 8.2/1,000, involving a total of more than 56,000 perinatal deaths and twice as many grieving parents. The support and assistance given to these parents is an important responsibility of their physicians and nurses.

Because deaths occur at all levels in the perinatal care system, each hospital's staff should carefully prepare policies and procedures for the management of families who have experienced a perinatal death. The multidisciplinary aspect of these procedures should be stressed, and the responsibilities of physicians, nurses, social workers, and consultants should be clearly delineated to ensure that the family receives the proper support and information. Such a program of support and counseling has two major components: 1) specific, practical management in the period immediately following the fetal or neonatal death and 2) responsibility for ongoing bereavement follow-up.

Specific practical management in the immediate perinatal period should be directed toward two goals: 1) learning as much as possible about the cause of death and implications for future pregnancies, and 2) helping the parents create a memory of the dead fetus or newborn.

MEDICAL MANAGEMENT AND EVALUATION OF THE NEONATE

When a stillbirth or neonatal death occurs, proper management includes documentation of clinical findings, evaluation of the remains, appropriate laboratory studies, and consultation with appropriate ancillary services. A thorough diagnostic workup is important and justified for the parents' emotional well-being, as well as for their guidance with regard to future pregnancies. Following is a suggested protocol for this process:

1. Prenatal history: This comprehensive evaluation should include details of the family history.
2. Autopsy: Fetus, placenta, and cord.
3. Photography: Total body photography is especially important if an on-site consultation concerning dysmorphology is not possible.
4. Total body roentgenograms: It is especially important to obtain roentgenograms of the skeleton if structural abnormalities or dysproportion is suspected.
5. Cytogenetics: Such studies should be undertaken when congenital anomalies are present. Although a sample of heparinized blood can be obtained from the umbilical cord, a peripheral vein, or the heart of fetuses or neonates who have died recently (within 12 hours), the yield of viable white cells may be quite small. A more reliable source is a fibroblast cell specimen obtained through sterile procedures up to 48 hours after death and placed in sterile saline, culture medium, or thyoglycolate broth.
6. Infections: Bacterial and viral cultures and serologic studies should be performed.

Autopsy is the only available means of confirming diagnoses and identifying previously unrecognized conditions. It is particularly important in the presence of congenital malformations that may not have been recognized before death, but may recur in subsequent pregnancies. In addition, the autopsy provides an important focus and starting point for follow-up meetings with parents several weeks after a perinatal death. Families who refuse permission for autopsy or who are not approached with this request by their physicians almost always ask questions in follow-up meetings that could have been answered or at least discussed in a more informed manner had an autopsy been performed. The failure to perform an autopsy is frequently due to the physician's benign but mistaken wish to spare the parents further stress or grief or to the parents' misunderstanding of the procedure and its implications. Parents are more likely to consent to an autopsy if the physician who managed the pregnancy or the newborn's care and who will also be involved in bereavement follow-up carefully explains the need for autopsy to both parents in a private, quiet setting at a time separate from the immediate death (eg, the next morning).

COUNSELING

Bereavement counseling of parents has a very important impact on the family's ability to adjust to their loss and continue with their lives. Each family and each individual react differently to a perinatal death based on their own life experiences (eg, ethnic, cultural, religious background; age; family; and extended family situation) and the circumstances surrounding the death. Health care staff should appreciate these differences. Nevertheless, there are a number of general considerations that hospital procedures can address. One of the most important aspects of care of a mother who has experienced perinatal death is her placement in the hospital during the postpartum stay. The care of these patients is best provided in units where the staff has an understanding of the grieving process.

In-Hospital Support and Counseling

The time in the hospital after the baby has died is unique in that it is the parents' only opportunity to create a memory of the child. Specific management procedures can help the parents achieve this:

- Encourage the parents to see, hold, and spend time with the baby in an environment conducive to privacy and respect. Physicians, nurses, and others should be available to help the parents during this difficult, but important, period.
- Obtain pictures and remembrances (eg, identification tags, locks of hair) of the baby. Even if they say initially that they do not want these mementos, parents frequently ask for them days or weeks later.

- Notify social workers who will provide practical information on funeral arrangements, as well as support and counseling.
- Encourage the family to name the baby, if they wish, and make funeral plans.
- Visit the parents daily while the mother is in the hospital, listen to them sympathetically, give them information as it becomes available.
- Ensure that the parents have access to support from their families, clergy, and friends. The physician should be available to help young parents explain what has happened to grandparents and siblings.
- Provide reliable preliminary information from the appropriate medical professionals concerning the cause and circumstances of death.
- Explain the process of grieving carefully and patiently. Parents frequently demonstrate reactions of acute grief, such as somatic disturbances, a preoccupation with the newborn's appearance or probable future appearance, guilt, hostility, and loss of ability to function. Mourning should be allowed and encouraged to proceed. Physicians should be aware that the staff's potential reactions—guilt, a sense of failure, and uncertainty—may cause them to avoid the parents, thereby impeding discussion of the deceased infant with the family.
- Provide written materials for the parents to read in the hospital and after discharge. The period after a fetal or neonatal death always has an element of confusion because of the continuing grief, the need to inform relatives and friends, and the need to attend to practical details of the funeral. Although there can be no substitute for a multidisciplinary group of professionals carefully organized to provide support, written material can provide concrete information about specific procedures, such as autopsy and funeral arrangements, as well as guidance on long-term issues, such as grief, marriage, explanations for young children, and consideration of another pregnancy. These materials can be designed by the individual hospital or obtained through various associations.
- Finally, because families may come from a distance and, thus, may not know their attending physicians well, it is especially important that tertiary care referral centers designate an individual to be responsible for documenting the management and

follow-up for each perinatal death. Too often, families from afar are lost to follow-up as physicians, nurses, and families avoid the sadness of bereavement.

Counseling After Discharge

The responsibility for ongoing bereavement counseling depends on the specific circumstances of the death and on the family's relationship to the physician. It is primarily the obstetrician's responsibility in the case of stillbirth and the neonatologist's responsibility in the case of neonatal death to ensure that the family has received counseling. The ongoing responsibility to the family includes an arrangement for future visits within six months after the death. These visits provide important opportunities for the parents to ask questions and for physicians and nurses to determine whether grieving is appropriate or pathologic. This may be an appropriate time to review the findings of the autopsy and to counsel patients about genetic implications.

Parents should be reassured that loss of appetite, sleep disturbances, loss of interest in sex, spontaneous crying, and frequent thoughts of their dead baby are normal in the grieving process and will become gradually less intense. Referral to bereavement support groups can be very helpful for many families. Pathologic grief is characterized by a more intense and consuming focus on the loss; it may be manifested as an inability to return to work, a loss of interest in self-care and hygiene, severe insomnia, or a desire to stay in bed for most of the day. Referral to a psychiatrist, psychologist, or social worker is appropriate for these patients. It may be helpful to enlist the aid of the family's pediatrician or school counselor if the other children in the family show signs of difficulty.

In order to optimize their ability to counsel families that have experienced a perinatal death, hospital departments of obstetrics and gynecology, newborn medicine, nursing, and social services should have an ongoing program of education in the normal grieving process surrounding fetal and neonatal loss. A system of monitoring the effectiveness of this program should also be established.

RESOURCES AND RECOMMENDED READING

American College of Obstetricians and Gynecologists: Grief Related to Perinatal Death (ACOG Technical Bulletin 86). Washington DC, ACOG, 1985

THE RELATIONSHIP BETWEEN PRENATAL AND PERINATAL FACTORS AND NEUROLOGICALLY IMPAIRED BABIES

The cause of chronic neurologic disorders in childhood, specifically with regard to cerebral palsy, is a topic of great medical uncertainty. It simply is not known what causes most cerebral palsy. The same is true for epilepsy, much of mental retardation, and most learning disorders. Questions about causation are not unique, of course, but uncertainties in the knowledge of causation are pervasive in the medical issues surrounding cases of poor outcome. The extremely unsatisfactory status of medical knowledge in this area, and the degree to which medical testimony lags behind that knowledge, are seldom acknowledged.

In the past, disorders of the brain that affected young children and had no clearly defined cause were assumed to have originated during parturition. These disorders fall into three major categories: 1) cerebral palsy, 2) mental retardation, and 3) epilepsy. Of these, cerebral palsy, defined as a chronic motor disability present since early in life, is the neurologic problem that has been linked most convincingly to the events of birth. More recently, however, it has been found that several previously implicated obstetric events (ie, oxytocin administration for either induction or augmentation of labor, nuchal cord, midforceps use, and duration of labor) cannot be related individually to cerebral palsy. On the other hand, some factors associated with labor and delivery are reliable predictors of cerebral palsy: gestational age less than 32 weeks, lowest fetal heart rate less than or equal to 60 beats/min, breech presentation (not breech delivery), chorioamnionitis, low placental weight, placental complications, and birth weight less than or equal to 2,000 g. Some of the difficulties in establishing reliable connections between antecedents and outcome in cerebral palsy result from the heterogeneity of the clinical syndromes, the low prevalence of the disorder, and the long delay between many of the putative causal events and clinical recognition of the disorder. This is equally true for childhood seizure disorders. Data from the National Collaborative Perinatal Project (NCPP), consistent with data from the British National Child Development Study, suggested that labor and delivery factors contribute very little to the incidence of mental retardation and childhood seizure disorders. Maldevelopment, rather than injury at birth, appears to be a more common cause of these disorders. Mental retardation and seizure disorders have a substantial association with birth asphyxia only if cerebral palsy is also present.

Despite rapid advances in obstetric and neonatal medicine during the past several decades, physicians, patients, and attorneys continue to believe that the major causes of brain disorders are related to birth trauma and labor complications. One of the most striking findings of the NCPP, however, was that most children with cerebral palsy had neither a low birth weight nor evidence of birth asphyxia.

Perinatal asphyxia, which causes respiratory depression, can cause brain injury and interfere with subsequent development, but its role in producing long-term neurologic impairment should not be overestimated. The evidence obtained in follow-up studies of depressed infants does not support the conclusion reached by some obstetric authorities that perinatal asphyxia is the major cause of cerebral palsy and severe mental retardation. Less than 15% of depressed infants develop chronic brain impairment that can be attributed to asphyxia.

Apgar scores at 1 and 5 minutes correlate poorly with either cause or outcome. Several conditions are required before a causal relationship between intrapartum asphyxia and cerebral palsy can be established:

1. Asphyxia must be severe and prolonged.
2. Evidence of the effects of asphyxia must be apparent in the delivery room.
3. Evidence compatible with hypoxic/ischemic encephalopathy (eg, hypotonia, poor feeding, problem with respiratory control, and seizures) is usually present in the neonatal period.
4. The resultant cerebral palsy is usually severe.

The absence of the findings listed strongly suggests that asphyxia was not the cause of the effect. Although the presence of these signs and symptoms is compatible with an anoxic insult, other causes for them should be considered.

RESOURCES AND RECOMMENDED READING

National Institutes of Health, Task Force on Joint Assessment of Prenatal and Perinatal Factors Associated with Brain Disorders: Report on causes of mental retardation and cerebral palsy. Pediatrics 76(3):457-458, 1985

Nelson KB, Ellenberg JH: Antecedents of cerebral palsy: Multivariate analysis of risk. N Engl J Med 315(2):81-86, 1986

Nelson KB, Ellenberg JH: Predisposing and causative factors in childhood epilepsy. Epilepsia 28(x s), 1987

Paneth N: Birth and the origins of cerebral palsy, editorial. N Engl J Med 315(2):124-126, 1986

Paneth N: Cerebral palsy and mental retardation in relation to indicators of perinatal asphyxia. An epidemiologic overview. Am J Obstet Gynecol 147(8):960-966, 1983

Stanley F, Alberman E (eds): The Epidemiology of Cerebral Palsies. Spastics International Medical Publications, 1984

THERMAL REGULATION

Thermoregulatory control mechanisms should balance heat production and heat loss so that body core temperature remains constant at approximately 36.5°C to 37°C. The high surface area:body mass ratio makes the newborn, especially the low-birth-weight newborn, particularly prone to heat loss. Heat or cold stress readily overwhelms the thermoregulatory control system of the sick low-birth-weight neonate with serious, even lethal, consequences.

When cold-stressed, a neonate rapidly depletes essential stores of fat and glycogen and grows more slowly or fails to thrive. Skin temperature receptors signal the neonate's central hypothalamic region, resulting in general sympathetic nervous system arousal and a rapid rise in the level of circulating norepinephrine. This catecholamine surge mediates several important thermal responses. First, lipolysis and reesterification of specialized brown fat stores release heat. Second, the heart rate rises, delivering more oxygen to fuel nonshivering thermogenesis. Third, peripheral vasoconstriction diverts blood from the skin toward the more metabolically active organs that drive thermogenesis. The resultant increased metabolic rate warms the neonate, but also depletes the endogenous substrate.

A neutral thermal environment is one that requires a minimum metabolic expenditure of energy, as measured by oxygen consumption. Temperature in such an environment can be variously defined. At best, the suggested temperature range for the thermoneutral zone (environment or skin) for neonates in the nursery is an approximation of the thermal conditions most likely to maintain normal body temperature at minimal metabolic cost to the neonates. Because cold response is skin temperature-mediated, any set of environmental conditions that maintains skin temperature in the range of 36.3°C to 36.8°C produces minimal oxygen consumption in premature neonates.

The site selected for estimating a neonate's core temperature should be recorded and used consistently in serial measurements. Moreover, because of inconsistencies in the accuracy of clinical thermometers, the same thermometer should be used for serial measurements in an individual neonate. Thermometers should be tested periodically.

Axillary temperature has been shown to reflect rectal temperature if taken properly, and axillary determinations of temperature are less hazardous than are rectal determinations. In preterm neonates, axillary temperature generally ranges 0.1°C-0.2°C cooler than rectal temperature. A normal axillary temperature in the preterm neonate probably ranges 36.3°C to 36.9°C. In order to produce accurate results, the neonate's arm should be adducted with the thermometer bulb deep in the axilla. It takes 5 full minutes to obtain repeatable equilibrium temperatures within 0.1°C. Deep body temperature can also be measured in the rectum, esophagus, or auditory canal by means of an appropriate flexible thermister probe.

The body temperature of vigorous full-term neonates should be determined when they are admitted to the nursery and at 4-hour intervals until it is in the normal range and stable. Thereafter, temperature should be determined and recorded on each 8-hour shift. The body temperature of low-birth-weight neonates should be monitored continuously by thermistors or determined at intervals of 1-3 hours. Critically ill infants should be continuously monitored for skin temperature, and an appropriate alarm for over- or underheating. In addition, the core temperature (eg, axillary or rectal) of these neonates should be determined every 1-2 hours.

DELIVERY ROOM CARE

Most neonates suffer some cold stress at the time of delivery because of large radiant, convective, and evaporative heat losses from their warm, wet skin. Their skin temperature may fall precipitously by 0.3°C/min; rectal temperature decreases more slowly. Most contemporary delivery rooms are air-conditioned; room temperature may have to be adjusted in consideration of the neonate.

Hypoxia, anesthesia, maternal sedation, infection, and birth injury may all have adverse effects on the thermal stability of the newborn. The surface area:body mass ratio is exaggerated in low-birth-weight neonates; their tissues have increased thermal conductivity, and heat loss per unit of surface area is enhanced. Neonates should not be bathed or washed until thermal stability has been ensured. The following steps can reduce heat loss during the first minutes following delivery:

1. Dry the neonate with prewarmed towels. It is particularly important to dry the head and face, which constitute a large surface area.

2. Use a radiant heater above the neonate to create a heat-gaining environment during the first minutes following delivery.
3. Wrap the full-term neonate in a dry, warm blanket or aluminum swaddler. A transparent plastic blanket may be used under a radiant warmer to reduce heat loss in a preterm neonate.
4. Cover the head.

THERMAL ENVIRONMENT AFTER DELIVERY

Bassinets

Normal, full-term neonates in bassinets should be dressed and blanketed. Table 10-2 shows the room air temperature necessary to provide adequate warmth for neonates kept clothed and well covered in a bassinet in a draught-free room of moderate (35-60%) humidity.

Convection Warmed Incubators

Enclosed incubators may be used routinely for thermal regulation of the premature neonate's ambient air. The traditional guidelines for selection of the ambient air temperature, given an individual neonate's size (ie, gestational age) and postnatal age, are presented in Table 10-3. Recently, these guidelines have been revised to recommend slightly higher (+0.5°C -1°C) ambient air temperatures for the extremely premature neonate (ie, born at less than 29 weeks of gestation) during the first week of life.

The use of a second wall (double-walled design) in an incubator reduces radiant heat loss from low-birth-weight infants, thus reducing their air temperature demands. Plastic blankets or heat shields inside incubators also reduce convective and evaporative heat loss from neonates. The administration of warmed/humidified respiratory

Table 10-2. Air Temperature Required to Provide Adequate Warmth for Neonates

Birth Weight (kg)	Air Temperature		
	29.5°C (85°F)	26.5°C (80°F)	24°C (75°F)
1.5-2*	For 2 days	After 2 days	After 2 weeks
2-3		For 1 week	After 1 week
3		For 1 day	After 1 day

*It is not recommended that neonates who weigh less than 1,750 g be nursed routinely in bassinets.

Table 10-3. Neutral Thermal Environmental Temperatures

Age and Weight	Starting Temperature (°C)	Range of Temperature (°C)
0-6 Hours		
Under 1200 g	35.0	34.0-35.4
1200-1500 g	34.1	33.9-34.4
1501-2500 g	33.4	32.8-33.8
Over 2500 (and > 36 weeks)	32.9	32.0-33.8
6-12 Hours		
Under 1200 g	35.0	34.0-35.4
1200-1500 g	34.0	33.5-34.4
1501-2500 g	33.1	32.2-33.8
Over 2500 (and > 36 weeks)	32.8	31.4-33.8
12-24 Hours		
Under 1200 g	34.0	34.0-35.4
1200-1500 g	33.8	33.3-34.3
1501-2500 g	32.8	31.8-33.8
Over 2500 (and > 36 weeks)	32.4	31.0-33.7
24-36 Hours		
Under 1200 g	34.0	34.0-35.0
1200-1500 g	33.6	33.1-34.2
1501-2500 g	32.6	31.6-33.6
Over 2500 (and > 36 weeks)	32.1	30.7-33.5
36-48 Hours		
Under 1200 g	34.0	34.0-35.0
1200-1500 g	33.5	33.0-34.1
1501-2500 g	32.5	31.4-33.5
Over 2500 (and > 36 weeks)	31.9	30.5-33.3
48-72 Hours		
Under 1200 g	34.0	34.0-35.0
1200-1500 g	33.5	33.0-34.0
1501-2500 g	32.3	31.2-33.4
Over 2500 (and > 36 weeks)	31.7	30.1-33.2
72-96 Hours		
Under 1200 g	34.0	34.0-35.0
1200-1500 g	33.5	33.0-34.0
1501-2500 g	32.2	31.1-33.2
Over 2500 (and > 36 weeks)	31.3	29.8-32.8
4-12 Days		
Under 1500 g	33.5	33.0-34.0
1501-2500 g	32.1	31.0-33.2
Over 2500 (and > 36 weeks)	31.0	39.5-32.6
4-5 days		
5-6 days	30.9	29.4-32.3
6-8 days	30.6	29.0-32.2
8-10 days	30.3	29.0-31.8
10-12 days	30.1	29.0-31.4
12-14 Days		
Under 1500 g	33.5	32.6-34.0
1501-2500 g	32.1	31.0-33.2
Over 2500 (and > 36 weeks)		

(continued)

Table 10-3. Neutral Thermal Environmental Temperatures *(Continued)*

Age and Weight	Starting Temperature (°C)	Range of Temperature (°C)
2-3 Weeks		
Under 1500 g	33.1	32.2-34.0
1501-2500 g	31.7	30.5-33.0
3-4 Weeks		
Under 1500 g	32.6	31.6-33.6
1501-2500 g	31.4	30.0-32.7
4-5 Weeks		
Under 1500 g	32.0	31.2-33.0
1501-2500 g	30.9	29.5-32.2
5-6 Weeks		
Under 1500 g	31.4	30.6-32.3
1501-2500 g	30.4	29.0-31.8

Data from Scopes JW, Ahmed I: Minimal rates of oxygen consumption in sick and premature infants. Arch Dis Child 41:407-416, 1966; Scopes JW, Ahmed I: Range of critical temperatures in sick and premature newborn babies. Arch Dis Child: 417-419, 1966. For his table, Scopes had the walls of the incubator 1° to 2° warmer than the ambient air temperatures.

Generally speaking, the smaller infants in each weight group require a temperature in the higher portion of the temperature range. Within each time range, the younger the infant, the higher the temperature required.

gases may provide supplemental heat, necessitating a decrease in the incubator air temperature. Because so many factors now influence incubator requirements for the sick, premature neonate, many physicians prefer to use an anterior abdominal wall temperature servocontrol mechanism to regulate skin temperature within a thermoneutral range skin (36.5°C-37°C) by automatic air temperature control. Core temperature should be measured frequently during servocontrol regulation, because incubation can result in overheating if the skin sensor becomes loose.

High humidity tends to reduce insensible water loss and evaporative heat loss; however, high ambient humidity also tends to encourage the growth of gram-negative bacilli on the skin, including *Escherichia coli* and *Pseudomonas*. A moderate relative humidity of approximately 50% provides optimal conditions for the neonate.

Radiant Warmers

The use of radiant warmers facilitates the care of the neonate, particularly the care of a critically ill neonate who requires cardiorespiratory support and monitoring. Radiant warmers promote insensible water loss and a small increase in metabolic rate. These changes vary with a neonate's weight and gestational age, and the fluid requirements should be regulated according to clinical and biochemical criteria. Infection has not been found to be a significant problem for neonates nursed under these conditions.

Radiant warmers should be used in the servocontrol mode with the abdominal skin temperature maintained at 36.5°C-37°C. The thermistor should be securely taped to the anterior abdominal wall in the supine patient and covered with an aluminum patch to prevent the radiant heat source from heating the probe directly. The servocontrol skin temperature should be reduced 0.2°C-0.5° C for mild neonatal core hyperthermia (ie, temperature above 37.5°C). Bundling the neonate may interfere with the proper function of temperature alarms. If used, shields should be very thin, pliable plastics that do not adhere to the neonate's skin. Surgical drapes may interfere with radiant warming, resulting in either severe hyperthermia or hypothermia.

HYPERTHERMIA

Infection, dehydration, and excessively high environmental temperatures in improperly regulated incubators and radiant warmers can produce hyperthermia in neonates. Radiant heat from phototherapy lights and sunlight can overheat the neonate without (initially) warming the air in the surrounding environment. Measurement of extremity skin temperature simultaneously with the core temperature helps to differentiate pyrexia due to environmental overheating from that due to disease. Hyperthermia increases metabolic demands and, thus, increases oxygen requirements; it causes sweating in the full-term and older premature neonate.

Hyperthermia is treated by cooling the neonate rapidly. When the skin temperature is 37.5°C-39°C, undressing and exposing the neonate to room temperature is usually all that is necessary. If the skin temperature is above 39°C, the neonate should be undressed and sponged with tepid water at approximately 35°C until the skin temperature is below 38°C.

HYPOTHERMIA

An abnormally low body temperature (ie, less than 36°C truncal skin temperature and less than 36.5°C deep rectal or axillary temperature) compromises neonates. Severely hypothermic neonates appear red and edematous, and they may have sclerema. Chronic cold stress, even if it is mild, in the newborn increases metabolic rate and oxygen requirement, decreases growth rate, and may contribute to mortality.

The rate at which hypothermic neonates should be warmed is controversial. Fast warming has been shown to increase oxygen consumption, possibly causing apnea. During the warming process, blood pressure, blood glucose, and blood gases should be monitored closely, because neonates who are undergoing this procedure may develop metabolic acidosis, hypoglycemia, shock, clotting disorders, and hypoxia.

TEMPERATURE CONTROL IN SPECIAL CIRCUMSTANCES

Very low birth weight neonates (ie, those who weigh less than 1,000 g) present special problems. First, their small size alone results in a geometrically larger surface area relative to the smaller metabolically active body mass. Second, the very low birth weight neonate does not have sufficient stores of glycogen and brown fat to mount a sustained response to cold stress. As a result, very low birth weight neonates are almost completely dependent on artificial thermal maintenance. Excessive heat and water losses should be avoided, and core temperature/skin temperature should be monitored in order to select a properly tailored set of environmental conditions. No one air temperature can suffice in these patients.

The temperature of respiratory gas delivered to the neonate should be similar to the temperature of the incubator. Gases delivered directly via endotracheal tubes should be warmed to 35°C-36°C.

Neonates should be transported to and from in-hospital facilities, such as the operating room or radiology department, in a transport incubator or in a regular incubator with the neonate lying on a heated mattress and covered by a thermal blanket. If a transport incubator is used, the air temperature should be set to approximate a thermoneutral environment. In cold environments, it is helpful both to use a double-walled incubator and to cover the neonate with a thermal blanket. Transport incubators with radiant warming hoods are also effective. A similar system (or a circulating warm water mattress) can be used to keep the neonate's temperature stable during surgical procedures or computed tomography scans, radiologic procedures, and cardiac catheterizations.

Because death and injuries have resulted from hyperthermia and hypothermia, alarm systems and range controls of all equipment used for neonatal thermal regulation should be tested regularly. Nursery policies and procedures should specifically address this issue, and the time of testing should be documented.

RESOURCES AND RECOMMENDED READING

Baumgard S: Reduction of oxygen consumption, insensible water loss, and radiant heat demand with use of a plastic blanket for low-birth-weight infants under radiant warmers. Pediatrics 74(6):1022-1028, 1984

Day RL, Caliguiri L, Kamenski C, et al: Body temperature and survival of premature infants. Pediatrics 34(2):171-181, 1964

Hey EN: Thermal regulation in the newborn. Br J Hosp Med 8(1):51-64, 1972

Malin SW, Baumgart S: Optimal thermal management for low birth weight infants nursed under high-powered radiant warmers. Pediatrics 79(1):47-54, 1987

Marks KH, Lee CA, Bolan CD Jr, et al: Oxygen consumption and temperature control of premature infants in a double-wall incubator. Pediatrics 68(1):93-98, 1981

Pleet H, Graham JM Jr, Smith DW: Central nervous system and facial defects associated with maternal hyperthermia at four to 14 weeks' gestation. Pediatrics 67(6):785-789, 1981

Pomerance JJ, Brand RJ, Meredith JL: Differentiating environmental from disease-related fevers in the term newborn. Pediatrics 67:485-488, 1981

Sauer PJ, Dane HJ, Visser HA: New standards for the neutral thermal environment of healthy very low birthweight infants in week one of life. Arch Dis Child 59(1):18-22, 1984

TOCOLYSIS

Despite significant advances in obstetric care
during the past 10 years, the rate of preterm
delivery has remained constant. Although only
approximately 7% of pregnancies end before term, approximately
75% of perinatal deaths in the United States are secondary to preterm
delivery.

In 1980, the Food and Drug Administration approved the drug
ritodrine hydrochloride, a sympathomimetic adrenergic drug, for use
in attempts to inhibit labor. Although randomized studies have
established the efficacy of ritodrine, only a small percentage of
patients at risk for preterm labor can potentially benefit from its use.
Its effectiveness is limited in some circumstances, including advanced
preterm labor, premature rupture of the membranes, and certain
underlying obstetric conditions (eg, infections or abruptio placenta).
Furthermore, treatment with ritodrine has resulted in a number of
life-threatening complications. Therefore, it is imperative for the
physician who uses ritodrine to have a full understanding of its
pharmacologic effects on the mother and fetus.

While ritodrine is the first and only drug approved by the FDA
specifically for treatment of preterm labor, other drugs have been
used for this purpose. Terbutaline, also a sympathomimetic adrenergic drug, and magnesium sulfate have been found to be as safe and
effective as ritodrine. Terbutaline and ritodrine are pharmacologically
comparable. The combination of sympathomimetic adrenergic drugs
with magnesium sulfate has been reported to increase their efficacy,
but it may increase their toxicity as well; therefore, combined simultaneous usage should be reserved for single agent failure. Calcium
channel blockers are currently under investigation as tocolytic agents.

Contraindications to tocolysis include severe hemorrhage, severe
pregnancy-induced hypertension, intrauterine fetal demise, and
chorioamnionitis. Because sympathomimetic adrenergic drugs may
be contraindicated in selected cases of diabetes mellitus, cardiac
disease, and hyperthyroidism, magnesium sulfate is a suitable alternative.

TOCOLYTIC PROCEDURES

Administration of Ritodrine

Sympathomimetic adrenergic drugs act by increasing the intracellular production of cyclic adenosine monophosphate (cAMP), which reduces the intracellular free calcium concentration in smooth muscle. A low calcium environment inhibits activation of the contractile proteins, actin and myosin, thus inhibiting smooth muscle contractions.

Intravenous therapy with ritodrine is initiated at 0.1 mg/min and increased by 0.05 mg/min every 10 minutes until contractions cease, until unacceptable side-effects (eg, significant maternal tachycardia) occur, or until a maximum rate of 0.35 mg/min is reached. Maternal blood pressure, pulse, and respiratory rate are measured every 10 minutes until the maintenance dosage is reached; after that, the mother's vital signs are obtained at 30-minute intervals while the fetal heart rate and uterine activity are continuously monitored electronically. The dosage is reduced if side-effects are poorly tolerated. After labor has been arrested, the infusion should be continued for 12 hours. Before the infusion is terminated, oral treatment is initiated. Oral treatment continues until inhibition of labor is no longer indicated or until preterm labor recurs and intravenous therapy is again indicated.

A randomized, prospective study has shown that ritodrine significantly decreases the incidence of preterm delivery in patients treated for preterm labor when compared with appropriate controls. In addition, the neonates of ritodrine-treated patients had significantly less respiratory distress and a greater birth weight. All patients in this trial had cervical dilatation equal to or less than 3 cm with intact membranes.

Administration of Magnesium Sulfate

The mechanism by which magnesium sulfate, a non-beta-mimetic, affects preterm labor is unclear, but it may involve the displacement of calcium from receptor sites within the uterine muscle, which increases the amount of free intracellular calcium. After a loading dose by intravenous infusion of 4-6 g magnesium sulfate, a constant infusion of 2 g/hour is indicated. In some instances, a higher dosage may be needed. If tocolysis is inadequate, measurements of serum magnesium levels may indicate when the infusion rate can be increased safely. Measurement of serum magnesium levels is also of value in avoiding toxicity at infusion rates at 2 g/hour or more or when there is decreased maternal renal function. If treatment with magnesium sulfate is successful, oral therapy with sympathomimetic adrenergic drugs may be initiated as outlined earlier.

COMPLICATIONS OF TOCOLYSIS

An ideal sympathomimetic adrenergic drug for tocolysis would stimulate only the beta-adrenergic receptors in the myometrium. Unfortunately, because tocolytic drugs stimulate sympathomimetic adrenergic receptors in other tissues, treatment affects other systems. The intravenous infusion of ritodrine uniformly causes an elevation of the maternal and fetal heart rates, a widening of pulse pressure, a moderate decrease in the serum potassium level, and a transient elevation in the levels of blood glucose, plasma insulin, and free fatty acids. Blood glucose levels of patients with diabetes mellitus require careful monitoring, as ketoacidosis has occurred with beta-mimetic treatment in these patients. For this reason, some physicians initially use magnesium sulfate to inhibit preterm labor in their diabetic patients.

Tremors, palpitations, nervousness, restlessness, and chest pain have all been reported fairly commonly in association with sympathomimetic adrenergic tocolysis. Severe hypotension is rare in the absence of hemorrhage or hypovolemia; however, myocardial ischemia and cardiac arrhythmias have been noted in some of these patients. In particular, premature ventricular contractions, premature nodal contractions, and atrial fibrillation have all occurred. These cardiac arrhythmias usually respond to the discontinuation of treatment and the administration of oxygen.

Because hypokalemia results from the movement of potassium from the extracellular to the intracellular space rather than from an increase in the urinary excretion of potassium, the amount of total body potassium does not change. Therefore, potassium supplementation is not recommended unless levels fall to unacceptably low levels.

Pulmonary edema, the most frequently reported major complication of parenteral sympathomimetic adrenergic drug treatment, has been associated with fluid overload in a number of cases. The risk increases when steroids are administered to prevent respiratory distress syndrome. Fluid overload can occur by two mechanisms: 1) excessive hydration during therapy and 2) decreased renal excretion of sodium, potassium, and water as a direct result of beta-sympathomimetic therapy. The increased blood volume in mothers with multiple gestations may explain the increased incidence of pulmonary edema associated with tocolysis in this group of patients. In order to avoid fluid overload, intravenous fluid administration should be limited.

Pulmonary edema has also been noted in tocolysis with magnesium sulfate suggesting that the specific pharmacologic actions of the sympathomimetic adrenergic drugs are not the only variables in the development of pulmonary edema. Careful management of fluid intake is the key to prevention of this complication.

CONCLUSION

Tocolytic drugs should be used only when the physician, staff, and institution are capable of monitoring and treating side-effects in both mother and fetus, as well as dealing with the consequences of a therapeutic failure. Although tocolysis is a valuable approach to controlling preterm labor and delivery, it demands careful selection of patients, continuing observation of these patients, and attention to the pharmacologic effects of the drugs involved.

RESOURCES AND RECOMMENDED READING

Barden TP, Peter JB, Merkatz IR: Ritodrine hydrochloride: A betamimetic agent for use in preterm labor. Obstet Gynecol 56(l): 1-6, 1980

Beall MH, Edgar BW, Paul RH, et al: A comparison of ritodrine, terbutaline, and magnesium sulfate for the suppression of preterm labor. Am J Obstet Gynecol 153(8): 854-859, 1985

Benedetti TJ: Maternal complications of parenteral β-sympathomimetic therapy for premature labor. Am J Obstet Gynecol 145(l): 1-6, 1983

Caritis SN, Edelstone DI, Mueller-Heubach E: Pharmacologic inhibition of preterm labor. Am J Obstet Gynecol 133(5): 557-578, 1979

Creasy RK, Golbus MS, Laros PK, et al: Oral ritodrine maintenance in the treatment of preterm labor. Am J Obstet Gynecol 137(2): 212-219, 1980

Elliott JP: Magnesium sulfate as a tocolytic agent. Am J Obstet Gynecol 147(3): 277-284, 1983

Ferguson JE, Hensleigh PA, Kredenster D: Adjunctive use of magnesium sulfate with ritodrine for preterm labor tocolysis. Am J Obstet Gynecol 148(2): 166-171, 1984

Hollander D, Nagey DA, Pupkin MJ: Magnesium sulfate and ritodrine hydrochloride: A randomized comparison. Am J Obstet Gynecol 156(3):631-637, 1987

Hatjis CG, Nelson LH, Meis PJ, et al: Addition of magnesium sulfate improves effectiveness of ritodrine in preventing premature delivery. Am J Obstet Gynecol 150(2): 142-150, 1984

Merkatz IR, Peter JB, Barden TP: Ritodrine hydrochloride: A betamimetic agent for use in preterm labor: II. Evidence of efficacy. Obstet Gynecol 56(l): 7-12, 1980

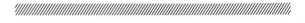

APPENDIX

A

ILLUSTRATIVE CATEGORIZATION OF PERINATAL SERVICES

The following matrix is offered as a guide in the organization of individual regional programs. The broad goals identified in Chapter 1 (ie, reduction of perinatal mortality and morbidity, efficient utilization of resources) should be linked to specific service, education, research, and administrative objectives that are locally determined. Parts of the matrix can be modified according to local needs and resources. The guidelines given here and, in greater detail, in Chapters 2 and 3 are probably attainable in most regions.

Table A-1. Perinatal Care Programs

	Level I	Level II	Level III
Function	Risk assessment Management of uncomplicated perinatal care Stabilization of unexpected problems Initiation of maternal and neonatal transports Patient and community education Data collection and evaluation	*General* Level I plus: Diagnosis and treatment of selected high-risk pregnancies and neonatal problems Initiation and acceptance of maternal-fetal and neonatal transports Education of allied health personnel Residency education (affiliation)	Levels I and II plus: Diagnosis and treatment of all perinatal problems Acceptance and direction of maternal-fetal and neonatal transports Research and outcome surveillance Graduate and postgraduate education System management
Types of patients	Uncomplicated, emergency, and remedial problems such as lack of progress in labor, immediate resuscitation of asphyxiated neonates, uterine atony, nursery care of large premature neonates (>2,000 g) without risk factors, physiologic jaundice	Level I plus: Selected problems such as preeclampsia, premature labor at 32 weeks and later, mild to moderate respiratory distress syndrome, suspected neonatal sepsis, hypoglycemia, neonates of diabetic mothers, postasphyxia without life-threatening sequelae	Levels I and II plus: Premature rupture of membranes at 24-26 weeks, severe maternal medical complications, pregnancy with concurrent cancer, complicated antenatal genetic problems, prematurity at 26-32 weeks (500-1,250 g), severe respiratory distress syndrome, sepsis, severe postasphyxia, symptomatic congenital cardica and other systems disease, neonates with special needs (eg, hyperalimentation), prolonged mechanical ventilation
Location and number of births, neonatal beds	Located within Level II or III hospital or in sparsely populated or isolated areas; at least 1 birth/day unless in isolated area	Medium and large communities, may be part of Level III facility; several births/day; 3-4 neonatal beds/1,000 births served	Medium and large communities, usually in academic centers; several births/day; 1 intensive care neonatal bed/1,000 births served in addition to Level II

(continued)

Table A-1. Perinatal Care Programs (*Continued*)

Personnel

	Level I	Level II	Level III
Chief of service	One physician responsible for perinatal care (or codirectors) from obstetrics and pediatrics	Joint Planning: Ob: Board-certified obstetrician with certification, special interest, experience, or training in maternal-fetal medicine. Peds: Board-certified pediatrician with certification, special interest, experience, or training in neonatology	Codirectors: Ob: Full-time board-certified obstetrician with special competence in maternal-fetal medicine. Peds: Full-time board-certified pediatrician with certification in neonatal medicine
Other physicians	Physician (or certified nurse-midwife) at all deliveries Anesthesia services Physician care for neonates	Level I plus: Board-certified director of anesthesia services Medical, surgical, radiology, pathology consultation	Levels I and II plus: Anesthesiologists with special training or experience in perinatal and pediatric anesthesia Obstetric and pediatric subspecialists
Supervisory nurse	RN in charge of perinatal facilities	Separate head nurses with educational preparation and advanced skills for maternal-fetal and neonatal services	Director/supervisor of perinatal services with educational preparation and advanced skills for maternal-fetal and neonatal services
Staff nurse/patient ratio	Normal labor 1:2 Second stage of labor 1:1 Oxytocin and augmentation 1:2 Cesarean delivery 1:1 Normal nursery 1-6 Admission nursery 1:4 LPN, assistants under direction of an RN	Level I plus: Complicated labor/delivery 1:1 Intermediate nursery 1:3-4	Levels I and II plus: Intensive neonatal care 1:1-2 Critical care of unstable neonate 2:1
Other personnel		Level I plus: Social service, biomedical respiratory therapy, laboratory as needed	Levels I & II plus: Designated and often full-time social service, respiratory therapy, biomedical engineering, laboratory technician, ultrasound technician Nurse-clinician and specialists Nurse program and education coordinators

		Obstetric Units
Admission /observation	Close to labor and delivery, comfortable, room to ambulate	Level I plus: Beds, space for diagnostic procedures, possible emergency	Levels I and II plus: Other beds designated for observation
Family waiting	Nearby/adjacent	Level I	Level I
Labor	Beds adjustable and movable to delivery bed may be used as birthing bed Full utilities, including auxiliary electrical, oxygen, suction Communication system Full routine patient care and CPR equipment Secure medication area Monitoring capabilities	Level I	Level I
Combined birthing	Combined equipment for labor and delivery, may be concealed Adequate space for ambulation, support person	Level I	Level I
Delivery (vaginal and operative)	Contiguous to labor; at least two available, with one equipped for cesarean delivery Operating room in design Equipment/supplies necessary for normal delivery and management of complications, including surgical intervention	Level I (actual number of delivery rooms depends on total births plus: Intensive care room in labor/delivery area for patients with significant complications	Levels I and II plus: Intensive care area
Antepartum and postpartum area	Contiguous with nursery Large enough to accommodate mother, baby, visitors Maximum two mothers/room Communication system Hospital standard utilities	Level I plus: Intensive care room for observing patients with postpartum complications	Level I plus: Intensive care area

(continued)

Table A-1. Perinatal Care Programs (*Continued*)

	Level I	Level II	Level III
		Nursery	
Resuscitation	100 foot-candles illumination Overhead radiant heat Wall clock Resuscitation and stabilization equipment Designated area or room Full utilities, including suction, oxygen, compressed air, electrical outlets	Level I	Level I
Admission/observation	Near or adjacent to delivery/cesarean birth room, may be part of maternal recovery area Equipment as in resuscitation area	May be located in newborn or continuing care area	Level II
Newborn nursery	Close to postpartum area Beds and equipment to exceed obstetric beds by 10% Resuscitation equipment 1 electrical outlet/2 beds, 1 O_2, air suction/5-6 beds	Level I	Level I
Continuing care	For reverse transport from Level II or III Resuscitation equipment 4 electrical outlets, 1 O_2, 1 air, 1 suction/neonate	Near intermediate nursery	Level II
Intermediate care	Not present	Near delivery and intensive care nurseries Full life support and monitoring in addition to resuscitation equipment 8 electrical, 2 O_2, 2 compressed air, 2 suction outlets/neonate	Level II

	Not present	Present in some hospitals	
Intensive care			Near delivery/cesarean birth rooms 16-20 electrical, 3-4 O_2, 3-4 compressed air, 3-4 suction outlets/neonate. Full life support, monitoring and resuscitation equipment
		Ancillary Support	
Operating room	Technicians on call 24 h/day, available within 15-30 min	Technicians immediately available for emergency situations	Level II, may be in delivery room area
Laboratory (microtechnique for neonates)			
Within 15 min	Hematocrit	Blood gases, blood type, and Rh	Level II
Within 1 h	Glucose, BUN, creatinine, blood gases, routine urinalysis	Level I plus: Electrolytes, coagulation studies, blood available from type and screen program	Levels I and II plus: Special blood and amniotic fluid tests
Within 1-6 h	CBC, platelet appearance on smear, blood chemistries, blood typed and cross-matched, Coombs' test, bacterial smear	Level I plus: Coagulation studies, magnesium, urine, electrolytes, and chemistries	Levels I and II
Within 24-48 h	Bacterial cultures and antibiotic sensitivity	Level I plus: Liver function test Metabolic screening	Levels I and II
Within hospital or facilities available	Viral cultures	Level I	Level I plus: Laboratory facilities available

(continued)

Table A-1. Perinatal Care Programs (Continued)

	Level I	Level II	Level III
Radiography and ultrasound	Technicians on call 24 h/day, available in 30 min Technicians experienced in performing abdominal, pelvic, and OB ultrasound examinations Professional interpretation available on 24-h basis Portable x-ray and ultrasound equipment available to labor, delivery, and nursery areas	Experienced radiology technicians immediately available in hospital ultrasound on call) Professional interpretation immediately available Portable x-ray equipment Ultrasound equipment available in labor, delivery, and nursery areas	Level II plus: Computed tomography Cardiac catheterization Sophisticated equipment for emergency GI, GU, or CNS studies available 24 h/day
Blood bank	Technicians on call 24 h/day, available in 30 min, performance of routine blood banking procedures	Experienced technicians immediately available in hospital for blood banking procedures and identification of irregular antibodies Blood component therapy readily available	Level II plus: Resource center for network Direct line communication to labor, delivery, and nursery areas
Examination and treatment room	Pelvic examination Culture of tissue from cervix and uterus	Level I plus: Amniocentesis Equipment for removal of suture for cerclage	Levels I and II plus: Services within unit
Auxiliary areas	Parent education Conference room Locker room (may be remote) Physician on-call room nearby	Level I plus: Breast-feeding area within unit Parent waiting room for intensive care	Levels I and II plus: All areas within unit Conference/lecture rooms as necessary for professional/regional education commitments
	Laboratory within unit for hematocrit, centrifuge for dip stick for urine, albumin, glucose microscope	Level I plus: Refrigerator to hold cultures, materials Gram stain material	Levels I and II

B

PRECONCEPTIONAL CARE INVENTORY

Patient name _____ Age _____ Husband _____
Patient address _____ Telephone _____
Referring physician _____
Referring physician address _____ Telephone _____
Religion _____ Ethnic background _____ Blood type _____
Receives regular health care by _____
Reason for seeking preconception counseling _____

Family history

_____ Diabetes (relationship to patient) _____
_____ Hypertension (relationship to patient) _____
_____ Epilepsy (relationship to patient) _____
_____ Multiple pregnancies (relationship to patient) _____
_____ Other (specify) _____

Genetic history

Has the patient been screened for special disease relating to ethnic background?
_____ yes _____ no   If yes, explain _____
Is there any family history of: (Include previous children by either parent)
_____ Muscular dystrophy (relationship to patient) _____
_____ Hemophilia (relationship to patient) _____
_____ Cystic fibrosis (relationship to patient) _____
_____ Mental retardation (relationship to patient) _____
_____ Birth defects (relationship to patient) _____
_____ Short stature (relationship to patient) _____
Is there anything that the patient is especially concerned about? _____
_____
_____
_____

Medical history

_____ Diabetes: Onset? _____
_____ Hypertension: Onset? _____ Range? _____
_____ Epilepsy: Onset? _____
_____ Anemia: For how long? _____
_____ Rubella: When? _____
_____ Menses: Onset? _____ Regular _____
_____ Surgery: If so, what type? _____
_____ Contraception: Methods used? _____
_____ Accidents: What type? _____
_____ Allergies: What type? _____
_____ Immunizations: _____

(continued)

Preconceptional Care Inventory *(Continued)*

Current medication

General: (including over-the-counter drugs) _____

_____

Specific:

_____ Oral contraceptives: Type _____ Duration _____
_____ Sedatives or Tranquilizers: _____
_____ Drugs: _____
_____ Alcohol: _____ Beer _____ Wine _____ Liquor _____
_____ Smoking: _____ Packs per day _____
_____ Snuff: _____
_____ Appetite suppressants: _____
_____ Diuretics: _____
_____ Antibiotics: _____
_____ Caffeine: _____

Nutrition

Present status:

Height _____ Weight _____
Does the patient make an effort to control weight? _____ yes _____ no
Does the patient take vitamins? _____ yes _____ no
If yes, which ones? _____
Is the patient a vegetarian? _____ yes _____ no
If yes, what type? _____

Environmental factors

Occupation _____
Hobbies _____
Source of water supply _____
Pets _____ Exercise _____

Obstetric history

Gravida _____ Para _____
Deliveries _____ Management _____
Surgery _____
Pregnancy complications _____

Counseling

Specialized _____

Comments

_____

_____

C

SAMPLE LIST OF PERINATAL CONDITIONS THAT INCREASE THE RISK FOR NEONATAL MORBIDITY OR MORTALITY

Conditions Requiring the Availability of Skilled Resuscitation at Delivery

1. Fetal distress
   a. Abnormalities of fetal heart rate
   b. Scalp pH less than or equal to 7.20
   c. Meconium-stained amniotic fluid
   d. Cord prolapse

2. Operative delivery
   a. Cesarean delivery (excluding uncomplicated repeats when fetal maturity has been ascertained)
   b. Midforceps delivery

3. Third trimester bleeding (ie, abruptio placenta, placenta previa)

4. Multiple gestation

5. Estimated birth weight less than or equal to 2,000 g or small for gestational age infants

6. Estimated gestational age less than or equal to 36 weeks

7. Abnormal presentation

8. Prolonged, unusual, or difficult labor

9. Insulin-dependent diabetes

10. Rh isoimmunization

11. Major anomalies detected antenatally

Conditions Requiring an Immediate Assessment and Initiation of Care Plan

1. Congenital disease or anomalies (polyhydramnios, oligohydramnios)

2. Respiratory distress

3. Apgar score of 5 at 5 minutes

4. Signs of depression in the neonate

5. Maternal infection
   a. Increased temperature
   b. Greater than 24 hours since rupture of membranes
   c. Foul-smelling amniotic fluid
   d. History of transmissible infection (eg, syphilis)

6. Maternal chronic illness
   a. Hypertension
   b. Diabetes (including gestational)
   c. Renal disease
   d. Thyroid disease
   e. Cardiovascular disease
   f. Alcohol or narcotic addiction
   g. Severe anemia

7. Suspected intrauterine fetal growth retardation, or excessive size

8. Prematurity, postmaturity, dysmaturity

9. Previous fetal wastage/neonatal death

10. No prenatal care

D

PREVENTION OF
NEONATAL OPHTHALMIA*

At the present, 1% silver nitrate, 0.5% erythromycin, and 1% tetracycline given topically are equally acceptable for prophylaxis of ocular gonorrheal infection in newborn infants. Silver nitrate may still be the best agent in areas where the incidence of chlamydial infection is low, especially if penicillinase-producing *Neisseria gonorrhoeae* (PPNG) are present, as published data on the efficacy of erythromycin or tetracycline prophylaxis against PPNG are not available. However, in areas of the United States where chlamydial infection is common and is a greater concern than gonococcal infections, erythromycin or tetracycline ointments are preferable. In the prevention of neonatal chlamydial conjunctivitis, the effectiveness of 0.5% erythromycin ophthalmologic ointment, in contrast to silver nitrate, has been demonstrated in one study. *Chlamydia* organisms also are susceptible to tetracyclines, but the clinical efficacy of tetracycline ointment in the prophylaxis of chlamydial conjunctivitis has not been adequately evaluated and comparative studies of the efficacy of tetracycline with that of erythromycin ointment are needed. Both erythromycin and tetracycline ointment are available now in single-dose tubes. Erythromycin ointment is favored by some, but the lack of conclusive evidence of superiority precludes a definitive recommendation for a single agent of choice for the prevention of chlamydial conjunctivitis. Pending further studies, specific recommendations by the Committee for the prevention of neonatal ophthalmia are the following:

- Choice of Drugs. For prophylaxis of gonococcal ophthalmia neonatorum, a 1% silver nitrate solution in single-dose ampules, single-use tubes of an ophthalmic ointment containing 0.5% erythromycin, or 1% tetracycline are each effective and acceptable regimens. The effectiveness of erythromycin or tetracycline in the

*From American Academy of Pediatrics: Report of the Committee on Infectious Disease, 20 ed. Elk Grove Village IL, AAP, 1986

prevention of ophthalmia caused by penicillinase-producing *N. gonorrhoeae* is not established. For penicillin-sensitive gonococcal ophthalmia, intramuscular penicillin G (50,000 U for full-term and 20,000 U for low-birth-weight infants) also is effective for prophylaxis.

Neonatal chlamydial conjunctivitis, although not as severe as gonococcal conjunctivitis, is common in the United States. In many areas of the United States, it is equal to or greater than gonococcal ophthalmia in frequency. Topical erythromycin or tetracycline may be preferable to silver nitrate or parenteral penicillin for the prophylaxis of conjunctivitis in patients in these localities, particularly if chlamydial conjunctivitis is clearly a greater problem than gonococcal ophthalmia.

- Administration. Prior to administration of local prophylaxis, each eyelid should be wiped gently with sterile cotton. Two drops of a 1% silver nitrate solution or a 1 to 2 cm ribbon of antibiotic ointment are placed in each lower conjunctival sac. The eyelids then are massaged gently to spread the ointment. After 1 minute, excess solution or ointment can be wiped away with sterile cotton. None of the prophylactic agents should be flushed from the eye following installation. Critical studies have not evaluated the efficacy of silver nitrate prophylaxis with and without flushing, but anecdotal reports suggest that flushing may reduce the efficacy of prophylaxis. In addition, flushing probably does not reduce the incidence of chemical conjunctivitis. Prophylaxis should be given shortly after birth. Although some suggest prophylaxis may be administered more effectively in the nursery than in the delivery room, no studies have evaluated the effect on efficacy of delaying prophylaxis. However, delaying prophylaxis for up to 1 hour after birth probably is not likely to affect efficacy. Hospitals in which prophylaxis is delayed should establish a check system to ensure that all infants are treated.
- Infants born by cesarean section also should receive prophylaxis against gonococcal and chlamydial ophthalmia. Although gonococcal and chlamydial infections usually are transmitted to the infant during passage through the birth canal, infection by the ascending route also occurs. The precise risk of these infections occurring in untreated infants born by cesarean section has not been determined.
- The identification of women who have gonococcal infections by routine cultures and then subsequent treatment is essential.

Gonococcal infections in pregnant women, including those that are asymptomatic, may be associated with fetal wastage, early and prolonged rupture of membranes, premature labor, and delivery of low-birth-weight infants. These infections also may result in sepsis or scalp abscesses if intrauterine fetal monitoring is used. Failure to treat an infected woman before or at delivery may result in postnatal transmission of gonococcal infection to infants.

- Newborn infants whose mothers have gonorrhea at the time of delivery should receive a single dose of penicillin G (50,000 U for full-term or 20,000 U for low-birth-weight infants), intravenously or intramuscularly, as occasional cases of gonococcal ophthalmia may occur in infants managed by any of the current modes of prophylaxis. In geographic areas where PPNG infections are occurring, ceftriaxone (125 mg), intramuscularly, is recommended in place of penicillin.

- Neonates with clinical evidence of gonococcal ophthalmia or complicated (disseminated) gonococcal infection should be hospitalized, placed in isolation, and treated appropriately. The emergence of strains of *N. gonorrhoeae* resistant to penicillin necessitates cultures from the mother and determination of antibiotic susceptibilities so appropriate antimicrobial therapy can be given.

- Treatment of pregnant women who have chlamydial cervicitis also may prevent neonatal chlamydial infection. Oral erythromycin is the only recommended treatment for these women; tetracyline is contraindicated. Women whose infants develop chlamydial conjunctivitis also should be tested and treated if test results are positive. Their sexual partners also should receive treatment to prevent reinfection.

- Identification of chlamydia-positive women can be accomplished by screening with fluorescent antibody techniques, culture, or detection of chlamydia antigen by enzyme-linked immunosorbent assay (ELISA). Testing is warranted in areas of high prevalence and in women found to have other sexually transmitted diseases.

- Treatment of Chlamydial Conjunctivitis. Orally administered erythromycin is recommended. Topical therapy is successful in the treatment of conjunctivitis, but does not eradicate nasopharyngeal colonization or prevent subsequent development of pneumonia.

E

MATERNAL CONSULTATION/TRANSFER RECORD

Date of referral call _____ Time _____
Person receiving call _____
Patient's name _____
Referring physician _____
Primary physician _____
Referring hospital _____
Person calling _____
Reason for admission _____

Maternal History

1. Age _____
2. Gravida _____
3. Para _____
4. Abortion _____
5. Weeks of gestation _____
6. Last menstrual period _____ Estimated date of confinement _____
7. Onset of contractions _____
8. Frequency of contractions _____
9. Cervical dilation _____
10. Evidence of vaginal bleeding _____
11. Rupture of membranes? Yes _____ No _____ Time _____
12. Fetal heart rate: Infant 1 _____ Infant 2 _____ Other _____
13. a. Temperature _____ b. Blood pressure _____ c. Pulse _____
14. Blood type _____
15. Referral history _____
    Relevant health problems _____
    _____
    _____

    Perinatal history _____
    _____
    _____

    Reason for transfer _____
    _____
    _____

16. Referral plan _____
    _____

17. Transported by _____
    _____

18. Assessment by _____
    Date _____

F

NEWBORN CONSULTATION/TRANSFER RECORD

DATE OF REF CALL:___ / ___ / ___

INFANT'S LAST NAME   FIRST NAME

PERSON RECEIVING CALL

TIME CALL RECEIVED _____

SEX (circle one):
1. female
2. male
3. other

INSURANCE

PATIENT IDENTIFICATION

REFERRING MD NAME

(   )
PHONE

MD WHO DELIVERED INFANT
("X" over Dr. if not appropriate)

(   )
PHONE

PRIMARY MD NAME

(   )
PHONE

HOSPITAL DELIVERED AT   DELIV. CITY, STATE   ZIP

REFERRING HOSPITAL NAME

CITY, STATE   ZIP

BIRTHDATE: __ / __ / __ BIRTHWT: _____ gm EGA:_____

NAME OF PERSON CALLING

(   )
REF. HOSP. PHONE

REF. APGARS
1 min _____
5 min _____

MATERNAL HISTORY
1. Age:_____
2. Grav:_____
3. Para:_____
4. Abo:_____

OTHER SIGNIFICANT INFORMATION
REFERRAL HISTORY (incl. lab & x-ray results):

PRELIMINARY DIAGNOSIS:

OXYGEN DELIVERY:

1. Nasotrach
2. Orotrach
3. Nasal prongs
4. Mask
5. Tracheostomy
6. Nasopharyngeal
8. Other
9. Unknown
0. None

VENT MODE:
1. Bagging
2. Respirator
8. Other
9. Unknown
0. None

VENT MODE/BLOOD	Gas	Site
Time		
CPAP		
PIP		
PEEP		
Rate		
IT		
Fio2		
Po2		
Pco2		
pH		
BE		
Site		

FLUID LINES PLACED? (Circle all that apply.)

	Solution	Rate
1. Peripheral		
2. U/A		
3. U/V		
4. Other (specify)		
5. None		

REF TEMP:_____°C
REF DEXTROSTIX:_____ MG%
REF GLUCOSE:_____ MG%
REF HCT:_____ %
REF BLOOD PRESSURE ___ / ___

	Yes	No
1. Apnea?		
2. X-rays taken?		
3. Blood cultures?		
4. Antibotics given?		
5. OG tube?		

HOUSE OFFICER ASSESSMENT AND INSTRUCTIONS

	Yes	No
1. Temp adequate?		
2. Monitoring adeq?		
3. Blood volume adequate?		
4. Glucose adequate?		
5. Ventilation adequate?		
6. Sepsis suspected?		
7. Meds appropriate?		
8. Other (instructions)		

RECOMMENDATIONS:

TYPE OF REFERRAL

DATE _____

ASSESSMENT BY (last name only)

ATTENDING CONSULTANT (last name only)

G

EQUIPMENT AND MEDICATION FOR MATERNAL-NEONATAL TRANSPORT

Equipment and medication for maternal or neonatal transport must be individualized for each transport service. Additions or deletions from this list are appropriate.

I. Maternal

  A. Obstetric delivery equipment (OB case)

Gloves: #'s 7, 7-1/2, 8	Cord clamps
10/pkg 4 x 4's	Chromic suture (3-0)
Bulb syringe	Y connector
Silver swaddlers	Disposable OB kit
DeLee suctions with	Needles
mucous trap	Scissors (one with long
Neonate electrodes	handles)
Plastic bag	Needle holder
Disp. scalpels	Pick-up forcep
Pediatric drips	Kling 2"
Thermometers	Hemostat
Scalp vein 25 gauge	Examination gloves, large,
pHisoHex	single, sterile
Alco wipes	

  B. Standard adult resuscitation equipment and drugs

II. Neonatal

  A. Essential equipment

Transport incubator	Compressed air
Oxygen supply (including	Oxygen analyzer
delivery tubing flow-	Oxygen hood
meter and humidifier)	Ventilation bag and masks

Endotracheal tubes
  2.5, 3, 3.5, 4, 4.5
Laryngoscope
Suction apparatus
Thermometer
Stethoscope
Heart rate monitor
Blood pressure unit

Emergency drugs
Intravenous set-up and solutions (plastic bags, ideal for IV solutions)
Constant infusion pump
Thoracocentesis set
Dextrostix
Small stylet for ET tube

B. Optional but desirable equipment

Silver swaddler
Electronic thermometer
Oxygen-air blender
Constant positive airway pressure unit
Mechanical ventilator (capable of running off compressed gas)

Transcutaneous O$_2$ monitor
Direct line arterial pressure monitor
Umbilical catheterization tray
Thoracostomy tray
Heimlich valves
Oximeter

C. Neonatal transport kit equipment and medications inventory

1. Laryngoscope
Laryngoscope blades (Miller 0, Miller 1)
Spare laryngoscope bulb (small size)
Spare laryngoscope batteries (size AA)
Packet sterile lubricant
Scissors

Anesthesia bag
Face masks (sizes 1 and 0)
Magill forceps
Gauze swabs (2 x 2)
Needle electrodes
Chest electrodes
Stylet
Tank key
Heart monitor lead wires

2. Thermometer
Feeding tubes (8 Fr)
Stopcock plugs
3-way stopcocks
Christmas trees
Needles (18, 20, 22, 25 gauge)
Saran wrap
Limb restraints
Safety pins

Rubber bands
Alcohol swabs
Corks
Cotton balls
Beta dine swabs
Sutures with curved needles (4-0)
Bandaids
Lancets
Capillary tubes

Dextrostix reagent strips
Tincture benzoin
Alcohol
Betadine

Pacifier
Umbilical tape
Blunt adaptors, 17, 19, 20
    gauge

3. Tuberculin syringes with
        needles
    3-ml syringes (20, 22, 25
        gauge needles)
    12-ml syringes
    20-ml syringes
    Scalp vein needles (3 each
        of 25 gauge; 1 each of
        21, 23, 27 gauge)
    Rolls adhesive tape
        ($\frac{1}{2}$ and 1 inch)
    Roll paper tape (1 inch)
    Rolls dermiclear tape
        ($\frac{1}{2}$ inch)
    Q-tips
    Wooden tongue blade
    Paper tape measure
    Disposable razor
    Arm board

Plastic medicine cups
    (IV caps)
22-gauge quik caths and
    27- gauge quick cath
IV "Medication Added"
    labels
Drugs:
    Heparin 1,000 u/ml
    Saline (10-ml vial)
    Sterile H_2O (10-ml vial)
    Flush solv D5 1/4 NS =
        2 u Heparin/ml
    NaCL 2.5 mEq/ml
        (30 ml)
    $NaHCO_3$ 8.4% (30 ml)
    Ampicillin 250-mg vial
    Gentamicin (2- ml vial
        [10 mg/ml])
    Aspirin and dramamine

4. Suction catheters and glove
        pace; 5/6 Fr, 8 Fr, 10 Fr
    Milli-pore filter
    12 Fr sump tube
    Sterile glove packs
        (sizes 6, $6\frac{1}{2}$, 7, $7\frac{1}{2}$)
    Metriset
    Pediatric IV set
    500-ml bag $D_{10}W$
    Extension tubing (20 inch)
    Stethoscope
    Arterial catheters ($3\frac{1}{2}$, 5 Fr)
    Heimlich set-ups:
        Heimlich valves
        16-g medicuts
        3-way stopcocks
        Extension tubing

Thoracocentesis set-ups:
    60-ml syringes
    3-way stopcocks
    23-g butterflies
DeLee Suction with mucus
    trap
Pump tubings
Bowel bag
Red rubber catheter (10 Fr)
Sphygmomanometer with
    2 cuffs (infant and
    newborn)
Jelly for BP transducer
24-hour urine bags,
    newborn, pediatric
Trocar cannulas
    (10 Fr, 12 Fr)

5. NaHCO₃ 4.2%
   (10-ml syringes)
   Aquamephyton (pediatric);
   phenobarbital; 5%
   albumin; calcium glu-
   conate; narcan; digoxin
   (pediatric); furosemide;
   dexamethasone; epine-
   phrine (10-ml syringe);
   lidocaine; isoproterenol;
   dopamine; prisocline;
   prostaglandin
   Dilantin
   Blood culture bottles
   Steridrape

T-connector
Platelet infusion set
Blood filter
Mini UA/thoracotomy set
1. Sterile drapes
2. Iris forceps
3. Needle holder
4. Scissor
5. Curved forceps
6. Tongue tissue forcep
7. Sterile 2 x 2
8. Catheter adaptor
9. Umbilical tape
10. Scalpel and blade

H

STANDARD TERMINOLOGY FOR REPORTING OF REPRODUCTIVE HEALTH STATISTICS IN THE UNITED STATES

The definitions, formulae, and reporting requirements presented here were prepared, reviewed, and approved by representatives of the American Academy of Pediatrics, the American College of Obstetricians and Gynecologists, the American Medical Association, the American Medical Record Association, the Association of Maternal and Child Health Programs, the Association for Vital Records and Health Statistics, the Centers for Disease Control, the National Center for Health Statistics, and the Office of Maternal and Child Health to promote uniform collection procedures and the proper use and interpretation of reproductive health statistics.

We believe that the adoption of these recommended definitions and reporting requirements will provide an improved basis for standardization and uniformity in the design, implementation, and evaluation of intervention strategies. The reduction of maternal and infant mortality and the improvement of the health of our nation's mothers and infants is our ultimate goal. The collection and analysis of reliable statistical data are an essential part of in-depth investigations which incorporate casefinding, individual review and analysis of risk factors. These studies could then yield valuable clinical information for practitioners to aid them in improved case management for high risk patients, resulting in decreased morbidity and mortality.

This standardization represents an attempt to enhance communication between those in the medical community who provide the data, those who are responsible for collecting the data, and those who analyze and interpret the data to plan and evaluate perinatal programs.

Both collection and use of statistics have been hampered by lack of understanding of differences in *definitions, statistical tabulations,* and *reporting requirements* among state, national, and international bodies. Misapplication and misinterpretation of data may lead to erroneous comparisons and conclusions. For example, specific requirements for reporting of fetal deaths have frequently been misinterpreted as implying a weight or gestational age for viability. Distinctions can and should be made among 1) the definition of an event, 2) the reporting requirements for the event, and 3) the statistical tabulation and interpretation of the data. The definition indicates the meaning of a term (for example, live birth, fetal death, or maternal death). A reporting requirement is that part of the defined event for which reporting is mandatory or desired. Statistical tabulations connote the presentation of data for the purpose of analysis and interpretation of existing and future conditions. The data should be collected in a manner that will allow them to be presented in different ways for different users. Adjustments should be made for variations in reporting before comparisons among data are attempted.

If information is collected and presented in a standardized manner, comparisons between the new data and the data obtained by previous reporting requirements can be delineated clearly and can contribute to improved public understanding of reproductive health statistics.

For ease in assimilating this information, it is divided into three sections: definitions, statistical tabulations, and reporting requirements/recommendations. Some of the definitions and recommendations are a departure from those currently or historically accepted; however, these recommendations were agreed upon by the interorganizational group that was brought together to review terminology related to reproductive health issues.

DEFINITIONS

Live Birth: The complete expulsion or extraction from the mother of a product of human conception, irrespective of the duration of pregnancy, which, after such expulsion or extraction, breathes or shows any other evidence of life, such as beating of the heart, pulsation of the umbilical cord, or definite movement of voluntary muscles whether or not the umbilical cord has been cut or the placenta is attached. Heartbeats are to be distinguished from transient cardiac contractions; respirations are to be distinguished from fleeting respiratory efforts or gasps.

Birth Weight: The weight of a neonate determined immediately after delivery or as soon thereafter as feasible. It should be expressed to the nearest gram.

Gestational Age: The number of completed weeks that have elapsed between the first day of the last normal menstrual period (not the presumed time of conception) and the date of delivery, irrespective of whether the gestation results in a live birth or a fetal death.

Neonate:

Low Birth Weight: Any neonate, regardless of gestational age, whose weight at birth is less than 2,500 g.

Preterm:* Any neonate whose birth occurs through the end of the last day of the 37th week (259th day), following onset of the last menstrual period.

Term:* Any neonate whose birth occurs from the beginning of the first day (260th day) of the 38th week, through the end of the last day of the 42nd week (294th day), following onset of the last menstrual period (Fig. A-1).

Postterm: Any neonate whose birth occurs from the beginning of the first day (295th day) of the 43rd week following onset of the last menstrual period.

Fetal Death: Death prior to the complete expulsion or extraction from the mother of a product of human conception, fetus and placenta, irrespective of the duration of pregnancy; the death is indicated by the fact that, after such expulsion or extraction, the fetus does not breathe or show any other evidence of life, such as beating of the heart, pulsation of the umbilical cord, or definite movement of voluntary muscles. Heartbeats are to be distinguished from transient cardiac contractions; respirations are to be distinguished from fleeting respiratory efforts or gasps. This definition excludes induced terminations of pregnancy.

---

*These definitions are for statistical purposes and not intended to affect clinical management. Appropriate assessment of fetal maturity for purposes of clinical management is delineated in Chapter 4.

Statisticians making a determination of the status of a neonate, namely preterm or term, should define preterm as less than 259 days and term as 259 to less than 294 days in order to insure comparable calculations with the medical community. Statisticians, by formula, subtract the date of the first day of the last menstrual period from the date of birth, whereas physicians include the first day, thus accounting for the difference.

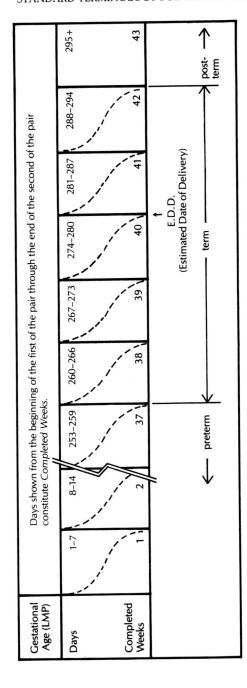

Fig. A-1. Gestational age of the term neonate.

Neonatal Death: Death of a liveborn neonate before the neonate becomes 28 days old (up to and including 27 days, 23 hours, 59 minutes from the moment of birth).

Infant Death: Any death at any time from birth up to, but not including, one year of age (364 days, 23 hours, 59 minutes from the moment of birth).

Maternal Death:* The death of a woman from any cause related to or aggravated by pregnancy or its management (regardless of duration or site of pregnancy), but not from accidental or incidental causes.

Direct Obstetric Death: The death of a woman resulting from obstetric complications of pregnancy, labor, or the puerperium; from interventions, omissions, or treatment; or from a chain of events resulting from any of these.

Indirect Obstetric Death: The death of a woman resulting from a previously existing disease or a disease that developed during pregnancy, labor, or the puerperium that was not due to direct obstetric causes, although the physiologic effects of pregnancy were partially responsible for the death.

Induced Termination of Pregnancy: The purposeful interruption of an intrauterine pregnancy with the intention other than to produce a live-born infant, and which does not result in a live birth. This definition excludes management of prolonged retention of products of conception following fetal death.

STATISTICAL TABULATIONS

Statistical tabulations for vital events related to pregnancy provide the medical and statistical community with valuable information on reproductive health, as well as generating data on trends apparent in this country and worldwide. This information often is disaggregated and used to examine specific events over time or within selected geographic locations. In informing the public about health issues, media sources often report various statistical measures. Heightened

*Death occurring to a woman during pregnancy or after its termination from causes *not* related to the pregnancy nor to its complications or management is *not* to be considered a maternal death. Nonmaternal deaths may result from accidental causes (eg, auto accident or gunshot wound) or incidental causes (eg, concurrent malignancy).

public interest in health related issues, makes it essential that the medical community understand and have the capacity to interpret these statistics.

The following explanations of statistical tabulations provide the reader with a better understanding of measures used for events related to reproduction.

Rate is a measure of the frequency of some event in relation to a unit of population during a specified time period such as a year; events in the numerator of the rate occur to individuals in the denominator. Rates express the risk of the event in the specified population during a particular time. Rates are generally expressed as units of population in the denominator (per 1,000, per 100,000, etc.). For example, the 1982 teenage birth rate was 52.9 live births per 1,000 women 15-19 years of age.

Ratios, on the other hand, express a *relationship* of one element to a *different* element (where the numerator is not necessarily a subset of the denominator). A ratio is generally expressed per 1,000 of the denominator element. For example, the sex ratio of live births for 1982 was 1,051 males per 1,000 females.

In the formulae that follow, "period" refers to a calendar year.

Live Birth Measures

These measures are designed to show the rate at which childbearing is occurring in the population. The crude birth rate, which relates the total number of births to the total population, gives an indication of the impact of fertility on population growth. The general fertility rate is a more specific measure of fertility since it relates the number of births to the population at risk, women in the childbearing ages (assumed to be ages 15-44 years). An even more specific set of rates, the age-specific birth rates, relates the number of births to women of a specific age directly to the total number of women in that age group. Formulae for these measures are shown below.

Crude Birth Rate = $\dfrac{\text{Number of live births to women of all ages during a calendar year}}{\text{Total estimated mid-year population}} \times 1{,}000$

General Fertility Rate = $\dfrac{\text{Number of live births to women of all ages during a calendar year}}{\text{Estimated mid-year population of women 15-44 years of age}} \times 1{,}000$

General Pregnancy
Rate

$=$

Number of live births +
number of fetal deaths +
number of induced
terminations of pregnancy
during a calendar year $\times$ 1,000

Estimated mid-year population
of women 15-44 years of age

Age-Specific Birth
Rate

$=$

Number of live births to
women in a specific age group
during a calendar year $\times$ 1,000

Estimated mid-year population
of women in the same age group

Total Fertility Rate

$=$

The sum of age-specific birth rates of women
at each age group 10-14 through 45-49.
Since 5-year age groups are used, the sum
is multiplied by 5. This rate can also be
computed by using single years of age.

Because the birth weight of the infant is included on the birth certificate, it is possible to tabulate and focus an analysis on selected groups of live births, for example, those weighing 500 grams or more.

Births can be tabulated by where they occur. Thus, they can be shown by place of occurrence, by place of residence, and by kind of setting of delivery such as at a hospital or at home. Most vital statistics tabulations are routinely tabulated by place of residence of the mother but they could be tabulated on another basis as well. What is essential, however, is that the classification be the same for all events under consideration for a specific measure.

Fetal Mortality Measures

The population at risk for fetal mortality is the number of live births plus the number of fetal deaths in a year. Alternatively, the number of live births alone is sometimes used as the population at risk. Fetal death indices indicate the likelihood that pregnancies in a population group would result in fetal death.

It is recognized that most states report fetal deaths based upon gestational age. However, birth weight can be more accurately measured than gestational age. Therefore, minimum reporting requirements of fetal deaths based upon and labeled as to specific birth weight rather than gestational age are recommended for adoption by states (see Fetal Death under Reporting Requirements/Recommendations). In addition, *statistical tabulations* of fetal deaths should include, at a minimum, fetal deaths of 500 grams or more.

Fetal Death Rate   = $\dfrac{\substack{\text{Number of fetal deaths} \\ \text{(of \_\_\_ weight or more)} \\ \text{during a period}} \times 1{,}000}{\substack{\text{Number of fetal deaths} \\ \text{(of \_\_\_ weight or more) +} \\ \text{number of live births} \\ \text{during the same period}}}$

Fetal Death Ratio   = $\dfrac{\substack{\text{Number of fetal deaths} \\ \text{(of \_\_\_ weight or more)} \\ \text{during a period}} \times 1{,}000}{\substack{\text{Number of live births} \\ \text{during the same period}}}$

It is recognized that states will not be able to translate data from gestational age to weight immediately, and, for comparative purposes, it may be desirable to know fetal death rates for varying gestational time periods. Therefore, the collection of both weight and gestational age is recommended to allow for these comparisons. When calculating fetal death rates based upon gestational age, the number of weeks or more of stated or presumed gestation can be substituted for weight in the above formulae.

Perinatal Mortality Measures

These indices combine fetal deaths and live births which survive only briefly (up to a few days or weeks) on the assumption that similar factors are associated with these losses. The population at risk is the total number of live births plus fetal deaths, or alternatively, the number of live births. Perinatal mortality indices can vary as to age of the fetus and the infant that is included in the particular tabulation. However, the concept itself cuts across all the calculations.

It is recommended that perinatal mortality measures be based upon and labeled as to specific weight rather than gestational age (see Reporting Requirements/Recommendations).

Perinatal Mortality Rate   = $\dfrac{\substack{\text{Number of infant deaths of} \\ \text{less than \_\_\_ days + number of} \\ \text{fetal deaths (with stated or} \\ \text{presumed weight of \_\_\_ or more)} \\ \text{during a period}} \times 1{,}000}{\substack{\text{Number of live births + number of} \\ \text{fetal deaths (with stated or} \\ \text{presumed weight of \_\_\_ or more)} \\ \text{during the same period}}}$

Perinatal Mortality Ratio $=$ $\dfrac{\begin{array}{c}\text{Number of infant deaths of}\\ \text{less than \_\_\_ days + number of fetal}\\ \text{deaths (with stated or}\\ \text{presumed weight of \_\_\_ or more)}\\ \text{during a period}\end{array} \times 1{,}000}{\text{Number of live births during the same period}}$

It is recognized that states will not be able to translate data from gestational age to weight immediately, and, for purposes of comparability, knowledge of gestational age (based on last menstrual period) may be required and should be collected. When calculating perinatal death rates based upon gestational age, the number of weeks of a stated or presumed gestational age can be substituted for weight in the above formulae. When comparisons are desired based upon gestational age, the generally accepted breakdown is as follows: Perinatal Period I includes infant deaths of less than 7 days and fetal deaths with a stated or presumed period of gestation of 28 weeks or more; Perinatal Period II includes infant deaths of less than 28 days and fetal deaths with a stated or presumed period of gestation of 20 weeks or more; Perinatal Period III includes infant deaths of less than 7 days and fetal deaths with a stated or presumed gestation of 20 weeks or more (Fig. A-2).

Perinatal measures can be specific for race and other characteristics. Perinatal events can be tabulated by where they occur. Thus, they can be shown by place of occurrence, by place of residence and by place of delivery such as at a hospital or home. Most vital statistics tabulations are routinely tabulated by place of residence of the mother but they could be tabulated by place of occurrence. What is essential, however, is that the classification be the same for all events under consideration for a specific measure.

Infant Mortality Measures

Indices of infant mortality are designed to show the likelihood that live births with certain characteristics will survive the first year of life, or, conversely, will die during the first year of life. For infant mortality, the "population at risk" is approximated by live births that occur in a calendar year. One can compare the infant mortality rate of different population groups, such as between white and black infants. Interest sometimes focuses on two different periods in the first year of an infant's life: the very early period before the infant becomes 28 days old (up through 27 days, 23 hours, 59 minutes from the moment of birth), called the "neonatal period", and the later period starting at the end of the 28th day up to but not including one year of

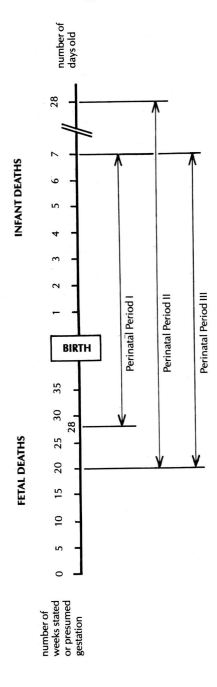

Fig. A-2. Perinatal periods.

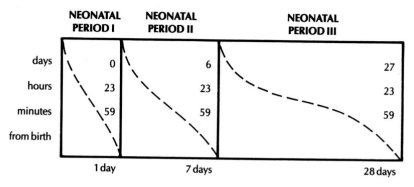

Fig. A-3. Neonatal periods.

age (364 days, 23 hours, 59 minutes), called the "postneonatal period". Accordingly, two indices reflect these differences, namely, the neonatal mortality rate and the postneonatal mortality rate. The neonatal period can be broken down further for statistical tabulations as follows: Neonatal Period I is from the moment of birth through 23 hours and 59 minutes; Neonatal Period II starts at the end of the 24th hour of life through 6 days, 23 hours, and 59 minutes; Neonatal Period III starts at the end of the 7th day of life through 27 days, 23 hours, and 59 minutes (Fig. A-3).

$$\text{Infant Mortality Rate} = \frac{\text{Number of infant deaths (neonatal + postneonatal) during a period} \times 1{,}000}{\text{Number of live births during the same period}}$$

$$\text{Neonatal Mortality Rate} = \frac{\text{Number of neonatal deaths during a period} \times 1{,}000}{\text{Number of live births during the same period}}$$

$$\text{Postneonatal Mortality Rate} = \frac{\text{Number of postneonatal deaths during a period} \times 1{,}000}{\text{Number of live births during the same period}}$$

The denominator for the postneonatal mortality rate can also be calculated by subtracting the number of neonatal deaths from the number of live births. This denominator more accurately defines the population at risk of dying in the neonatal period. In addition, it should be noted that infant deaths can be broken down into birth weight categories, if desired, for comparative purposes when birth and death records are linked (see Reporting Requirements/ Recommendations).

Maternal Mortality Measures

These measures are designed to indicate the likelihood that a pregnant woman will die from complications of pregnancy, childbirth, or the puerperium. Accordingly, the population at risk is an approximation of the population of pregnant women in a year: the approximation is usually taken to be the number of live births. Maternal mortality can be examined in terms of characteristics of the woman such as age, race, and cause of death. The maternal mortality rate measures the risk of death from deliveries and complications of pregnancy, childbirth, and the puerperium.

The group exposed to risk consists of all women who have been pregnant at some time during the period. Thus, the population at risk should theoretically include all fetal deaths (reported and unreported), all induced terminations of pregnancy, and all live births. Because most states do not require the reporting of all fetal deaths and there are still a large number of states that do not require reporting of induced terminations of pregnancy, the entire population at risk can not be included in the denominator. Therefore, the total number of live births has become the generally accepted denominator. It is recommended that when complete ascertainment of the denominator (that is, the number of pregnant women) is achieved, that a modified maternal mortality rate be defined, in addition to the traditional rate.

The rate is most frequently expressed per 100,000 live births, as follows:

$$\text{Maternal Mortality Rate} = \frac{\text{Number of deaths attributed to maternal conditions during a period}}{\text{Number of live births during the same period}} \times 100,000$$

Cause of death rates for specified maternal causes are computed by restricting the numerator to the specified cause. The maternal mortality rates specific for race and age groups are computed by appropriately restricting both the numerator and denominator to the specified group. Caution should be used in interpreting rates in small geographic areas; it may not be possible to generate race and age specific rates.

For statistical comparisons with the World Health Organization, it is recommended that two tabulations of statistics be prepared: 1) maternal deaths within 42 days of the end of pregnancy (WHO), and 2) with no time limitation for comparison within the United States.

Induced Termination of Pregnancy Measures

These measures parallel those of fetal deaths, but they refer to "induced" events. The population at risk for induced termination of pregnancy is taken to be live births in a year, which is used as a surrogate measure of pregnancies. Because this is not actually the total population at risk, this measure is generally considered a ratio.

$$\text{Induced Termination of Pregnancy Ratio I} = \frac{\text{Number of induced terminations occurring during a period} \times 1{,}000}{\text{Number of live births occurring during the same period}}$$

Another measure (Induced Termination of Pregnancy Ratio II) is one which, by also including an estimate of pregnancies which do not result in live births, more closely approximates the population at risk.

$$\text{Induced Termination of Pregnancy Ratio II} = \frac{\text{Number of induced terminations occurring during a period} \times 1{,}000}{\text{Number of induced terminations of pregnancies} + \text{live births} + \text{reported fetal deaths during the same period}}$$

Still a third measure is a rate which provides information on the *probability* that women of a certain age or race will have an induced termination of pregnancy.

$$\text{Induced Termination of Pregnancy Rate} = \frac{\text{Number of induced terminations occurring during a period} \times 1{,}000}{\text{Female population age 15-44 years}}$$

Sometimes induced termination indices are specific for certain characteristics of the woman: that is, they can refer to women of particular age or race groups.

REPORTING REQUIREMENTS/RECOMMENDATIONS

Reporting requirements for vital events related to reproductive health enable the collection of data essential to the calculation of statistical tabulations which look at trends and changes at the local, state, and national levels. The data which are used in statistical tabulations may only be a portion of those which are collected, due to the need for consistency in a tabulation, and the variations in reporting requirements from state to state. For instance, while a few states require that all fetal deaths, regardless of length of gestation, be reported, statistical tabulations of fetal death rates by the National Center for

Health Statistics (NCHS) only utilize fetal deaths of 20 weeks or more gestation.

Live Birth

It is generally recognized that all states report all live births as defined in the definitions section of this document. It is recommended that all live births be reported regardless of birth weight, length of gestation, or survival time.

Fetal Death

Reporting requirements for fetal deaths now vary from state to state. At present, most states require reporting of fetal deaths by gestational age. It is generally recognized that birth weight can be more accurately measured than gestational age.

It must be emphasized that a specific birth weight criterion for reporting of fetal deaths does not imply a point of viability and should be chosen instead for its feasibility in collecting useful data.

Current statistical tabulations of fetal deaths, include, at a minimum, fetal deaths of 500 grams or more. Furthermore, all but three states now require either reporting of all fetal deaths or reporting of some fetal deaths below 500 grams, for example, those which fall below 500 grams because of the variation in birth weights at a given required gestational age such as 20 weeks. Therefore, it is recommended that

- Statistical tabulations for comparisons of perinatal mortality rates within the United States exclude fetal deaths of less than 500 g.
- Each state adopt a specific birth weight criterion for reporting of fetal deaths which will result in continued collection of data on as close as possible to 100% of the population of fetal deaths currently reported in that state. When birth weight is unknown, an estimate of gestational age should be utilized to determine whether or not this event is required to be reported.
- All state fetal death report forms include birth weight and gestational age.

Perinatal Mortality

Perinatal mortality indices generally combine fetal deaths and live births which survive only briefly (up to a few days or weeks). Since reporting requirements on fetal deaths vary from state to state, perinatal mortality reporting will also vary (see previous section on Perinatal Periods).

As with fetal deaths, it is recommended that perinatal mortality be weight specific. However, for purposes of comparability, knowledge of gestational age (based on last menstrual period) should be collected.

Infant Mortality

All states require that all infant deaths (neonatal plus postneonatal) as defined in the definitions section of this document be reported.

Infant deaths by birth weight are not routinely available for the U.S. as a whole since birth weight information is not collected on the death certificate. However, since birth weight is reported on the birth certificate, by linking together the birth certificate and the death certificate for the same infant, it is possible to obtain information on infant deaths by birth weight. At the present time, most states link birth and death certificates. It is recommended that this be encouraged to create a national data base for infant mortality by birth weight.

In addition, it is recommended that infant death reports include the exact interval from birth rather than categories such as neonatal or postneonatal. This too, will allow for more specific age-related death analyses.

Maternal Mortality

Every state is required to report all maternal deaths. Since annual deaths attributed to maternal mortality only approximate 300, emphasis must be placed on in-depth investigations. Case-finding, together with individual review and analysis of risk factors contributing to maternal deaths, is of the highest importance. Collection of data regarding these rare events is critical, when combined, as it should be, with educational review by those closest to the case, usually the obstetrician-gynecologists in the hospital and the surrounding region. Such analysis can yield clinical information about risk factors associated, for example, with detection and treatment of ectopic pregnancies, or with anesthesia. This clinical information can then be gathered and exchanged to help practitioners identify risk factors which contribute to maternal death and associated conditions.

Induced Termination of Pregnancy

The United States has no national system for reporting induced terminations of pregnancy. State health departments vary greatly in their approaches to the compilation of this data from compiling no data to: 1) periodically requesting hospitals, clinics and/or physicians performing the procedures to voluntarily report total number of procedures performed; 2) requiring (by legislative or regulatory authority) hospitals, clinics and/or physicians to periodically report aggregate level data on number or number and characteristics of procedures; or, 3) requiring (by legal or regulatory authority) hospitals, clinics, and/or physicians to periodically report individual level data on each procedure performed.

Since 1969, the Division of Reproductive Health (DRH), Centers for Disease Control (CDC), has published an annual Abortion Surveillance Report based upon data provided from state health departments, when available, and from data voluntarily provided to CDC from hospitals and clinics in states with no data available from health departments. In addition to information on the number and characteristics of induced terminations of pregnancy, the Abortion Surveillance Report contains information from CDC's abortion mortality surveillance, which was begun with the cooperation of state health departments in 1972. Investigation and review of each related death by DRH epidemiologists result in improved detailed nosological identification of abortion mortality by type of risk.*

Since 1977, the National Center for Health Statistics has analyzed the induced terminations of pregnancy occurring in up to 13 states in which individual reports of induced terminations are submitted to state vital registration offices. In addition, the Alan Guttmacher Institute, a private organization, publishes information on induced terminations that it obtains from a nationwide survey of induced termination providers.

Collecting information on the number of induced terminations of pregnancy, the characteristics of women having such procedures, and the number and characteristics of all deaths related to induced termination of pregnancy would be extremely valuable in identifying and evaluating risk factors for specific population groups and for the public in general. By gathering these data, studies could be instituted which would examine clinical issues and then results could be shared with practitioners. Knowing the outcomes could further the body of knowledge and ultimately reduce the risks.

Therefore, we urge state health departments that compile statistics on induced terminations of pregnancy to evaluate and improve the

---

*The CDC Abortion Surveillance Report includes information on events categorized by CDC as abortions (legal, illegal, and spontaneous). While this terminology preexisted the recommendations in this paper and is at variance with the definition herein, it has been commonly used and understood to include induced termination of pregnancy.

quality of their data. Furthermore, we urge state health departments that do not compile such statistics to explore mechanisms for initiating their collection.

The following General Fetal Death Reporting Requirements, as of January 1988, should be brought into conformity with the recommendations in this report:

20 weeks or more gestation

Alabama	Indiana	North Dakota
Alaska	Iowa	Ohio
Arizona*	Maryland*	Oklahoma
California	Minnesota	Oregon*
Connecticut	Montana	Texas
Delaware	Nebraska	Utah
Florida	Nevada	Vermont*
Guam	New Jersey	Washington
Illinois	North Carolina	West Virginia
		Wyoming

20 weeks or more gestation or birth weight of 500 grams or more
District of Columbia

20 weeks or more gestation or birth weight of 350 grams or more

Idaho	Massachusetts	New Hampshire
Kentucky	Mississippi	South Carolina
Louisiana	Missouri	Wisconsin

Birth weight in excess of 350 grams
Kansas

20 weeks or more gestation or birth weight of 400 grams or more
Michigan

Birth weight of 500 grams or more

New Mexico	South Dakota	Tennessee*

5 months or more gestation
Puerto Rico

16 weeks or more gestation
Pennsylvania

All products of human conception

American Samoa	Hawaii	Rhode Island
Arkansas	Maine	Trust Territory of the
Colorado	New York City	Pacific Islands
Georgia	New York State	Virginia
		Virgin Islands

---

*Specific modifiers apply

I

ADOPTION
COMMUNICATION SHEET

Completed by: _____

Mother's Name _____ EDC _____ DOB _____

Hospital Record # _____

The woman named above has planned an adoptive placement of her infant. Her wishes prior to birth are that she:
_____ wishes to assume regular care of her infant until discharge
_____ wishes to hold her infant one or more times
_____ wishes to see her infant only
_____ wishes to be told about her infant only
_____ authorizes these other persons to see the infant
_____ wishes to be off the OB floor

Agency Adoption
Caseworker _____
Agency _____
Phone #_____

Private Adoption
Attorney _____
Phone # _____

Prospective Adoptive Family
Name _____
Address _____
Phone # _____

A consent has been signed to authorize this family to:
_____ see infant
_____ hold and care for infant
_____ be told about the infant

Relinquishment Signed _____
(date)
Foster Family
Name _____
Address _____
Phone # _____ .

J

ADOPTION DATA BASE

Child's Birth Name_____ DOB _____ Loc. of Birth___
Amended Name(s) _____ Hosp. Record #_____
Mother's Name _____ DOB _____ Ethnic Origin_____
Father's Name _____ DOB _____ Ethnic Origin_____
Pregnancy: Gravidity _____ Parity _____ SAB _____ TAB _____ Living Children ____
1st Prenatal visit at: _____ Alcohol _____ Nicotine _____ Drugs _____
Complications of Pregnancy_____

Delivery: Vag _____ C-Sec. _____ Fetal Distress _____ Apgars _____ / _____
BW _____ Length _____ HC _____ Gestational Age _____
SGA _____ LGA _____ AGA_____

Resuscitation _____ Perinatal Complications_____
D/C Date _____ Placed with_____
Follow-up Appointments/Plans:_____

Family History	Maternal Family	Paternl Family
Allergies		
Heart Disease		
Endocrine		
Pulmonary		
Anemia		
Blood Problems		
Cancer		
Mental Retardation		
Seizures		
Vision/Hearing Problems		
GI Disease		
Mental Illness		
Chemical Dependency		
High Cholesterol/Triglycerides		
Obesity		
Strokes/Hypertension		

K

SAMPLE PRENATAL GENETIC SCREEN*

Name _____ Patient# _____ Date _____

1. Will you be 35 years or older when the baby is due? Yes _____ No _____
2. Have you, the baby's father, or anyone in either of your families ever had any of the following disorders?

   • Down syndrome (mongolism) Yes _____ No _____
   • Other chromosomal abnormality Yes _____ No _____
   • Neural tube defect, ie, spina bifida (meningomyelocele or open spine), anencephaly Yes _____ No _____
   • Hemophilia Yes _____ No _____
   • Muscular dystrophy Yes _____ No _____
   • Cystic Fibrosis Yes _____ No _____

   If yes, indicate the relationship of the affected person to you or to the baby's father: _____

3. Do you or the baby's father have a birth defect? Yes _____ No _____
   If yes, who has the defect and what is it? _____

4. In any previous marriages, have you or the baby's father had a child, born dead or alive, with a birth defect not listed in question 2 above? Yes _____ No _____

   If yes, what was the defect and who had it? _____

5. Do you or the baby's father have any close relatives with mental retardation? Yes _____ No _____

   If yes, indicate the relationship of the affected person to you or to the baby's father: _____

   Indicate the cause, if known: _____

6. Do you, the baby's father, or a close relative in either of your families have a birth defect, any familial disorder, or a chromosomal abnormality not listed above? Yes _____ No _____

   If yes, indicate the relationship of the affected person to you or to the baby's father: _____

---

*Any patient replying "YES" to questions should be offered appropriate counseling. If the patient declines further counseling or testing, this should be noted in the chart. Given that genetics is a field in a state of flux, alterations or updates to this form will be required periodically.

(American College of Obstetricians and Gynecologists: Antenatal Diagnosis of Genetic Disorders (ACOG Technical Bulletin 108). Washington DC, ACOG, 1987)

7. In any previous marriages, have you or the baby's
father had three or more first-trimester spontaneous
pregnancy losses or a stillborn child?   Yes _____ No _____

   Have either of you had a chromosomal study?   Yes _____ No _____

   If yes, indicate who and the results: _____

8. If you or the baby's father are of Jewish ancestry, have
either of you been screened for Tay-Sachs disease?   Yes _____ No _____

   If yes, indicate who and the results: _____

9. If you or the baby's father are black, have either
of you been screened for sickle cell trait?   Yes _____ No _____

   If yes, indicate who and the results: _____

10. If you or the baby's father are of Italian, Greek,
or Mediterranean background, have either of you
been tested for Beta-thalassemia?   Yes _____ No _____

   If yes, indicate who and the results: _____

11. If you or the baby's father are of Phillippine or
Southeast Asian ancestry, have either of you been
tested for Alpha-thalassemia?   Yes _____ No _____

   If yes, indicate who and the results: _____

12. Excluding iron and vitamins, have you taken any
medications or recreational drugs since being pregnant
or since your last menstrual period? (Include
nonprescription drugs.)   Yes _____ No _____

   If yes, give name of medication and time taken during pregnancy: _____

L

SAMPLE OBSTETRIC DATA BASE

Name _____ Patient # _____ Date _____

Infections

1. Are you of Asian, Pacific Island, or Alaskan
   Eskimo descent?   Yes _____ No _____

2. Were you born in Haiti or sub-Saharan Africa?   Yes _____ No _____

3. Do any of the following factors apply to you:

   - A history of acute or chronic liver disease   Yes _____ No _____
   - Work or receive treatment in a hemodialysis unit   Yes _____ No _____
   - Work or live in an institution for the mentally retarded   Yes _____ No _____
   - A history of rejection as a blood donor   Yes _____ No _____
   - A history of you or your partner having had a blood
     transfusion   Yes _____ No _____
   - Occupational exposure to blood in a medicodental
     setting   Yes _____ No _____
   - Household contact with a hepatitis carrier or
     hemodialysis patient   Yes _____ No _____
   - A history of multiple episodes of sexually
     transmitted disease   Yes _____ No _____
   - A history of you or your partner using injectable
     "street drugs"   Yes _____ No _____
   - A bisexual partner   Yes _____ No _____
   - A history of you or your sexual partner having
     had multiple sexual partners   Yes _____ No _____

4. Do you have a cat?   Yes _____ No _____

5. Have you had a rash since your last menstrual period?   Yes _____ No _____

6. Have you received rubella vaccination within three
   months prior to your last menstrual period?   Yes _____ No _____

7. Has your partner ever had a genital herpes infection?   Yes _____ No _____

   If yes, indicate who and date of last lesion _____

General Screen

1. Do you ever smoke?   Yes _____ No _____

   If yes, quantity _____ (cigarettes/day)

2. Do you ever drink alcohol?   Yes _____ No _____

   If yes, quantity (drinks/week) _____

Diabetes mellitus

1. Do you have a history of any of the following?

   - Parents or siblings with diabetes   Yes _____ No _____
   - A child with a birth weight of 9 lb or more   Yes _____ No _____
   - A malformed or stillborn child   Yes _____ No _____
   - Hypertension (high blood pressure)   Yes _____ No _____
   - Glycosuria (sugar in your urine)   Yes _____ No _____

2. Are you over 30 years old?   Yes _____ No _____

INDEX

Abortion
  induced, 312
    reporting requirements in,
      322-323
    statistical measures of, 324
  repetitive, 235
Abuse
  of child, 108-109
    in decisions for nontreatment
      of newborn, 254-255
  of drugs, HIV infection and
    AIDS in, 151, 155
Accreditation of health care
  organizations, 227
Acidemia, glutaric type II, 92, 93
Acidosis, neonatal, 8-79, 80
Acoustic characteristics of neonatal
  care areas, 37, 89
Administration of perinatal care, 9,
  10
Admission/observation areas, 291,
  292
  in obstetric unit, 18-19
  in pediatric unit, 27-28
Admission procedures
  intrapartum, 61-63
  in nursery, and infection control,
    114-115
Adolescents, recommended daily
  dietary allowances for, 193,
  194
  in pregnancy, 195-196
Adoption, 229-234
  counseling in, 230, 231, 232
  examination of neonate in,
    231-233
  legal issues in, 230, 231, 233
  medical records in, 231-232, 233,
    325, 326
    communication sheet, 232,
      325
    data base, 326
  procedure of, 229-231
  responsibility to adoptive parents
    in, 233

Age
  gestational. *See* Gestational age
  maternal, and risk for Down
    syndrome, 236
  and neutral environmental
    temperatures, 278-279
AIDS, 149-158. *See also* HIV
  infection and AIDS
Airborne transmission of infections,
  control of, 136
Aircraft in interhospital transport,
  215, 216
Albumin
  bilirubin bound to, 259, 260
  in resuscitation of newborn, 80
Alcohol-containing hand-washing
  agents, 120
Alcohol use in pregnancy, 55, 59
Ambulances in interhospital
  transport, 215, 216
Ambulation, postpartum, 82
Ambulatory services, 8
Amethopterin contraindicated in
  breast-feeding, 200
Amino acid metabolism, inborn
  errors of, 92
Ammonia, and neonatal
  hyperammonemia, 93
Amniocentesis, in diagnosis of
  genetic disorders, 238
Amniotic fluid, α-fetoprotein levels
  in, 240, 241
Analgesia in labor and delivery,
  63-64
Anemia
  of neonates, 102
  sickle cell, antenatal detection of,
    235, 237
Anesthesia in labor and delivery,
  63-65, 70
  and aspiration of gastric
    contents, 64,66
  personnel in, 41, 42, 64-65
Antepartum care, 51-60
  area in hospital for, 18, 291

331

Assessment of perinatal care
(continued)
induced termination of
pregnancy in, 312, 320,
322-323
infant mortality in, 312,
316-319, 322
live births in, 309, 313-314,
321
in local hospital, 225-226
maternal mortality in, 312,
319, 322
misapplication and
misinterpretation of data
in, 309
neonatal mortality in, 255,
312, 315-316, 321
outcome assessment in, 227
in quality assurance, 226-227
and reporting requirements,
309, 320-324
in transport program, 221
of risks. *See* Risk assessment
Audiometric assessment of infants,
102, 109
Autopsy in perinatal death, 267-268
Auxiliary areas, 32-36, 294
Axillary temperature of neonates,
275

Bacille Calmette-Guérin vaccine in
tuberculosis, 170-171
in pregnancy, 174
Bacteria levels in breast milk, 201
Bacterial colonization of newborn,
114
staphylococcal, 177, 178
streptococcal, 164, 165
Bacterial infections
neonatal, 134-135, 177-184
streptococcal, 164-165, 183-184
in pregnancy, 172-173
Bacteriuria in pregnancy, 172-173
Barium enema in newborn, 250
Bassinets
cleaning and disinfection of, 188
number required in newborn
nursery, 28-29
thermal environment of, 276

Bathing
of mother, postpartum, 83
of neonate, 90, 127, 128, 275
area for, 34-35
thermal environment of, 34,
90, 127, 275
Bayley Scales of Infant
Development, 106
BCG vaccine in tuberculosis,
170-171
in pregnancy, 174
Bed rest, postpartum, 82
Behavioral status of infant, 106-107
Benzyl alcohol, as preservative in
intravascular flush
solutions, 126
Bereavement in perinatal death, 266
counseling in, 268-270
Bicarbonate therapy in resuscitation
of newborn, 80
Bilirubin
albumin-bound, 259, 260
crossing blood-brain barrier, 260,
261
serum levels
in breast-fed infants, 262-263
and hyperbilirubinemia,
259-265
in premature neonates, 260
Bioethics committees, use of,
255-256
Biopsy of fetal skin, in detection of
genetic disorders, 237
Birth control methods, postpartum,
101
tubal ligation in, 83
Birth rate, 309, 313-314
compared to neonatal mortality
rate, 266
Birth records, 84-85
Birth weight, 86-88
definition of, 310
low. *See* Low birth weight
Birthing rooms, 291. *See also*
Delivery rooms
infection control in, 121, 122-123
Bladder, postpartum care of, 82-83
Blood banks, 294
personnel of, 45

Organization of perinatal care
  (continued)
  problem areas in, 3, 11-13
  risk assessment in, 3, 11
Osmolality of infant formulas,
  204-205
Outreach education, 47-48
  on regional transport system,
  220-221
Oximetry, pulse, in monitoring of
  oxygen therapy, 245
Oxygen
  arterial partial pressure of
  in oxygen therapy, 245,
  246-247
  and retinopathy of
  prematurity, 244, 245, 246
  therapy with, 244-248
  administration of, 245
  emergency, 245, 246, 247
  facilities for, in newborn care
  area, 37
  monitoring of, 245-246, 247
  and retinopathy of
  prematurity, 103, 244-245,
  246
Oxytocin
  in induction and augmentation
  of labor, 70
  postpartum use of, 81

Pain relief
  intrapartum, 63-65
  postpartum, 82
Palsy, cerebral, 271, 272
Papillomavirus infection, human,
  158-159
Parenteral nutrition, infection
  control in, 125-126
Pasteurization of equipment, 185
Pediatric units
  facilities of, 25-38
  neonatal care in. See Neonatal
  care
Pelvic examination, intrapartum, 62
Pelvimetry in pregnancy, radiation
  exposure in, 250
Penicillin
  in gonorrhea, 163, 164

Penicillin in gonorrhea (continued)
  and ophthalmia neonatorum,
  300, 301
  in streptococcal infections of
  neonates, 183
Personnel in perinatal care, 5, 9-10,
  39-48, 290
  in anesthesia, 41, 42, 64-65
  dress codes for, 120-122
  hand-washing of, 115, 119-120
  121, 122
  health standards for, 117-119
  herpes simplex infection in,
  117-118
  in-service and continuing
  education of, 46-47
  in interhospital transport, 213,
  215
  medical staff, 9, 40-42, 46-47, 290
  nursing staff, 9-10, 42-45, 46-47,
  119, 290
  precautions preventing
  transmission of
  blood-borne pathogens,
  129-130
  radiation exposure of, 252
  responsibilities in patient
  education, 59-60
  in outreach programs, 47-48
  support staff, 45-46
Pertussis in premature infants,
  128-129
pH, capillary, fetal, 68
Phenindione contraindicated in
  breast-feeding, 200
Phenylketonuria
  neonatal screening for, 90, 91
  preconceptional care in, 51
Phosphorus, recommended daily
  dietary allowances for, 194,
  195-196, 197
Phototherapy in
  hyperbilirubinemia, 260,
  261, 263-265
  toxicity of, 264-265
Physical examination
  maternal
  antepartum, 53-54
  intrapartum, 62, 63
  postpartum, 104

Prenatal care, 51-60. *See also*
Antepartum care
Preterm infants
bilirubin serum levels in, 260
in convection warmed
incubators, 276
definition of, 310
historical development of care
for, 2-3
immunization of, 128-129
nutrition for, 203, 206
oxygen therapy in, 244, 247
and retinopathy, 103, 244-245,
246
temperature of, 275, 276
Preterm labor and delivery, 57-58,
68-69
assessment of risk for, 57-58
tocolytic drugs in, 282-286
Protein
in infant formulas, 204-205
recommended daily dietary
allowances for, 194, 195,
197
Psychosocial factors
in follow-up care, 107-109
in postpartum period, 104-105,
107-109
in pregnancy, 60
Pyelography, intravenous, in
pregnancy, radiation
exposure in, 249
Pyelonephritis in pregnancy,
172-173

Quality assurance in perinatal care,
226-227

Rabies vaccine in pregnancy, 174
Radiant warmers in neonatal care,
38, 277
Radiation exposure, 249-253
maternal-fetal, 249-250
in neonatal intensive care unit,
250-252
of personnel, 252
Radiography, 294
radiation exposure in

Radiography, radiation exposure in
(continued)
of neonates, 250
of personnel, 252
in pregnancy, 249, 250
Radioisotope studies in pregnancy,
250
Recovery area, postpartum care in,
23, 81-82
Rectal temperature of neonates, 275
Referrals, 8, 9
and interhospital transport of
patients, 209-222
Reflex irritability of neonate, 75
Regional perinatal care
interhospital transport in,
209-222
organization of, 1-15
Reporting requirements, 309,
320-324
in child abuse, 109
in fetal death, 321, 324
in HIV infection and AIDS, 157
in induced termination of
pregnancy, 322-323
in infant death, 322
in live birth, 321
in maternal death, 322
in neonatal death, 321
standard terminology in, 308-324
in tuberculosis, 168
Research component of perinatal
care, 8, 11
Respirations of neonate, 75, 77
Respiratory depression of neonate,
narcotic-induced, 80
Respiratory syncytial virus
infection, neonatal, 135,
136
Respiratory tract infections,
maternal, contact with
neonate in, 132
Resuscitation
facilaites for, 26-27, 292
of neonate, 26-27, 74-75, 76,
77-80, 297-298
conditions requiring, 74,
297-298
drug therapy in, 78-80

Staff in perinatal care, 39-48. *See also*
    Personnel in perinatal care
Stanford-Binet Intelligence Test, 106
Staphylococcal infections, neonatal,
    177-179
Statistical evaluation of perinatal
    care, 223, 224-225, 309,
    312-321
    rates and ratios in, 313
Steam autoclaving in sterilization of
    equipment, 185
Sterilization of equipment, 184-190
    compared to disinfection, 184
    methods of, 185
Sterilization procedures, tubal
    ligation in, postpartum, 83
Stillbirth, 235, 266-270. *See also*
    Fetus, death of
Stimulation programs for high-risk
    infants, 110-111
Stomach, aspiration of contents in
    obstetric anesthesia, 64, 66
Storage areas, 33
    cleaning of, 187
Streptococcal infections
    group A, 176
        isolation procedures in, 131
        in neonates, 183-184
    group B, 164-165
Suctioning of neonates, 76, 122
    infection control in, 122
    for meconium, 76
Support services
    facilities for, 32-36, 294
    in follow-up care, 105
    personnel in, 45-46
Surgical therapy
    fetal, 257-258
    infection control in, 123
Surveillance programs
    in antepartum care, 51-59
    in infection control, 115-117
Syphilis, 166-168
    congenital, 135, 166, 167
    in pregnancy, 54, 166, 167
    tests for, 54, 88, 166, 167

Tay-Sachs disease, 235

Team approach. *See*
    Multidisciplinary approach
Temperature
    of environment, neutral, 274,
        278-279
    of mother, in postpartum fever,
        83, 131, 132, 175
    of neonate, 38, 274-281
        adequate warmth in, 276
        in bassinets, 276
        in bathing, 34, 90, 127, 275
        in delivery room, 76, 275-276
        in hyperthermia, 279, 280
        in hypothermia, 279-280
        in incubators, 276, 277, 280
        in low birth weight, 274, 275,
            280
        measurement of, 274-275
        radiant warmers increasing,
            38, 277
        regulation of, 274-275
        in transport, 280
    of respiratory gas delivered to
        neonate, 280
Terbutaline, as tocolytic agent in
    preterm labor, 282
Term neonate, definition of, 310
Term pregnancy, labor management
    in, 65-68
Tetanus vaccine
    in pregnancy, 174
    in premature infants, 129
Tetracycline, in gonococcal
    ophthalmia neonatorum,
    88, 299
Thalassemia, antenatal detection of,
    235, 237
Thermal regulation, 274-281
Thiamin, recommended daily
    dietary allowances for, 194
Thiouracil contraindicated in
    breast-feeding, 200
Thyroid disorders, neonatal
    screening for, 90, 91
Tocolysis, 282-286
    contraindications to, 282
    complications of, 284-285
    magnesium sulfate in, 282,
        283-284, 285
    ritodrine in, 282, 283, 284